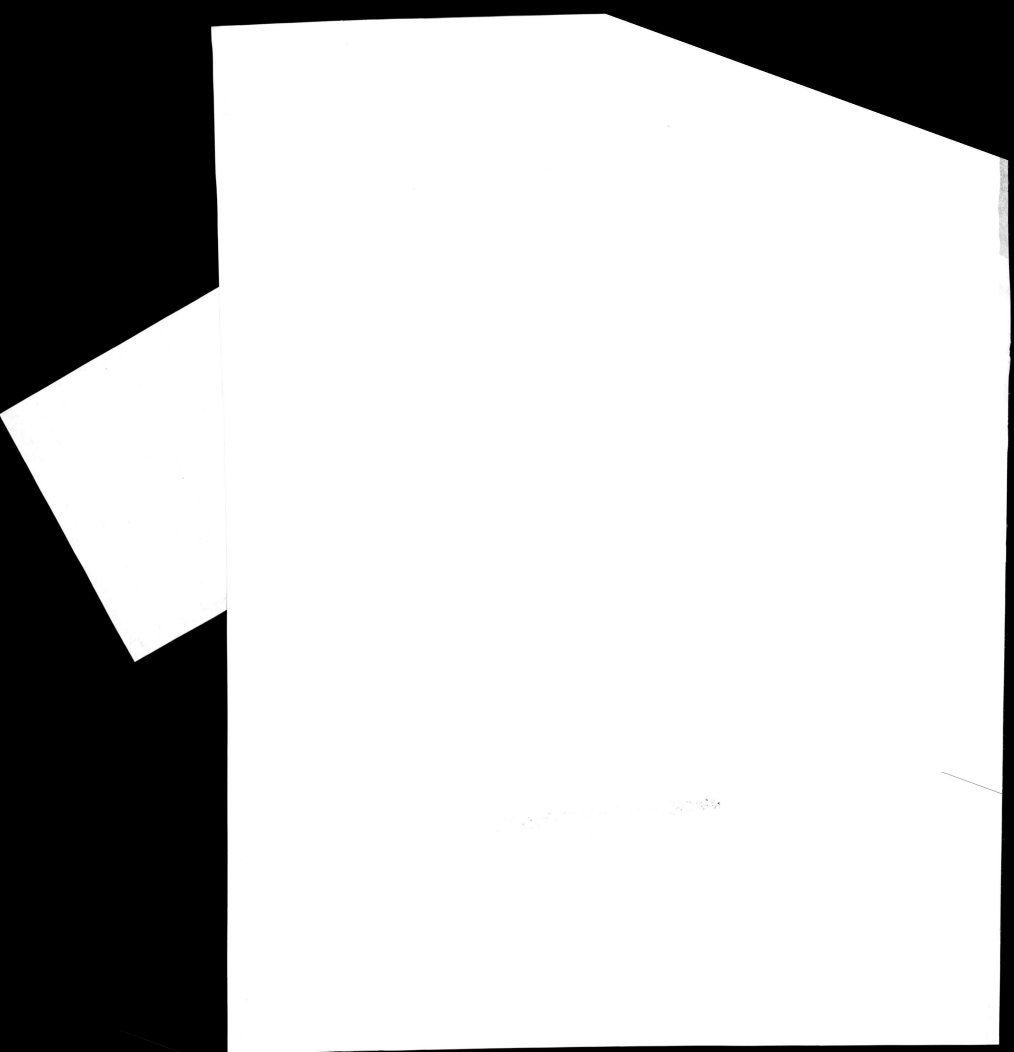

Complications of Gynecologic Endoscopic Surgery

Keith Isaacson, MD

Associate Professor of Obstetrics and Gynecology
Harvard Medical School
Boston, Massachusetts

Director of Minimally Invasive Gnyecologic Surgery and Infertility
Associate Chair of Obstetrics and Gynecology
Newton Wellesley Hospital
Newton, Massachusetts

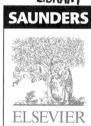

SAUNDERS

ELSEVIER

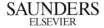

SAUNDERS
ELSEVIER

1600 John F. Kennedy Blvd.
Ste 1800
Philadelphia, PA 19103-2899

Notice

Knowledge and best practice in this field are constantly changing. As new research and experience broaden our knowledge, changes in practice, treatment, and drug therapy may become necessary or appropriate. Readers are advised to check the most current information provided (i) on procedures featured or (ii) by the manufacturer of each product to be administered to verify the recommended dose or formula, the method and duration of administration, and contraindications. It is the responsibility of practitioners, relying on experience and knowledge of their patients, to make diagnoses, to determine dosages and the best treatment for each individual patient, and to take all appropriate safety precautions. To the fullest extent of the law, neither the Publisher nor the Editor assumes any liability for any injury and/or damage to persons or property arising out of or related to any use of the material contained in this book.

The Publisher

Library of Congress Cataloging-in-Publication Data

Complications of gynecologic endoscopic surgery [edited by] Keith B. Isaacson.
    p. ; cm.
  Includes bibliographical references and index.
  ISBN 0-7216-0669-5 (alk. paper)
    1. Generative organs, Female—Endoscopic surgery—Complications.   2. Endoscopic surgery—Complications.   I. Isaacson, Keith B.
    [DNLM: 1. Endoscopy—adverse effects.   2. Genital Diseases, Female—surgery.
WP 660 C7363 2006]
RG104.C562 2006
618.1′0597—dc22

                                                         2005057455

Acquisitions Editor: Todd Hummel
Publishing Services Manager: Frank Polizzano
Project Manager: Lee Ann Draud
Design Direction: Karen O'Keefe Owens

Printed in Canada

Last digit is the print number: 9 8 7 6 5 4 3 2 1

To my wife, Jennifer, and to my children, Leigh and Casey, who
have shown tremendous support and patience.

To all of the contributing authors and their families for the numerous
hours spent researching, writing, and editing their chapters. This book is
for you.

Contributors

Dennis R. Anti, JD
Partner, Morrison Mahoney LLP, Springfield, Massachusetts

Physician, Heal Thyself: Malpractice Prevention and Treatment

Heather G. Beattie, RN, JD
Associate, Morrison Mahoney LLP, Springfield, Massachusetts

Physician, Heal Thyself: Malpractice Prevention and Treatment

Andrew I. Brill, MD
Professor and Director, Gynecologic Endoscopy, Department of Obstetrics and Gynecology, University of Illinois at Chicago College of Medicine, Chicago, Illinois

Reducing Risk and Maximizing Efficacy with Thermal Modalities

Simon Chau, BM, BS
Specialist Registrar in Anaesthesia, Bradford Teaching Hospitals NHS Foundation Trust, Bradford, United Kingdom

Physiologic and Metabolic Complications

Stephen M. Cohen, MD
Associate Professor of Obstetrics and Gynecology, Albany Medical College; Chief of Infertility and Minimally Invasive Surgery, Albany Medical Center, Albany, New York

Preventing Complications before the Operation

Paul Cramp, BSc, MBChB
Consultant in Anaesthesia and Intensive Care, Bradford Teaching Hospitals NHS Foundation Trust, Bradford, United Kingdom

Physiologic and Metabolic Complications

Ellis Downes, SMBChB
Honorary Senior Lecturer, University College Hospital; Consultant Gynaecologist and Obstetrician, Chase Farm Hospital, Middlesex, United Kingdom

Complications of Endometrial Ablation

Roger J. Ferland, MD
Associate Clinical Professor of Obstetrics and Gynecology, Brown Medical School; Chief, Gynecology Attending Team, Women & Infants' Hospital of Rhode Island, Providence, Rhode Island

Pelvic Adhesions

Gary Frishman, MD
Associate Professor of Obstetrics and Gynecology, Brown Medical School; Acting Director, Division of Reproductive Medicine and Infertility, Department of Obstetrics and Gynecology, Women & Infants' Hospital of Rhode Island, Providence, Rhode Island

Laparoscopic Training and Education

Keith Isaacson, MD
Associate Professor of Obstetrics and Gynecology, Harvard Medical School, Boston; Director of Minimally Invasive Gynecologic Surgery and Infertility and Associate Chair of Obstetrics and Gynecology, Newton Wellesley Hospital, Newton, Massachusetts

Unusual Complications during Gynecologic Laparoscopic Surgery; Complications Related to Hysteroscopic Distention Media

Sandra Abadie Kemmerly, MD
Associate Head, Department of Infectious Diseases, and Medical Director, Clinical Practice Improvement, Ochsner Clinic Foundation, New Orleans, Louisiana

Perioperative and Postoperative Infection

Charles H. Koh, MD, FACOG, FRCOG
Co-Director, Milwaukee Institute of Minimally Invasive
    Surgery, Milwaukee, Wisconsin

Laparoscopic Bowel Injuries

Neeraj Kohli, MD, MBA
Director, Division of Urogynecology, Harvard Medical School
    and Brigham and Women's Hospital, Boston,
    Massachusetts

*Complications of Minimally Invasive Urogynecologic
Surgery*

Barbara Levy, MD
Medical Director, Women's Health and Breast Center, St.
    Francis Hospital, Federal Way, Washington

Vascular Injuries

Ali Mahdavi, MD
Fellow in Minimally Invasive Surgery, Division of Gynecologic
    Oncology, Mount Sinai School of Medicine, New York,
    New York

*Complications of Laparoscopic Surgery in Gynecologic
Oncology*

Madhavi Manoharan, MD
Specialist Registrar, Chase Farm Hospital, Middlesex, United
    Kingdom

Complications of Endometrial Ablation

John R. Miklos, MD
Atlanta Urogynecology Associates, Alpharetta, Georgia

*Complications of Minimally Invasive Urogynecologic
Surgery*

Rob Moore, DO
General Surgeon; Staff Member, Anne Arundel Medical
    Center, Annapolis, Maryland

*Complications of Minimally Invasive Urogynecologic
Surgery*

Stephanie N. Morris
Clinical Instructor of Obstetrics and Gynecology, Harvard
    Medical School, Boston; Associate in Minimally Invasive
    Gynecologic Surgery, Newton Wellesley Hospital,
    Newton, Massachusetts

Laparoscopic Bowel Injuries

Malcolm G. Munro, MD, FRCS(C), FACOG
Professor, Department of Obstetrics and Gynecology, David
    Geffen School of Medicine at UCLA; Kaiser Permanente
    Southern California, Los Angeles Medical Center, Los
    Angeles, California

Complications of Laparoscopic Access

Farr Nezhat, MD, FACOG
Professor of Obstetrics and Gynecology and Director of
    Gynecologic Minimally Invasive Surgery, Mount Sinai
    School of Medicine, New York, New York

*Complications of Laparoscopic Surgery in Gynecologic
Oncology*

Peter J. O'Donovan, MBBCh
Consultant Obstetrician and Gynaecologist, Bradford
    Teaching Hospitals NHS Foundation Trust, Bradford,
    United Kingdom

Physiologic and Metabolic Complications

Resad Pasic, MD, PhD
Associate Professor, Department of Obstetrics and
    Gynecology and Women's Health, University of Louisville
    School of Medicine, Louisville, Kentucky

*Reducing Risk and Maximizing Efficacy with Thermal
Modalities*

Charles R. Rardin, MD
Assistant Professor, Brown Medical School; Associate,
    Division of Urogynecology and Reconstructive Pelvic
    Surgery, Women & Infants' Hospital of Rhode Island,
    Providence, Rhode Island

Laparoscopic Training and Education

James K. Robinson III, MD, MS
Fellow, Gynecologic Endoscopy, Newton-Wellesley Hospital,
    Newton, Massachusetts

*Unusual Complications during Gynecologic Laparoscopic
Surgery*

Peter L. Rosenblatt, MD
Assistant Professor of Obstetrics, Gynecology, and
    Reproductive Biology, Harvard Medical School, Boston;
    Director of Urogynecology and Reconstructive Pelvic
    Surgery, Mount Auburn Hospital, Cambridge,
    Massachusetts

Urologic Injuries in Laparoscopic Surgery

Warren S. Sandberg, MD, PhD
Assistant Professor of Anesthesia, Harvard Medical School;
    Assistant in Anesthesia, Department of Anesthesia and
    Critical Care, Massachusetts General Hospital, Boston,
    Massachusetts

*The Role of the Anesthesia Team in the Avoidance,
Diagnosis, Management, and Genesis of Laparoscopic
Complications*

Joseph S. Sanfilippo, MD, MBA
Professor of Obstetrics, Gynecology, and Reproductive
    Sciences, University of Pittsburgh School of Medicine,
    Pittsburgh, Pennsylvania

Complications of Pediatric and Adolescent Laparoscopy

Andrea J. Singer, MD
Associate Professor of Medicine and Obstetrics and
  Gynecology, Georgetown University School of Medicine;
  Chief, Women's Primary Care, Georgetown University
  Hospital, Washington, DC

Preventing Complications before the Operation

Edward Stanford, MD, MS
Director of Urogynecology/Urodynamics, St. Mary's Good
  Samaritan Hospital, Centralia, Illinois

Urologic Injuries in Laparoscopic Surgery

Liza M. Swedarsky, MD
Chief Resident in Obstetrics and Gynecology, Massachusetts
  General Hospital and Brigham and Women's Hospital,
  Boston, Massachusetts

Complications Related to Hysteroscopic Distention Media

Michael P. Traynor, MD
Fellow in Advanced Laparoscopic and Hysteroscopic Surgery,
  Department of Obstetrics and Gynecology and Women's
  Health, University of Louisville School of Medicine,
  Louisville, Kentucky

*Reducing Risk and Maximizing Efficacy with Thermal
Modalities*

Rodger M. White, MD
Assistant Professor of Anesthesia, Harvard Medical School;
  Assistant in Anesthesia, Department of Anesthesia and
  Critical Care, Massachusetts General Hospital, Boston,
  Massachusetts

*The Role of the Anesthesia Team in the Avoidance,
Diagnosis, Management, and Genesis of Laparoscopic
Complications*

Morris Wortman, MD, FACOG
Clinical Associate Professor of Gynecology, University of
  Rochester School of Medicine, Rochester,
  New York

Complications of Hysteroscopic Surgery

Ryan J. Zlupko, MD
Instructor, University of Pittsburgh School of Medicine,
  Pittsburgh, Pennsylvania

Complications of Pediatric and Adolescent Laparoscopy

Preface

As surgeons, we have heard the mantra "If you have not had a complication during surgery, you are not doing enough surgery." Although there is a great deal of truth to this, it is also true that as surgeons we do our best to avoid complications and perform the safest surgical procedure possible. Part of being an excellent surgeon is not only being able to avoid complications but also being able to recognize and manage complications when they occur. It is within this framework that *Complications of Gynecologic Endoscopic Surgery* is organized. As editor, I have asked the chapter authors, who are experts in their fields, to write their chapters using the following general format:

1. What is the likelihood that a complication will occur for a given procedure?
2. What steps can be taken in advance to avoid a complication?
3. How can we recognize a complication when it occurs?
4. How is a complication best managed—both intraoperatively and postoperatively?

This book is organized to take a patient through the surgical process. The first chapter, written by two expert trial attorneys, is meant to educate the surgeon. It is not intended as a scare tactic to encourage physicians to practice defensive medicine. Instead, the authors discuss important measures that can be taken in advance to avoid the likelihood of litigation and then outline the appropriate steps to take once notice of litigation has been served and the trial begins. All of the steps described in this chapter ultimately lead to enhanced patient safety. Improved documentation and patient communication, in my mind, are important first steps.

Once the patient is deemed appropriate for surgery, the next step in the process is assessing the risk of anesthesia. I have chosen to look at this from three perspectives: the anesthesiologist's viewpoint, which includes preoperative evaluation and intraoperative team dynamics, and the laparoscopist's and hysteroscopist's viewpoints, which overlap the anesthesiologist's but also include subjects such as patient positioning and hysteroscopic distention media.

The majority of the text is written by surgical and medical experts who have had personal experience with the complications they describe. The chapters as written are evidence based. The authors not only review the literature but also convey as much personal experience as possible when data are scant. As a result, we are able to learn from the experience of the surgical "masters."

The reader will note several inconsistencies throughout the text regarding how a particular complication should be avoided and managed. I have purposely included these different approaches and have asked the authors to provide logical explanations for each approach. The individual reader can determine which management option best fits his or her medical philosophy.

In conclusion, it seems obvious that the best way to reduce the incidence of surgical complications is to enhance physician training. The old-fashioned way of "see one, do one, teach one" is no longer valid. Residents have reduced 80-hour work weeks and have less hands-on surgical time. Although we are in the infancy of this technology, we now can obtain "hands-on" experience using computer-simulated models. We don't have to learn a new procedure or use a new device on someone else's mother, sister, or daughter. Computerized simulation has become commonplace in the airline industry and in military training. As described in the concluding chapter by Drs. Rardin and Frishman, this technology will become an integral part of our ongoing surgical training and credentialing.

Keith Isaacson

Contents

Physician, Heal Thyself: Malpractice Prevention and Treatment

Heather G. Beattie and Dennis R. Anti

Obstetrician-gynecologists are frequent targets of malpractice actions, both because of the numerous risks associated with childbirth and because these physicians additionally perform surgery on the reproductive organs, which encompasses the risks associated with abdominal and pelvic surgery. Since the onset and acceptance of endoscopic gynecologic procedures, malpractice actions related to this seemingly less invasive but also risky approach may be undertaken as well. Unfortunately, a bad outcome following a laparoscopic gynecologic procedure frequently results in large-amount verdicts or settlements awarded because of organ damage or loss of fertility or other related complications. Like other types of surgery, endoscopic gynecologic surgery carries the risk of serious permanent injury; compounding factors include the impact of new technology, changes in the traditional physician-patient relationship, and unrealistic expectations by some patients for perfect results without complications.

Today's physician can mitigate the potential impact of medical malpractice litigation on his or her career in medicine. Foresight and some minor adjustments to administrative and clinical practices will not guarantee a career without a lawsuit but certainly will minimize the chances of malpractice litigation. This chapter provides a guide to the prevention of litigation for the obstetrician-gynecologist performing laparoscopic surgery. Recommendations for the physician's response to the recognition of a maloccurrence also are presented. The litigation process, starting from the initiation of a medical malpractice action, is then outlined, with the objective being to increase the physician's understanding of the process and his or her ability to participate in these sometimes mysterious proceedings.

PREVENTION OF LITIGATION

It frequently is said that a good physician-patient relationship is instrumental in preventing a medical malpractice action. Communication skills are a significant component of that relationship. The physician must communicate clearly and effectively not only with other health care providers regarding diagnosis and treatment but with the patient as well. As all physicians are aware, however, communication is easier with some patients than with others. In addition, physicians today lack the time to allow leisurely conversation with their patients because of financial constraints and the requirements of health maintenance organizations (HMOs) and other managed care programs. Although no magic exists to avert a potential communication deficit between physician and patient, the physician can do much to maximize professional and personal communication skills, improve the overall physician-patient relationship, and mitigate the risk of litigation.

Each physician embodies a unique combination of personal and professional qualities, and bedside manner and communication skills will be greatly influenced by personality. Notwithstanding these differences, any physician may make a conscious effort to listen, allowing the patient to see that he or she is the honest focus of the physician's attention and efforts. This simple measure will go a very long way toward improving communication, thereby fostering a good physician-patient relationship and assisting in preventing future litigation.

Obtaining and Documenting Informed Consent

Allegation of failure to obtain informed consent is perhaps one of the easiest of all malpractice claims to avoid. A majority of plaintiffs' lawyers will allege counts related to informed consent as a matter of course, so as not to waive their ability to argue the issue later in the litigation process. Adherence to certain mechanisms in the physician's practice and routine in discussing potential procedures with patients can successfully defend against such claims.

Most states use the "reasonable person standard" in determining the sufficiency of informed consent. As a professional who has superior knowledge of medicine and the patient's condition, the physician has a duty to reveal all facts that are necessary for the "reasonable person" to consent to the proposed treatment. Consent for a surgical procedure, including laparoscopic gynecologic procedures, should not be obtained on the day of surgery. A relaxed and less overwhelming atmosphere than that encountered in the clinic or hospital is preferable for this process. A discussion in the physician's office, a much less intimidating milieu, at least 1 day before the scheduled surgical procedure, will promote the patient's and family members' understanding of the procedure and any potential complications. This venue and timing for the exchange of information also will allow for more give-and-take with questions and answers.

An informed consent discussion just before surgery is almost never justifiable, especially if the patient has already been medicated. The only exception to obtaining informed consent occurs when the patient is unable to give consent, a representative for the patient is unavailable, and a risk of death without immediate surgery is recognized. The attending physician should always obtain the written consent in person from the patient. A consent form obtained by a nurse, resident, or covering physician who will not be performing the procedure in the only informed consent exchange does not meet the requirements of full disclosure, with an adequate opportunity for the patient to ask questions of the attending physician.

Contemporaneous documentation of the physician's discussion of the risks and benefits with the patient offers the defendant physician the best protection. The standard form typically used by hospitals to obtain consent for a surgical procedure most times is not sufficient to defend against a medical malpractice action alleging failure to obtain informed consent. Jury members who have been interviewed after serving on malpractice cases have consistently minimized the attention that they as patients have paid to standard consent forms. Their collective experience is that they rarely read the form and discount it as a pro forma process necessary for them to have the required surgery.

Optimal documentation is done in a progress note or office note format stating that a discussion of the risks and benefits of the procedure has in fact taken place. Enumeration of the more significant risks associated with laparoscopic procedures, including infection, bleeding, and injury to bowel, ureter, veins and arteries, and other structures, is essential. Documentation of the patient's questions and concerns, as well as the patient's ultimate decision, also is required. The possibility of alternative treatments, including open laparoscopy or laparotomy when appropriate, also should be documented. Finally, the presence of any family members should be documented, as well as their contribution to the discussion. Other information that should be included when appropriate includes informing the patient of resident or house officer participation in the procedure.

The patient should be encouraged to read and sign this note as part of the informed consent process. When a co-signed note is enlarged and used as an exhibit for trial, a claim for lack of informed consent is seriously undermined when the enlarged note has the signature of the plaintiff patient.

An alternative to the progress note format is a dictated progress note including the informed consent information, as described, in the presence of the patient and a family member. The dictated note should include mention that the note was dictated in the presence of the patient. Some physicians choose to create and use a detailed template of a consent form particular to the surgical procedure to be performed. Such a detailed consent form should list all risks including and specifically enumerating perforation of the bowel, ureter, and other organs, as well as injury to blood vessels. In addition to the patient's signature on the consent form, it also is necessary for the physician to sign the consent form, and the form or other

---

BOX 1–1   *INFORMED CONSENT*
• Obtain consent in person *before* the day of the procedure.
• Document discussion with patient and family contemporaneously with the discussion.
• Document the discussion in progress note format.
• Include enumeration of risks, presence of family members, and concerns of the patient in documentation.
• Encourage the patient to sign the progress note.

document should be witnessed by another person in the office.

Postoperative Communication with and about the Patient

THE OPERATIVE NOTE

The operative note, in accordance with most hospital policies and guidelines, usually is required to be written within 24 hours of the surgery. This timely documentation of the actual procedure will lend credibility to the content of the operative note some 5 or 6 years later, when the malpractice action is in progress. The operative note should contain sufficient detail regarding the procedure itself, with special attention to documentation of inspection for injury before withdrawal of the laparoscope. The operative note also should include accurate documentation of the identity of other physicians who were present for the procedure and whether or not any of them actually participated in the procedure, as opposed to just observing. If a resident physician dictates the operative note and the attending physician signs the resident's dictated note, the attending must read the note carefully and make any amendments or changes to the note he or she believes to be necessary at the time, initialing each change. By signing the resident's dictation, the physician as the attending or supervising resident is confirming everything written as being true and accurate; thus, the note is construed as the physician's own documentation during the litigation process.

Unfortunately, dictated operative notes may occasionally become lost in the system. It is not rare for the attorney for the defendant physician to discover, during the course of litigation, that an operative note is missing from the medical record. The attending physician has the responsibility to ensure that the operative note does eventually make it to the medical record. If the original dictation is lost and the physician must redictate the operative note at a later date, the operative note must indicate that it was redictated, with a brief explanation of why redictation was necessary.

BOX 1–2   *THE OPERATIVE NOTE*
• Document within 24 hours of the operative procedure.
• Provide sufficient detail of the procedure.
• Provide information regarding findings on inspection for injury before withdrawal of the endoscope.
• Identify others present for the procedure.
• Read the resident's operative note carefully before co-signing.

Postoperative Care

Good follow-up care of the postoperative patient, both in the hospital and after hospital discharge, is a cornerstone in preventing medical malpractice. Frequently, signs of laparoscopic gynecologic surgical complications are not obvious during the procedure or during the immediate postanesthesia recovery period. Often, after discharge of the patient from the hospital, vague symptoms begin to develop that require heightened suspicion of the possibility of a complication. Because post–laparoscopic surgery patients frequently will experience pain, including abdominal, chest, or shoulder pain, the patient's complaints must be taken seriously, investigated completely, and documented, whether the information is revealed by telephone conversation or during an office visit. Obtaining a complete set of vital signs with every visit is essential. During the course of litigation, documentation of vital signs, especially absence of fever, can be important evidence in defending a physician's decision to not initiate further work-up and investigate the possible existence of a complication such as bowel perforation.

Documentation of all postoperative contact with the patient and of the physician's follow-up plan is critical. As always, all documentation should contain the date and time of the interaction with the patient, because such documentation can be very helpful in defending a physician's day-to-day actions at trial. In addition to documenting postoperative office appointments, a physician also should make it a habit to document all patient telephone calls. Frequently, vital information is relayed from the patient to the physician during a telephone conversation. Without such documentation at the time of trial, the testimony resorts to the memory of the patient and the physician. Documentation of the telephone conversation, including the patient's specific complaint of symptoms and the physician's assessment and plan of follow-up and care, can be strong evidence that will frequently benefit the defense.

RECOGNITION AND DIAGNOSIS OF MALOCCURRENCE

Complications, or maloccurrence, are part of the practice of medicine and certainly part of surgical intervention. Whether the term *accepted complication* or *recognized complication* is used, complications and inadvertent outcomes do happen and frequently are not a result of negligence or any wrongdoing by the surgeon. When a complication has occurred and is recognized, it behooves the surgeon to take special care in interaction with the patient and family members and in documentation of the maloccurrence in the medical record.

Discussing the Complication with the Patient

The complication or maloccurrence must, of course, be explained to the patient. Whether or not the physician believes that he or she was in fact negligent or at fault in any way in causing the complication, the physician must take great care in explaining the complication to the patient and family members. The physician should express empathy but should not apologize for the maloccurrence nor expressly state personal responsibility for the outcome. An apology may be considered to be an admission of liability in the eyes of the law, and especially in the eyes of the patient's attorney. The physician can clearly, in lay terms as necessary, explain to the patient what occurred without admitting any personal fault for the adverse event.

It may be useful for the physician to consider this conversation to be a continuation of the informed consent discussion in which the actual risks associated with the procedure were reviewed. In this context, the maloccurrence is referred to as one of the previously discussed risks that has in fact occurred.

Documentation of Physician-Patient Discussions

The physician should always document discussions regarding the complication with the patient and the patient's family and should do so in a somewhat generalized fashion without citing specifics of the conversation. In keeping with the new federal HIPAA laws, as well as many state laws, issues of confidentiality must be recognized at that time, and no discussion with the patient's family or friends should occur without the consent of the patient.

Finally, the physician should not keep personal notes regarding the complications or maloccurrence experienced by the patient. Personal or ad hoc notes that are not kept in the medical record will always be requested during the discovery process in the litigation and will usually be harmful or at least troublesome to the defense of a case, especially when they contain very detailed information regarding the complication or error. Any documentation necessary should be done in the patient's medical record only.

Continuing Care of the Patient

Frequently the physician, after recognizing a complication, will have some intuitive feeling that the patient or the patient's family may be considering a lawsuit even while the postoperative patient remains under the physician's care. The patient

---

BOX 1–3	*POSTOPERATIVE CARE OF THE PATIENT*

- Consider all postoperative complaints carefully.
- Take complete vital signs on all postoperative visits.
- Document all postoperative contact with the patient, including telephone calls.

BOX 1–4	*INITIAL RECOGNITION OF MALOCCURRENCE*

- Explain occurrence of the complication in lay terms with empathy but without apology.
- Document this discussion with the patient without citing specifics of the conversation.
- Do not discuss these issues with the patient's family or friends without the patient's consent.
- Do not keep personal notes regarding the maloccurrence; document in the medical record only.

BOX 1–5   *CONTINUED CARE OF THE PATIENT*
• Continue to care for the patient unless the patient is noncompliant or demonstrates other behavior that interferes with postoperative care.
• Carefully document all interactions with the patient.
• Follow office policy, and without discussion, give the patient a copy of her medical record when requested.

BOX 1–6   *MASSAGING THE MEDICAL RECORD: IMPROPER AND POTENTIALLY COSTLY*
• Never add to or change documentation already entered into the medical record.
• Add information only by addendum with contemporaneous dating.
• Leave the massage to the masseuse!

should not be transferred to the care of another physician at this time unless the patient is clearly noncompliant or interfering with the physician's ability to provide good post-operative care. Such an action of transfer could be seen as an admission of liability or self-serving behavior on the part of the physician. If a patient, however, is continuously canceling or failing to keep office appointments, or is exhibiting clear drug-seeking behavior or other behaviors destructive to the physician-patient relationship, only then should the physician consider notifying the patient that these behaviors are unacceptable, and that if these behaviors continue, transfer of the patient to the care of another physician will become necessary.

It has been our experience that in almost all malpractice cases, a disparity between the physician's memory and the patient's memory is inevitable. Careful and accurate documentation of all conversations with the patient and her family, as well as of the patient's clinical symptoms and complaints, is very effective at the time of trial. Such "black-and-white" contemporaneous evidence can go a long way toward helping a jury to sort out the facts. It is important to avoid subjective wording that downplays the patient's manifestation of the complication in the documentation, because such wording may be construed as self-serving in the event of litigation.

If the patient requests her medical record, whether it be the hospital medical record or the physician office chart, the tendency of many physicians is to inquire about the reasons for her request. This is not advisable. The better approach is to follow whatever procedure is in place, either in the office or at the hospital, that allows the patient to obtain a copy of her medical record. Under federal and state laws, all patients are entitled to have access to their medical records, and a smooth and nonconfrontational delivery of the relevant documents is always preferred.

Alterations or Additions to the Medical Record

On recognition of a complication or bad outcome, the physician occasionally may be tempted to add information or signatures to the record that were inadvertently omitted before the surgery. Such an action constitutes an alteration of the record when done to look like the documentation occurred before the time actually documented. Alteration in any way of a patient's medical record poses grave dangers in a future medical malpractice case. The medical record is considered, in the eyes of the law, to be a business document and as such is readily admitted into evidence at the time of trial. Any alteration or addition to the medical record that is made to look

like it was documented at an earlier time contemporaneous with an event will always be injurious to the defense of a physician during a medical malpractice case.

The plaintiff or her family at times will request a copy of the medical record very early in the litigation process and sometimes even earlier, during the patient's hospital admission. A physician contemplating adding to or otherwise altering the medical record cannot know whether a copy of that record has already been obtained. If such an addition or alteration is in fact made, then at litigation, two separate copies of medical records will surface during the discovery process—clearly indicating that the medical record was altered for a self-serving purpose. In such instances, the physician's credibility is severely damaged, and cross-examination of the defendant physician at trial will be extremely painful for that physician and very effective for the plaintiff.

As an example, in one case a defendant physician altered the medical record after the incident to reflect documentation of informed consent. Unbeknownst to the defendant physician, the patient had requested a copy of her record before the alteration. After the lawsuit was initiated, the patient requested a second copy, thereby verifying the "massage" of the record. As a result of the physician's indiscretion, her counsel could not permit the physician to testify on her own behalf. Allowing the defendant physician to take the stand would have subjected her to a devastating cross-examination that would have ensured an adverse outcome. Inability of a defendant physician to testify at trial invariably affects how the jury perceives and judges that physician.

After recognizing a maloccurrence or the development of a complication, if the physician feels compelled to add a note or information to the record that was either inadvertently left out or not known at the time, that new documentation must be dated, timed, and labeled as an addendum to the medical record. No harm is incurred in completing such an addendum, and if it is done properly, the physician maintains both credibility and integrity.

THE LITIGATION "TREATMENT PLAN"

Service of the Complaint and Retention of an Attorney

Once the patient or members of her family have decided that they intend to sue the physician, they will contact an attorney. If that attorney, on review of the case, and perhaps with some review by a health care provider, believes that a remittable malpractice action is a possibility, the attorney will file a complaint with the court. Once the physician is served with the complaint, he or she should contact his or her insurance representative or, if employed by a hospital, the hospital risk manager. Physicians pay a great deal of money for malpractice insurance, and this is when that insurance policy and all of its privileges and benefits come into play.

In speaking with the insurance representative or the hospital risk manager, the physician should not discuss any of the specific details of the care of the patient until he or she has been assigned an attorney and that attorney is present for any of those conversations. At this time, the physician should also *not* contact the patient directly. Once the lawsuit is served, all communication between the physician and the patient should be through their attorneys.

At this point, the insurance representative will assign an attorney to represent the defendant physician. As the insured client, however, the physician has the right to have input into the selection of the defense attorney. The physician should question either the insurance representative or the attorney to determine that attorney's level of experience with medical malpractice cases and litigation in general. The field of medical malpractice defense is a very specialized, technical, and complicated area of the practice of law. The average, everyday litigator who tries small cases is not necessarily prepared to handle a major medical malpractice lawsuit. Many attorneys specialize in the area of medical malpractice defense, however, and are very capable of understanding the medicine involved in the case, as well as retaining the right experts to testify on behalf of their clients.

The physician is well within his or her rights to discuss potential conflicts of interest with the defense attorney. A conflict of interest is possible but not inevitable when the defense attorney is asked to represent more than one of the defendants in any given lawsuit. When two or more defendants have a common theme of defense, and neither is blaming the other for the plaintiff's bad outcome, usually no conflict is present. Sometimes, however, a conflict is not apparent in the initial stages of litigation but becomes known as defendants are answering interrogatories or preparing for deposition. The defense attorney has an ethical and legal duty to acknowledge this conflict and request that the defendants in question be afforded separate counsel. Retention of new counsel under these circumstances can take place at any time up to the start of trial.

Once the complaint has been served, the physician's immediate reaction may be a wish to discuss the case with others, to try to "flush out" concerns and the possibility that an error occurred that constituted negligence. The physician must not discuss the case, however, with any professionals or anyone other than the defense attorney and his or her spouse. During the course of litigation, the physician defendant will be deposed—that is, he or she will give testimony under oath before the trial. At that time, the physician defendant will be asked if he or she has discussed this case with any other physicians or individuals. The contents of those discussions must be disclosed at this deposition. In most states, however, conversations with an attorney or a spouse are protected as privileged conversations and not discoverable during the litigation process. This is, again, a very good reason for retaining an attorney who has experience in the field of medical malpractice litigation, to support the physician during this stressful

---

BOX 1–7	*RECEIPT OF A SUMMONS*

- Contact your insurance carrier immediately.
- Request an experienced medical malpractice attorney.
- Communicate with the patient only through this attorney.
- Do not discuss the case with anyone except the defense attorney.

---

process. An experienced attorney will be quite adept at addressing the physician's concerns and giving accurate advice to help steady the physician during this long process.

Initial Meeting with Counsel

Once the defendant physician is assigned an attorney, the attorney will arrange for an initial meeting with the physician. At this time, the physician should bring all original records and documents in his or her possession that pertain in any way to the care and treatment of the plaintiff patient. This usually means that the physician brings office documents, photographs, and test results kept in the office and not those documents kept at the hospital. Hospital medical records usually are not in the custody or control of the individual physician; therefore, owing to privacy regulations, the physician should not even attempt to obtain these.

At this initial meeting, the physician defendant should be honest and forthcoming with the attorney. The medical malpractice defense attorney will be most effective when armed with all of the available information. This meeting also is an appropriate time for the defendant physician to ask initial questions regarding the process, especially if this is the first time that he or she has been sued for malpractice.

This meeting will be the first of numerous meetings and contacts with the attorney over a number of years. Unfortunately, owing to the complexity of the court system and the vast numbers of civil lawsuits that are brought every day, a medical malpractice case can continue for approximately 3 to 6 years or longer before trial or settlement. During this period, the physician frequently feels that nothing is happening and that he or she is receiving no information. In fact, however, long periods of inactivity are typical in a medical malpractice case, especially during the discovery phase. Some of this apparent inactivity is attributable to the mechanisms of the legal process, and some to the tremendous backlog of civil cases in the court system.

Litigation Discovery Phase

The discovery phase of the litigation process begins after the complaint is served and ends at the time that a trial date is assigned by the court. This phase can last anywhere from 2 to 4 or 5 years or longer.

INITIAL JUDICIAL SCREENING

During the discovery phase, a number of events will take place. A few states still have what is referred to as a *tribunal*, or screening process after the complaint is filed, to try to prevent frivolous lawsuits from being continued. In the few states that do continue this process, however, a majority of cases do progress past the screening or tribunal process and are allowed to continue through litigation.

PAPER DISCOVERY

Throughout the discovery phase, the plaintiff's and the defendant's attorneys will exchange written *Requests for the Production of Documents*. This phase affords each side of the lawsuit to gain knowledge of any and all medical records, diaries, radiographic films, and other graphic or written materials in preparation for trial. The defense attorney will contact the defendant physician when the plaintiff's attorney has made such a request for documents in the physician's possession. On receipt of such a request, the physician must make a "diligent search" to find any and all documents that satisfy each of the requests made by the plaintiff's attorney. This search may include looking back through files, diaries, or datebooks or in the archives of physician office records. Compliance with these requests is mandated by law, and the physician should be forthcoming with the defense attorney regarding the existence of any documents, regardless of concern that they may be injurious to the defense of the case. Certain documents will not need to be produced if in the opinion of the defense attorney they are privileged for one legal reason or another. The defense attorney cannot make this determination, however, without access to all documents in the physician's possession that may pertain to the litigation.

The discovery phase includes an exchange of written questions called *interrogatories.* The plaintiff will serve the defense attorney with interrogatories that must be answered and signed under oath by the physician defendant. The defense attorney in turn will serve the plaintiff with interrogatories that he or she must answer under oath as well. Once the defense attorney receives these requests for interrogatories, he or she should contact the physician to ask for active participation in answering these questions.

The need for accuracy in answering interrogatories cannot be overstated. Answers to interrogatories, once signed under the pains and penalties of perjury, become the physician's sworn testimony and are essentially the equivalent of sworn testimony at trial. Because they are done early in the discovery process and usually a number of years before the trial, the physician's memory of the events will arguably be better and more accurate at the time that he or she answers the interrogatories.

Interrogatories are used by the plaintiff for a number of purposes. First, the plaintiff uses them to obtain additional information such as the identification of other persons who may have information regarding the facts of the case, the defendant physician's memory of conversations with the plaintiff patient that are not documented in the medical record, and the physician's recollection of statements or activities by the plaintiff patient that also are not documented in the medical record. The plaintiff also will prepare to use the physician's answers to interrogatories at the time of trial to cross-examine the physician on the witness stand. Any conflict between the physician's testimony at trial and the physician's answers to interrogatories will provide grist for the plaintiff's cross-examination mill. A new and conflicting memory brought up at trial, often a few years after sworn answers to interrogatories, presents the physician as lacking in credibility to the 12 to 14 members of the jury.

Accuracy in answering these interrogatories, therefore, is crucial, and the theme of the physician's defense must be at least preliminarily formulated at the time these documents are prepared, so that the physician's answers do not later injure the ultimate theory of defense at trial. The need for careful, well-thought-out answers cannot be overemphasized, and this is one phase in the discovery process in which the physician must actively participate and cooperate with the defense attorney.

Parties will, although less often, also serve each other with *Requests for Admissions*. These documents are similar to interrogatories but are statements made that must be either admitted or denied. Requests for admissions are extremely time sensitive and, again, are the equivalent of testimony under oath. The physician's timely contribution to information and completion of this document also are essential.

RETENTION OF EXPERT WITNESSES

As soon as the plaintiff's medical records are available, the medical malpractice defense attorney retains experts in the same field as that of the defendant physician, as well as in areas of medicine necessary to determine the exact cause of the plaintiff's injury. These expert witnesses are paid, usually an hourly rate, by the insurance company to review all records, radiographs, and legal documents and then to render an opinion regarding the defendant physician's compliance with the standard of care, as well as any causal link between the defendant physician's actions and the plaintiff's alleged injuries. The expert is not necessarily the top physician in any given field but is instead a qualified physician with experience in the field. Most important, the expert has an ability to explain the issues to a lay jury and teach the lay jury the basis of his or her opinion.

Usually, the defendant physician is not in contact with any of the retained experts. This avoidance of contact is to protect the defendant physician from knowledge regarding the identity and opinions of the defense experts that would require disclosure at his or her deposition before the defense team has solidified the theory of the defense and determined which experts will testify at trial. Information regarding defense expert opinions is usually shared to some extent between co-defense attorneys in a malpractice case. Such sharing is most frequent with expert testimony regarding issues of causation and damages, because the defense of causation and damages is often common to all defendants. Less often but not uncommonly, standard of care defense themes also are shared by co-defense attorneys, especially if the allegations against the defendants are identical in nature and in timing.

DEPOSITIONS

The last and perhaps most significant element of the discovery process is the taking of depositions. The plaintiff will take the depositions of the defendant physician and fact witnesses, and the defendant physician's attorney will take the depositions of the plaintiffs, family members, and other fact witnesses.

Plaintiff's counsel deposes the defendant physician with multiple purposes in mind. The attorney is always seeking information, to uncover previously unknown facts. He or she also tries to maneuver the defendant physician into verbalizing specific facts or opinions, with the hope of obtaining statements that can be used at trial to injure the defense. These statements are used to cross-examine the physician if he or she attempts to change his or her testimony at trial. Plaintiff's counsel also will attempt to use each defendant physician as a potential expert against any co-defendant physician or other health care provider. It is therefore easy to recognize that notwithstanding the physician's participation in answering interrogatories and gathering documents, the physician's most crucial role before the trial is in giving his or her deposition. The need for preparation for the defendant physician's deposition cannot be overstated. This preparation is akin to preparation for trial, because the deposition is testimony under oath, given over a period of perhaps hours, that is recorded by a stenographer and becomes the physician's sworn statement.

Many physicians believe they can convince plaintiff's counsel to dismiss the case if they can tell "their side of the story" at deposition. This is a critical mistake. The physician must guard against the instinct to be too forthcoming, trying to explain his or her actions in the case and in the treatment of the plaintiff. The defendant physician's only two obligations at the deposition are (1) to tell the truth and (2) to answer the question that is asked. A case is never won at the deposition stage, but many cases are lost. Failure to keep the answer focused on the attorney's question many times generates testimony that appears to be defensive or that can easily be taken out of context and injure the defendant.

The physician should insist that the defense attorney prepare him or her extensively for deposition testimony. The best preparation includes not only a discussion of the facts, issues, and theme of the defense but a mock or practice deposition, with the attorney playing the role of the plaintiff's attorney and putting the physician through a session of difficult questioning. Defense firms that conduct mock depositions of their client physicians also frequently videotape these sessions, which allows the defendant physician and the attorney to review the mock testimony process and then critique and improve the physician's performance.

Before discussing and practicing the deposition testimony with the attorney, the physician should have a thorough knowledge of the medical record, both the hospital record and the office record, as well as of his or her answers to interrogatories. Knowledge of the facts will assist the physician in supporting or refuting statements at the time of deposition. Notwithstanding the need to know the medical record, the physician is cautioned, however, not to do general research on the issues of the case nor to discuss the case with others, including co-workers and peers. Research into the medical issues of the case potentially subjects the physician to extensive questioning regarding the content of that research. Such outside investigation also increases the risk that the defendant physician may inadvertently testify to some scholarly source that plaintiff's counsel could argue is a proof of a standard of care contradictory to the defendant's theme of defense. Discussion with co-workers or peers about the case also subjects the physician to the possibility that plaintiff's counsel will then later depose those peers in an attempt to elicit information that may be construed as an admission of guilt by the physician.

At the time of the deposition, the physician defendant is cautioned to listen carefully to each question and then to answer only that question. Although it is well known that physicians are inherently teachers with a great desire to explain complex issues to lay people, this is not the time to teach or educate the plaintiff's attorney. To the contrary, the plaintiff's attorney should be made to work for any information that he or she obtains at a deposition.

A deponent physician may testify from three bases. First, he or she may testify from actual memory of the events. Second, the physician may testify to what he or she alone has documented. Last, the physician may testify, absent a memory and documentation, based on his or her usual custom and practice with respect to a given activity. The physician is cautioned to testify only to what he or she actually recalls, and never to guess or assume that information provided by the plaintiff's attorney in the question is, in fact, true.

The physician deponent should remain calm at all times and not allow himself or herself to be lulled by a friendly attorney or enraged by a confrontational attorney. The physician is being evaluated by plaintiff's counsel during the tenancy of the deposition for his or her potential courtroom appearance. If the physician can present himself or herself at a deposition as professional, caring, and articulate, plaintiff's counsel may recognize the potential difficulty in portraying the physician as less than competent to a lay jury.

On completion of the deposition and a number of weeks later, the physician will receive a copy of the transcript of the deposition. This deposition must then be reviewed for errors made in the transcription, and for minor errors made in the physician's articulation of answers, before signing the transcript. Once the physician signs the transcript, the deposition testimony becomes a sworn statement and essentially carries the same legal weight as that of testimony at trial.

Trial versus Settlement

After the completion of all discovery and before trial, a decision is made by the physician's insurers to either settle the case or proceed to trial. Some jurisdictions and some insurance companies request the defendant physician's consent to settle before entering settlement negotiations.

Trial versus settlement is a complex decision, dependent on a number of factors. These factors include (1) expert support on behalf of the defendant physician for his or her compliance with the standard of care, (2) expert support

---

BOX 1–8   *DISCOVERY PHASE OF LITIGATION*

- Make a diligent search for all pertinent documents and medical records.
- Work with your attorney to complete accurate answers to the plaintiff's interrogatories.
- Prepare thoroughly for deposition testimony to prevent potential cross-examination at trial.
- Present yourself as professional, caring, and articulate.

regarding the relationship between the physician's actions and the actual cause of the plaintiff's alleged injury, (3) sympathy factors, (4) assessment of the plaintiff as a witness, and (5) assessment of the defendant physician as a witness. These factors all are evaluated and a risk analysis is completed. Strong defendant expert support and willingness by the experts to testify are necessary before trial can even be considered. When contributing to the decision of trial versus settlement, the defendant physician should consider personal risks and benefits of settling versus trying a malpractice action. The experienced medical malpractice attorney is a valuable resource in assisting the physician in evaluating these risks and benefits.

A trial is mentally and emotionally taxing to the physician. Extensive preparation is necessary in light of the physician's need to give both direct testimony and cross-examination testimony. The physician also will be subject to sitting in the courtroom for days on end (usually 1 to 3 weeks) listening while the plaintiff's attorney and witnesses testify to the physician's "uncaring" attitude and "incompetent" diagnosis and treatment of the plaintiff. Win or lose, the physician defendant is emotionally and professionally taxed for this period of time.

Should the defendant physician lose the trial, the loss is reported to that state's Board of Registration in Medicine, as well as to the National Practice Data Bank, and becomes a public record as a plaintiff's verdict and a loss for the physician defendant. Another consideration is the negative publicity that frequently surrounds medical malpractice cases, especially the larger, more dynamic cases or any case that is tried in a small town.

Should the physician and the insurer decide that settlement is the appropriate method of resolution, numerous discussions then ensue among plaintiff's counsel, the insurance company, and defense counsel. Settlement, at times, can take place months before the trial, the evening before trial, or even after the trial has begun. A settlement also must be reported to the Board of Registration in Medicine for the individual state, as well as to the National Practice Data Bank, and again becomes part of a public record. Most settlement agreements, however, contain confidentiality agreements wherein the name of the physician may be kept confidential and not publicized.

Trial Preparation

Should a medical malpractice case go to trial, extensive preparation is necessary. The defense attorney will begin preparing months before the trial but may involve the defendant physician only as late as 3 to 4 weeks before trial. At that time, the defendant physician will need to start meeting with the defense attorney and preparing the specific theme of the defense. Included in this preparation is the identification of necessary witnesses, evidence, illustrations, and other visuals. The defendant physician can be instrumental in assisting the defense attorney in identifying evidence necessary for trial and in creating visuals or other displays necessary to teach the jury the intricacies of medicine. The defendant physician's participation and cooperation in trial preparation, including flexibility regarding time requirements for this process, are essential.

BOX 1–9	**TRIAL**

- Participate with your attorney in trial preparation.
- Speak directly to the jury and take the role of caretaker and teacher.
- Remain calm and professional under cross-examination.
- Convince the jurors that each of them would want you as his or her physician.

The defendant physician's attorney must prepare the physician extensively, both for direct examination and for cross-examination by the plaintiff's attorney. Again, such preparation is best done with mock or practice sessions, with the defense attorney playing the role of the plaintiff's attorney. This role playing allows the physician to experience the difficult questions and possible badgering anticipated at the time of trial.

When testifying, the physician must remember to speak to the jury. Eye contact and responsiveness to the jury will help create a line of communication with understanding and bonding between jury members and physician. When giving direct testimony, the physician should recognize that his or her role with the jury is that of teacher, because this is an opportunity to explain his or her reasoning and actions when caring for the plaintiff. Under cross-examination, the physician should remain calm and listen carefully to each question, enabling him or her to professionally point out any mischaracterizations of facts or suppositions made by the plaintiff's attorney in the question. The physician should at all times avoid intense emotion and maintain a calm, professional, and caring attitude, thereby convincing each member of the jury that they would potentially want him or her as their physician.

During preparation for the trial and pendancy of the trial, it is important for the physician to remember to let the defense attorney do the lawyering. The attorney needs and wants the physician's input into medical matters, including the facts and details of the medical case. When it comes to judgment calls in the courtroom and decisions regarding legal issues, however, the attorney is far more experienced than the physician in these areas.

SUMMARY

Medical malpractice lawsuits have become an unfortunate companion to the practice of medicine. Such lawsuits are expensive, time consuming, and emotionally painful to the physician. Some suits are avoidable, and the physician should make earnest attempts to structure his or her practice and communication style with patients to help prevent such litigation. Other lawsuits are, unfortunately, unavoidable. The pain and expense of the litigation process, however, may be greatly mitigated by the physician's conduct in caring for the patient, by timely recognition of the complication or unwanted outcome, and by knowledgeably participating in the litigation process. The physician who practices this form of "defensive medicine" can and does limit his or her ultimate exposure to the medical malpractice lawsuit.

The Role of the Anesthesia Team in the Avoidance, Diagnosis, Management, and Genesis of Laparoscopic Complications

2

Warren S. Sandberg and Rodger M. White

Preventable medical errors such as complications of surgery have become a central focus in health care. Public attention was drawn to this issue in 1999 by the Institute of Medicine (IOM).[1] In the IOM report, between 50,000 and 100,000 people were estimated to die every year in U.S. hospitals from preventable medical errors.

The perioperative period is one of particular significance for patient safety. More than 25 years ago, initial studies focusing on anesthesia practices identified multiple areas in which improvements could be made in these systems.[2] Through those efforts, many accomplishments were successfully made in augmenting fundamental processes in anesthesiology, and risks were reduced substantially in the operating room.[3] The primary areas for change to increase patient safety have been in teamwork and the culture of the operating room environment. Many programs have been developed to heighten training and increase the use of "checklists" before and during procedures, to diminish the likelihood of mistakes. These sociologic modifications enhance the patient's protection from harm and the precision with which health care providers work. When sociologic modifications depend solely on changing clinical practices and attitudes, the opportunity for human error persists.

System changes to reduce error each have an inherent power or robustness. In descending order of robustness, these changes are as follows[4]:

- Force function (i.e., explicit exclusion of dangerous items from a care path)
- Automation and computerization of functions
- Protocols and preprinted orders
- Checklists
- Rules and double-checks
- Education
- Information

The most powerful safety interventions complement human activity with a property that can be described as "augmented vigilance." For example, computerized provider order entry (CPOE) systems collect information about patient medication allergies, as well as previous orders, and issue warnings when incompatible and duplicate drugs are ordered.[5] The CPOE system has tremendous power in typical ward and intensive care unit (ICU) settings, bringing force function and automation features to pharmacy and treatment ordering. Unfortunately, many of the most powerful interventions for error prevention are not useful in the perioperative environment. The CPOE system is completely short-circuited in the operating room, where clinicians give drugs directly from the supply cabinet without any automated features.

Because of the immediacy of the environment, the compressed time frame, and the criticality of events, error reduction strategies that are highly effective in the rest of the hospital sometimes are impractical in the operating room. Instead, current approaches to minimizing errors and preventing complications involve the accumulation of perioperative procedures and redundant checks that add to the cognitive workload of operating room personnel and are still often ineffective. For example, most operating rooms have adopted a "time-out" procedure wherein, just before the procedure begins, the entire team stops to review information about the identity of the patient and the site, laterality, and nature of the surgical procedure. To be effective, this protocol requires each team member to become independently informed of the answers to these questions by directly querying the conscious patient. Such repeated investigations are neither efficient nor reassuring to the patient. The time-out procedure itself is an example of a double-check—and consequently a weak agent for system improvement.

The best perioperative systems highlight the potential for the application of basic principles of management and industrial design, coupled with emerging technologies, to smooth the flow of patients through the operating suite and to enhance their safety. It has not yet been possible, however, to assemble all of the available pieces in one project, and many pieces are missing altogether. Instead, preoperative, intraoperative, and postoperative environments are characterized by (1) an array of ergonomic deficiencies; (2) inefficient, ineffective, and redundant processes; (3) fragmented communications and team integration; (4) inflexible "systems" of operation; (5) staffing shortages (nurses and technicians); and (6) variable levels of competency among perioperative personnel. These factors contribute to an environment in which patient safety cannot be assumed. Within this context, laparoscopic surgery has developed in earnest over the past 2 decades and has come to be perceived as "safer" or less traumatic than conventional surgery, both by patients and increasingly by the medical community.[6]

Laparoscopic surgery has many advantages for patients. For example, laparoscopy is recognized to cause fewer intraabdominal adhesions than result with open surgery and to be associated with a quicker recovery of bowel function.[7,8] It also results in less pain,[9] shorter hospital stays,[10,11] lower hospital costs,[12] quicker return to activities of daily living,[13] improved postoperative pulmonary function,[14-18] and smaller incisional scars. As noted by several authors, however, "Minimally invasive surgery does not mean minimal surgery."[19,20] In fact, because even the simplest laparoscopy carries a risk of life-threatening complication requiring immediate laparotomy, it has been suggested that laparoscopy should be performed only in operating rooms "fully equipped to handle all aspects of open surgery including vascular suturing."[19]

It generally is accepted that the risk of complications is greater with more complex and difficult laparoscopic procedures than with simpler cases.[21] In a nationwide study of laparoscopic complications from Finland, both the study findings[22] and the literature review[23,24] confirmed that the rates of complications increased with the difficulty of the procedure. A later Finnish study documented a risk of complications that was more than 10 times greater for operative laparoscopy than for diagnostic or sterilization laparoscopy.[25]

Most discussions concerning complications of laparoscopic surgery take a surgical perspective. Complications are divided into immediate and delayed types, and the focus is on the prevention, recognition, and management of common and also less frequent complications of laparoscopy. This chapter presents a somewhat broader view that encompasses the role of the anesthesiologist in the prevention, recognition, and management of complications encountered during laparoscopy—specifically, those complications that occur and are managed primarily in the operating room. Accordingly, discussion begins with complications heretofore regarded as primarily surgical in nature, stressing the multidisciplinary approach to their prevention, recognition, and management. Included next is a section on complications managed primarily by anesthesiologists, as well as complications related to anesthesia that may affect the surgical result or could otherwise surface during postsurgical care. Then, some of the challenges impeding the reliable early recognition and effective management of complications that do occur are presented, and an effective approach to minimizing the likelihood of intraoperative complications is outlined. Finally, a suggested

framework is provided for actually rehearsing the management of the rare but life-threatening complications of laparoscopic surgery.

SURGICAL COMPLICATIONS

Acute complications of laparoscopic surgery occur fairly rarely and usually are recognized and managed in the immediate perioperative period. Surgical complications such as intestinal and vascular injuries, gas embolism, or pneumothorax, however, can cause severe physiologic derangements and frequently are fatal if not recognized and effectively managed. In many cases, the anesthesia team is involved in the diagnosis and management of complications that have primarily surgical origins, so they are in many senses shared. Thus, when appropriate, a team approach to prevention and management is recommended and is described in the following discussion.

Intestinal Injuries

Intestinal injuries have been reported to occur during laparoscopic surgery at a rate of between 0% and 0.5%.[26] Approximately half of these injuries are caused during entry into the abdominal cavity with a Veress needle or trocar, and the other half occur during the operative procedure itself,[26-28] with many of these from electrocautery.

Prevention

Hasson and colleagues[29] and other investigators[30] have suggested that intestinal injuries related to entry can be largely if not completely avoided by use of an open technique to gain access to the peritoneal cavity. Others have suggested that indications for open entry include a history of more than two previous lower abdominal surgeries, generalized peritonitis, and inflammatory bowel disease.[31] Trocar-related bowel injury often can be prevented by decompressing the stomach if distention related to induction of anesthesia is suspected and by carefully evaluating the patient for possible abdominal wall adhesions.[32] If presence of adhesions is likely, alternatives to closed entry include the open access described by Hasson and colleagues[29] and a left upper quadrant incision.[32] With respect to gastric decompression, many laparoscopic teams routinely use orogastric tubes for decompression.

In a review of 266 cases of intestinal injury, more than half were caused by electrocautery.[26,33] These injuries often can be prevented by meticulous technique with application of cautery contact points during tissue dissection.[26,33] In addition, because it has been shown that monopolar cautery can easily raise the temperature of tissue up to several centimeters from the operative site and that a temperature differential of 30° C for just 2 seconds can lead to tissue death,[34] monopolar cautery should not be used on duct-like strands of tissue that may be attached to bowel.[26,33]

Recognition

Because of the blind nature of the closed entry technique and the limited field of view of the surgeon during the procedure, most bowel injuries are not recognized intraoperatively.[26,32] Even postoperatively, the diagnosis may be complicated by the fact that most patients do not present with the typical signs and symptoms of a bowel perforation.[26] Instead of the ileus, abdominal rigidity, rebound tenderness, and leukocytosis that are traditionally associated with perforated viscus, most of these injuries manifest as increased pain at a single trocar site, without erythema or purulent discharge. During subsequent laparotomy, the injured bowel segment frequently is found near the painful trocar site. Signs and symptoms can progress from abdominal distention with diarrhea and normal bowel sounds to sepsis and death before overt peritoneal signs are apparent. Leukopenia is a more common finding than leukocytosis.[26,33] When the clinical picture in the postoperative period is suggestive of bowel perforation, computed tomography (CT) can help confirm the diagnosis.[35] Because most bowel injuries go unrecognized at the time of surgery and manifest atypically in the postoperative period, they rank as either the most common or the second most common cause of postoperative death related to laparoscopy.[36-38]

Why bowel injury caused by laparoscopy manifests differently from that caused by open surgery is not clear. One possibility may be that laparoscopic surgery, performed in the absence of a large skin incision, produces less of a metabolic and immune response than that observed with open surgery.[39] Subsequently, sepsis may supervene before natural homeostatic responses are clinically apparent.[26,33]

Management

When recognized intraoperatively, bowel injuries should be repaired immediately.[26,33] Repair often can be accomplished without the need for colostomy.[40,41]

Vascular Injuries

Injury to major vascular structures in the anterior abdominal wall can occur during trocar insertion and in the intraperitoneal and the retroperitoneal spaces during Veress needle or trocar insertion or during surgical dissection or resection.[32]

Prevention

Epigastric vessel injury usually can be prevented by placing accessory trocars lateral to the rectus muscles and by directly observing their placement through the endoscopic camera.[42] Minor intraperitoneal bleeding occurs during any abdominal procedure. It is prevented by meticulous surgical technique and managed by cautery, suture ligature, or application of vascular clips. Injury to major retroperitoneal vessels is nearly five times more likely to occur during Veress needle or trocar insertion than during the laparoscopic procedure.[32,43] These injuries occur infrequently (0.04% to 0.1% of laparoscopic procedures),[28,30,36,44,45] but they carry a 9% to 17% mortality rate.[36,44] These injuries are caused with almost equal frequency by needle and by trocar insertion.[28,43,46,47] The need for meticulous technique and constant vigilance is highlighted by the finding that greater than a third of trocar-related retroperitoneal vessel injuries are caused by insertion of secondary trocars.[47]

Recognition

Although major vascular injuries are easily recognized when they result in hemoperitoneum and hemodynamic instability, most entry injuries to retroperitoneal vessels result in the more subtle finding of retroperitoneal hematoma,[26,48] which accounts for the fact that these injuries sometimes are missed intraoperatively.[48] In one series from 1995, all patients whose major retroperitoneal vascular injuries were recognized and corrected intraoperatively survived, whereas almost half of those whose injuries were discovered in the postoperative period died. This group consisted almost entirely of young healthy women. The investigators noted that as more laparoscopic procedures are performed on older and sicker patients, the probability of surviving an unrecognized injury to a major retroperitoneal vessel probably will decrease.[48]

Management

Management of vascular injuries depends on the clinical stability of the patient and on the skill and experience of the laparoscopic surgeon. Options for management of epigastric vessel injury include balloon tamponade and suture ligature.[32] Major retroperitoneal vessel injuries historically required immediate laparotomy. With the development of more sophisticated endoscopic instruments, major retroperitoneal vessel injuries often can now be managed laparoscopically.[49] Nevertheless, in the event of a major vascular injury, immediate consultation in the operating room with a vascular surgeon is recommended.

The anesthesia team can do little to modify the risk of vascular injury during laparoscopy, but they contribute significantly to its management, starting with the initial intravenous access. A 20-gauge intravenous line is adequate for most uncomplicated laparoscopic procedures. Even the most minor procedure has the potential for major vascular injury, however, so consideration should be given to establishing supplemental large-bore intravenous access proactively if difficulty with intraoperative placement of additional intravenous lines is anticipated. In practice, we routinely place 18-gauge intravenous lines for most laparoscopic procedures and are quick to add 14-gauge catheters when potentially needed.

The anesthesia team will deal with resuscitation during the repair of a vascular injury, with attention to several details. First, in the instance of an arterial injury, a balance must be struck between keeping the blood pressure low enough to limit hemorrhage and high enough to provide organ perfusion. Second, pressors may be used to temporize while intravascular volume is being restored, but they are not substitutes for adequate circulating volume. With sufficient driving pressure, 1000 mL of warmed crystalloid can be given through an 18-gauge intravenous line in approximately 5 minutes. Such a volume challenge should restore normal hemodynamics during the early phase of all but the most severe vascular injuries. An ongoing pressor requirement during laparoscopy, especially in patients without intercurrent cardiovascular disease, is an indicator of a problem (typically with circulating volume) that needs to be identified and addressed. The anesthesiologist may bring this suspicion to the attention of the surgeon when no hemorrhage had been previously noted. Finally, in the instance of a venous injury, the anesthesia team must strike a balance between keeping the central venous pressure low to minimize hemorrhage and keeping the pressure normal to high to minimize the likelihood of CO_2 embolism. Because the vast majority of laparoscopy patients do not have central catheters in place, central venous pressure, which reflects the adequacy of intravascular volume, can be derived only very indirectly from the blood pressure.

Some vascular injuries can be repaired laparoscopically,[49] but a definitive repair should be completed by whatever method is most likely to lead to a good outcome for the patient. The anesthesia team should keep the surgical team apprised of the patient's hemodynamic and homeostatic status during attempts at laparoscopic repairs of vascular injuries. This is an important contribution to the overall management of the patient so that, if necessary, the decision to convert a laparoscopic to an open procedure can be made in a timely fashion.

Hemorrhage Not Related to Vascular Injury

Persistent bleeding from cut or cauterized surfaces (such as the gallbladder bed, the prostate bed, or cavities from uterine fibroids) can occur and may be severe. Such bleeding is an entity distinct from vascular injury involving a great vessel because its pathogenesis is related to a typical feature of the surgery.

Prevention

Meticulous surgical technique is key to preventing excessive postoperative hemorrhage. In some cases, patients may be coagulopathic, either by design or as a result of illness. Frequently these patients can be safely operated on with appropriate attention to surgical technique. Nevertheless, patients who are anticoagulated are at increased risk for postoperative hemorrhage, and anticoagulation should probably be reversed or allowed to remit before surgery. One exception to this approach is in the management of those patients who have recently had an intracoronary stent. Such patients should not undergo elective surgery in the immediate post-stent period (see later on).

Recognition

Postoperative hemorrhage can manifest as abdominal pain and hemodynamic instability in the postanesthesia care unit (PACU). The extent of the bleeding, perhaps due to tamponade from the insufflating gas, may not be appreciated in the operating room. Ongoing hemorrhage may possibly be recognized only as hemodynamic instability in the PACU. If the hemorrhage is brisk and volume resuscitation has been inadequate, the hematocrit remains normal. Typically, hypotension is treated with crystalloid loading, so dilutional anemia does develop during the course of resuscitation. A drop in hematocrit should raise concerns about hemorrhage, but a normal hematocrit in the setting of hemodynamic instability points more to inadequate resuscitation than to the absence of hemorrhage.

Management

Expectant management is possible, but reexploration, potentially by laparotomy, frequently is required. Marked postoperative hemodynamic instability in the setting of suspected ongoing hemorrhage requires urgent or emergent reexploration by laparotomy. The anesthesia team will insist on placing large-bore (16-gauge or greater in adults) intravenous access lines and will administer resuscitation fluids (warm crystalloid or blood), as appropriate, before reestablishing anesthesia in patients who are markedly unstable. It may be difficult to achieve skeletal muscle paralysis with nondepolarizing agents if anticholinesterases have been used. The patient also may be much less robust in the face of vasodilators (such as propofol) due to intravascular volume depletion, leading the anesthesia team to consider alternative induction agents such as etomidate.

Unrecognized, uncontrolled postoperative hemorrhage could be catastrophic for patients who are discharged home. Thus, it is important to observe patients at risk (particularly those with potentially elevated risk due to large exposed surfaces or coagulopathy, for example) for a reasonable period in the PACU, which may extend beyond that required to recover from anesthesia. Patients also should meet formally established and consistently applied criteria for discharge from the PACU.

Urinary Injuries

Prevention

The type of procedure largely determines which urinary structures are at greatest risk intraoperatively for injuries to the urinary tract. The bladder is particularly vulnerable during laparoscopically assisted vaginal hysterectomy, whereas the ureter is a greatest risk during endoscopic adnexectomy.[50] Regardless of procedure type, endometriosis and dense adhesions from previous surgery or pelvic inflammatory disease increase the risk of urinary injuries during laparoscopy.[32,50] As the complexity of operative cases performed laparoscopically increases, so too does the risk of serious urinary complications.[32] Although meticulous exposure, identification of anatomic landmarks, and careful dissection will reduce the risk, at present no technique completely devoid of risk for ureteral complications is available.[50]

Recognition

Urinary injuries are seen in 0.02% to 1.7% of laparoscopies. This is the same incidence as that seen with open gynecologic surgery.[26] Bladder injuries are both more common and more commonly recognized intraoperatively than ureteral injuries.[26,32,50-52] A review of urinary injuries showed that bladder injuries were recognized intraoperatively greater than 90% of the time, whereas ureteral injuries were recognized intraoperatively less than 7% of the time.[53] Bladder perforations account for greater than half of all urinary injuries, followed by fistula, ureter ligation, and ureter transection.[29] The bladder is especially vulnerable during insertion of Veress needles and trocars if not decompressed first with a Foley or straight catheter.[32]

Management

Anesthesiologists participate indirectly in the management of urinary injuries. When ureteral injury is suspected, intravenous injection of indigo carmine dye followed by observation for spillage into the surgical field and cystoscopy to confirm ureteral jets into the bladder can aid diagnosis.[26,32,50] Sufficient intravenous fluid volume should be given to ensure adequate urine flow, so that the dye may be visualized if a leak is present, but without subjecting the patient to volume overload. Most bladder injuries can be repaired primarily and drained for 7 to 10 days.[54] Ureteral injuries are managed by placement of a ureteral stent and urologic consultation.[32,50,55]

Pneumothorax

Prevention

Although pneumothorax is believed to be a rare complication of pneumoperitoneum of laparoscopy,[56-59] several cases are described in the literature.[57,60-65] These events most frequently are attributed to diaphragmatic defects, which may be either congenital or acquired.[59,62,64] Certainly, any procedure involving extensive dissection around the diaphragm carries a risk of diaphragmatic injury that could lead to pneumothorax. Again, low insufflation pressures, facilitated by optimal anesthetic conditions, as well as meticulous surgical technique, especially in anatomic areas close to the diaphragm, are key to preventing this complication.

Recognition

Because a pneumothorax can rapidly progress to a tension pneumothorax, a high index of suspicion must be maintained and corrective action should be undertaken quickly.[57,60,62,64] The most frequently reported signs of intraoperative pneumothorax related to entry of CO_2 through diaphragmatic defects are a decrease in oxygen saturation (SpO_2)[6,62,64-66] (Fig. 2–1), an increase in end-tidal CO_2 caused by increased CO_2 absorption,[59,65,66,68] an increase in airway pressures,[59,64-67] and, if hemodynamic instability develops, a decrease in arterial blood pressure.[65,66]

The literature contains at least one documented report of tension pneumothorax associated with use of the argon beam coagulator,[68] presumably caused by a sudden increase in intracavitary pressure from the rapid influx of argon gas. The authors of this case report recommend opening the trocar evacuation valves to avoid barotrauma.[68]

Management

When pneumothorax occurs during laparoscopy, it is essential to first establish the cause in order to guide treatment. Suspicion of pneumothorax prompts a discussion between the anesthesia and the surgical teams to pinpoint the likely cause and to plan management. Traditionally, intraoperative pneumothorax is managed with thoracentesis,[62,64,66,69,70] sometimes followed by tube thoracostomy.[59,66] In otherwise normal patients, especially when dissection involves the diaphragm, migration of CO_2 from the abdomen is a reasonable first assumption for the cause. In such instances, it is reasonable to

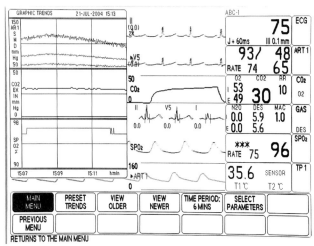

Figure 2–1 ▪ **Physiologic monitor with trends displayed.** The *left* side of the image displays key trend data for laparoscopy anesthesia. Arterial blood pressure (continuous in this case, because the patient has an intra-arterial catheter), end-tidal CO_2 ($ETCO_2$), and oxygen saturation (SpO_2) are displayed for the preceding 6 minutes. The *middle* section displays instantaneous waveform data for physiologic parameters, and the right side displays numeric data recapitulating and extending the middle section. The first two waveforms in the *middle* section are electrocardiogram (ECG) tracings used for rhythm monitoring. The heart rate derived from the ECG is given in the first box on the *right* side of the display. The heart rate also is derived from the arterial pressure waveform and SpO_2 plethysmograph (boxes 2 and 5 on the *right* side of the display); bradycardia is readily recognized both from waveform tracings and from the numeric rate information. The fourth waveform in the *middle* section of the display is an ST segment monitor for inferior and lateral ECG leads, useful for diagnosing myocardial ischemia. The third waveform in the *middle* section of the display (and the corresponding third box on the *right*) shows the $ETCO_2$. The anesthesiologist has adjusted the ventilation to lower the $ETCO_2$ to 30 mm Hg; the resultant arterial PCO_2 probably is somewhat less than the normal value of 40 mm Hg. The fifth and sixth *center* waveforms are the SpO_2 plethysmograph and arterial pressure, respectively. The fourth box on the *right* indicates that anesthesia is being maintained with desflurane, probably at an adequate concentration to suppress recall. The sixth box on the *right* displays temperature. The patient is hypothermic, the monitor image having been captured just after surgical preparation.

replace nitrous oxide (if it is being used) with oxygen and then to adjust ventilator settings to correct hypoxemia. Positive end-expiratory pressure (PEEP) should be applied and the intra-abdominal pressure lowered as much as possible. Application of PEEP decreases the pressure gradient between the peritoneal and the pleural cavities and reinflates the affected lung.[57] If these maneuvers prove efficacious, then thoracentesis and tube thoracostomy probably can be avoided, because the CO_2 will be rapidly reabsorbed in the early postoperative period.

PEEP is therapeutic for pneumothorax caused by passage of CO_2 from the abdominal cavity into the interpleural space only when airway integrity is intact.[57] If these initial maneuvers do not solve the problem, and the likely cause is airway or alveolar rupture, then PEEP should be discontinued. In cases in which pneumothorax is caused by airway or alveolar disruption, as by rupture of a preexisting pulmonary bulla, application of PEEP would exacerbate rather than alleviate pulmonary dysfunction and probably lead to tension pneumothorax, with decreased cardiac output and decreased end-tidal CO_2. Treatment is with thoracentesis, followed by tube thoracostomy.[57]

Gas Embolism

Gas embolism is a rare but often fatal complication of laparoscopic surgery.[26,71] Reported incidence rates for carbon dioxide embolism range from 0.002% to 0.016%.[72] Previous abdominal surgery has been proposed as an independent risk factor for gas embolism.[73] Although this complication occurs most frequently during or shortly after insufflation when CO_2 is injected under pressure,[26] cardiac arrest[74,75] and fatalities[76] due to gas embolism also have been associated with laparoscopic use of the argon beam coagulator. Furthermore, at least two case reports describe delayed cardiac arrest attributed to gas embolism. In one report, a patient died suddenly approximately 1 hour after CO_2 insufflation. X-ray studies and postmortem examination revealed gas in the portal circulation, the heart, the brain, and the coronary circulation, with a probe-patent foramen ovale.[77] In the second report, a patient suffered a sudden cardiac arrest (all other potential causes ruled out) 6 hours after the conclusion of laparoscopy.[78] Although CO_2 is approximately five times more soluble than air and therefore less toxic when injected intravascularly, the fact that it is injected under pressure can lead to rapid development of CO_2 embolism, with resultant obstruction of the right ventricular outflow tract and subsequent precipitous drop in cardiac output.[26]

Prevention

Because massive gas embolism is a result of insufflating directly into the circulation, prevention of this complication focuses on measures directed at minimizing the likelihood of intravascular insufflation. These measures include use of low initial insufflation rates (particularly when a Veress needle is used), open placement of the initial trocar if possible, and maintenance of low gas pressures intraoperatively. Aspiration of blood from the Veress needle before insufflation should reveal intravascular placement. Hence, routine aspiration before insufflation is a prudent step to prevent CO_2 embolism during initial establishment of pneumoperitoneum.[32]

Recognition

A high index of suspicion for this potentially catastrophic complication must be maintained during both insufflation and use of the argon beam coagulator. The earliest commonly available indicator of gas embolism is end-tidal CO_2, as displayed on a monitor (see Fig. 2–1 for typical normal CO_2 and SpO_2 tracings). If available, the CO_2 trend display should be set to include just a few minutes of trend history during insufflation (as shown in Fig. 2–1), so that the anesthesiologist may appreciate a precipitous drop in end-tidal CO_2 even without a specific value for the "near-current" end-tidal CO_2 in mind. A "mill wheel" murmur may be present, although appreciation of this abnormality would be unlikely in the midst of the crisis precipitated by sudden cardiovascular collapse. Transesophageal echocardiography (TEE) reveals the gas[79-81] and should be considered in concert with aggressive intervention.

Management

A rapid drop in SpO_2 and end-tidal CO_2 (see Fig. 2–1 for a normal tracing) followed by a drop in blood pressure must prompt an immediate and decisive response from the surgical and the anesthetic teams. If stopping insufflation does not correct the hemodynamic instability, the patient must be promptly placed in the left lateral decubitus position with the head down to shift the gas bubble away from the right ventricular outflow tract and restore cardiac output. A central line placed into the right atrium (usually through the right internal jugular vein) can be used to aspirate gas from the heart. These measures must be undertaken while other supportive measures including cardiopulmonary resuscitation (CPR) and fluid or pressor administration are being continued. Cardiopulmonary bypass has been used successfully in resuscitation and should be considered if initial measures are unsuccessful.[82]

The incidence of small-volume gas embolism during laparoscopy is unknown, but small-volume emboli are frequent during hysteroscopy.[83] Carbon dioxide is rapidly absorbed from blood, without formation of gas emboli when infused into a systemic vein at a rate less than 1 L per minute.[84] In an ongoing process, small-volume emboli lodge in the pulmonary circulation and are absorbed. If the embolic burden exceeds the ability for absorption, pulmonary vascular obstruction may lead to pulmonary hypertension.[79] In severe cases, pulmonary obstruction due to emboli and pulmonary vasoconstriction leads to underfilling of the left heart and a concomitant decline in systemic pressures, embarrassing right ventricular perfusion (and performance) at a very inopportune time. This vicious circle may not be recognized until cardiovascular collapse is imminent, because unexplained decline in systemic pressures may be the first warning sign of a problem. In such instances, inotropic support of the blood pressure with a drug that enhances contractility and maintains the systemic pressure (and hence the right ventricular perfusion pressure) should be promptly instituted. If the patient was not breathing 100% oxygen, all other gases should be turned off and 100% oxygen supplied to minimize further expansion and speed reabsorption of the CO_2.

Subcutaneous Emphysema

Prevention

Subcutaneous emphysema is almost unavoidable in extraperitoneal endoscopic procedures that involve gas insufflation. Preventative measures focus on minimizing gas pressures and minimizing unproductive exposure to gas distention.

Recognition

Subcutaneous emphysema is manifested by palpable crepitus and increased end-tidal CO_2. It develops frequently during laparoscopy.[26] When the emphysema begins to involve the chest wall (ascending from the abdomen), the surgical team should be made aware of the developing situation. Hence, identification and management of subcutaneous emphysema depend on frequent physical examination of the patient for crepitus. Rising end-tidal CO_2 is a less specific indicator.

Management

Although subcutaneous emphysema generally has few clinical consequences, it can herald more serious complications such as pneumomediastinum, pneumopericardium, or pneumo-thorax.[85] Subcutaneous emphysema can progress to involve laryngeal structures, but it usually does not prevent postoperative extubation.[6] If, however, cervical or facial crepitus suggesting laryngeal emphysema is combined with prolonged Trendelenburg position–induced facial or scleral swelling indicative of pharyngeal edema, airway compromise is likely after premature postoperative extubation. The safest course of action in such instances may be to keep the patient ventilated and sedated with the head up at least 30 degrees from horizontal until facial edema clinically resolves and hypercarbia is corrected. Subsequent cuff leak test or direct laryngoscopy to rule out pharyngeal or vocal cord edema may provide some reassurance of post-extubation airway patency. If concern for airway compromise persists, the patient may be extubated over a tube exchanger or fiberoptic bronchoscope, but even these precautions provide no guarantee that the trachea can be reintubated. Prudence dictates that someone with the skills and materials necessary to establish a surgical airway should be available if needed. If necessary, the patient can be left intubated until the clinical picture improves.

Deep Venous Thrombosis

Laparoscopic surgery increases the risk of deep venous thrombosis (DVT) because the procedures tend to be prolonged and because the requisite increased intra-abdominal pressure, often coupled with reverse Trendelenburg position, decreases venous return and promotes venous stasis and pooling of blood in the lower extremities.[20,86]

Trocar Site Herniation

Although the incidence of postoperative ventral hernia formation after laparoscopy is 10 to 100 times lower than that seen after laparotomy, when herniation does occur, the risk of bowel incarceration is nearly 20%.[26,87] Most surgeons do not close the fascia at 5-mm trocar wounds because it is extremely rare for herniation to occur at these sites.[26] Trocar site punctures larger than 5 mm do require fascial closure, to reduce the risk of postoperative hernia.[26] Such herniations at the time of emergence from anesthesia have been attributed to coughing and straining,[88] activities common in *all* patients in the postoperative period.

ANESTHESIA COMPLICATIONS

"Anesthesia complications" are the complications during laparoscopic surgery for which the anesthetic contributes to pathogenesis, or for which the anesthesiologist takes the lead in management. These complications are presented in rough chronologic order relative to a typical laparoscopic procedure.

Contributions to Bowel Perforation

Prevention

All anesthesiologists have had the experience of inducing anesthesia and then attempting to deliver a first controlled positive-pressure breath, only to encounter a glottic obstruction leading to delivery of some part of the breathing bag's gas into the stomach. Care must be taken during induction of anesthesia and intubation to avoid insufflation of air into the stomach, because this will increase the risk of gastric perforation during Veress needle or trocar placement. If gastric insufflation is suspected, the stomach should be decompressed with a nasogastric or orogastric tube before the start of surgery.[6,32]

Recognition

The anesthesia team has little in its armamentarium to aid in the recognition of a bowel perforation, except, perhaps, for the unlikely scenario in which the patient who begins to manifest the signs of sepsis during laparoscopy.

Management

If a bowel perforation is detected in the course of laparoscopy, the anesthesia team contributes to management of the complication by providing optimal operating conditions, maintaining normothermia and euvolemia. Broad-spectrum antibiotics with gram-negative and anaerobic efficacy should be administered as soon as the complication is recognized.

In reoperations to repair bowel perforation that had gone unrecognized until the patient decompensated, the anesthesia team plays a prominent role in management. Such patients frequently are critically ill, and the anesthesia team provides invasive monitoring, including central venous access for monitoring, and vasopressor administration, and generally strives to maintain homeostasis while the surgical team seeks to correct the underlying cause of the patient's problem. Postoperative admission to the ICU is likely.

Positioning Injuries

Positioning injuries caused by stretch or compression of nerves, leading to postoperative neuropathy, are potential complications of any surgical procedure. Particularly vulnerable are the brachial plexus, which is subject to stretching and the ulnar, femoral, and common peroneal nerves, because they are long and course superficially.

Prevention

Proper positioning and padding during prolonged laparoscopic surgical procedures are crucial to prevent these injuries.[6] Textbooks of anesthesiology describe the prevention of positioning injuries in detail. Because laparoscopy frequently requires extremes of Trendelenburg or reverse Trendelenburg position, the patient may fall off the table if not restrained. Such restraint is readily and safely accomplished with a footboard for reverse Trendelenburg position, but extreme head-down positions require shoulder supports or a beanbag hardened and secured to the table (Fig. 2–2).

In addition to positioning the patient carefully at the beginning of surgery, it is important to remember not to allow parts of the patient's body to be compressed or potentially crushed during surgery as a result of movements of the operating room table. Similarly, operating room personnel should

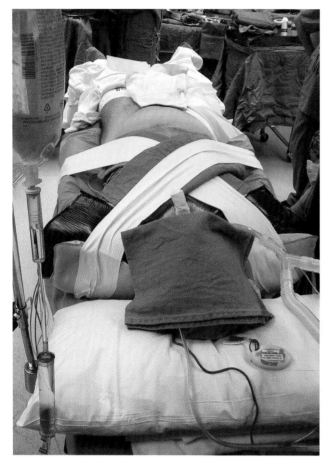

Figure 2–2 ▪ **A patient positioned for a laparoscopic procedure of approximately 3 hours' duration in steep Trendelenburg position.** The patient is in a body-conforming "sled" consisting of a gel pad on top of a vacuum-hardened beanbag molded to the body before air evacuation. The beanbag is then secured to the table with the wide strips of adhesive tape running prominently from the beanbag at the shoulders across the patient and secured to the bottom of the operating room table bed plate. The arms are padded and tucked at the patient's side before air evacuation of the beanbag. Many methods of positioning a patient are acceptable for prolonged extreme Trendelenburg position, but this one spreads the resistance to downhill movement over most of the patient's contact surface with the operating room table, rather than concentrating it on the shoulders (which would put the patient at risk for bilateral brachial plexus stretch injuries).

not lean heavily on the anesthetized patient, because this too can cause compression injuries.

Recognition

Positioning injuries can be recognized in the PACU if the patient is examined carefully. More frequently, they are recognized by the patient on awakening from anesthesia, when he or she becomes aware of pain or weakness at a site distant from the surgical site. Virtually no tools are available intraoperatively (beyond vigilance) to aid the recognition of a positioning injury developing during surgery. Positioning injuries also are difficult to predict: Such injuries do *not* develop in most patients who are found at the end of surgery to have slipped into some uncomfortable-appearing position, whereas such

injuries do develop in some patients who were apparently perfectly cared for.

Management

Typical positioning injuries are not immediately remediable, because they involve nerve injuries. Management focuses on assessment of the extent and likely prognosis of the injury and on counseling the patient. Accordingly, the initial approach to the patient should be to acknowledge the injury and obtain immediate consultation from an expert in peripheral nerve injuries, usually a neurologist, or sometimes a pain specialist. The specialist will be able to determine the extent of the injury, its probable cause, and the likely prognosis. Generally, positioning injuries resolve slowly, because peripheral nerves can regenerate so long as the axon sheath was not transected.

Identifying a potential cause of the injury is useful for attempting to prevent future incidents, but "assigning blame" is not a useful exercise, particularly in front of the patient. Because positioning injuries usually are not detected in the operating room, most members of the team can potentially remain unaware of their occurrence. All members of the operating room team involved in the occurrence of a positioning injury, however, should be made aware of the complication as soon as possible. This facilitates post-event debriefing and may aid the identification of a root cause, allowing future injuries to be avoided.

Hypothermia

Moderate hypothermia is an almost inevitable consequence of general anesthesia. The pathogenic mechanism is redistribution of heat from the body core to the surface (and vice versa) secondary to vasodilation of surface capillaries caused by the anesthetic agents used. The incidence and severity of hypothermia are the same for patients undergoing the identical operation performed using a laparoscopic and an open approach, so long as basic steps are taken to preserve normothermia.[89-91] This is because most of the initial heat loss from surgery occurs during steps common to both laparoscopic and open procedures: induction of anesthesia, followed by surgical skin preparation of the naked patient with cold solutions. Significant hypothermia is much less common, although the incidence increases with the duration of anesthesia and surgery. Significant hypothermia delays discharge, contributes to potential patient misery in the postoperative period and, in extreme cases, can precipitate myocardial ischemia in at-risk persons who shiver severely to generate heat.

Prevention

Loss of body heat during induction of anesthesia can be averted by actively warming patients before anesthesia,[92] although in practice this is rarely done. Intraoperative warming to prevent hypothermia is now quite common. Some methods are more effective than others.

Laparoscopy usually does not require large-volume fluid administration. At the flow rates used during laparoscopy (i.e., 100 to 200 m per hour), intravenous fluid passed through a fluid warmer exits the tubing and associated extension just proximal to the intravenous entry site at room temperature. Thus, intravenous fluid warmers for maintenance are not cost-effective in our view, because they do not actually contribute significant warming. On the other hand, warming liter bags of crystalloid intended for bolus infusion to 104° F overnight is highly effective in providing warm fluid (when high infusion rates are used) at the distal intravenous site, with virtually no cost. Similarly, using warmed irrigation fluid during laparoscopy aids in the prevention of hypothermia.[93] Forced-air warming for procedures of greater than 1 hour's duration is highly effective in preventing hypothermia.[89] For patients undergoing laparoscopy, forced-air warming is sufficient for prevention of hypothermia, even as the sole preventive modality. By contrast, heating and humidifying the insufflating gas do not appear to be particularly effective for warming (although these measures may provide other benefits). For example, in a small number of patients undergoing laparoscopic Nissen fundoplication, heating and humidification of CO_2 used for insufflation, when added to forced-air warming, had no effect on core body temperature or postoperative pain scores and opioid use.[94] Outcomes are the same for heating the insufflating gas as a sole warming intervention and for no warming effort at all.[95]

Management

When significant hypothermia occurs, it should be treated aggressively in the operating room, usually by applying a forced-air warmer. Forced-air warming accomplished with the patient under anesthesia is effective because the cutaneous capillaries are dilated in anesthesia. It is important to apply the blanket designed to be used with the warming system, because the output of the warming unit applied to the patient's skin without diffusion can cause burns. Hypothermia also can be treated in the PACU using forced-air warming. Shivering is effectively treated with meperidine, 12.5 to 25 mg given intravenously. Ablation of shivering is an effect unique to meperidine among all opioids.

Awareness

Minimally invasive surgery with the goal to fast-track patients through perioperative processes and on to home leads anesthesiologists to use light anesthesia techniques. Awareness has been reported for all general anesthesia techniques.[96] Use of total intravenous anesthesia (TIVA) may increase the risk of awareness, owing to the "fussy" nature of the infusion pumps in common use.[97] Of course, patients expect to be asleep for surgery. Although a universal goal is to ensure unconsciousness during surgery, it is important to adjust the patient's expectations in this regard, because 1 to 2 patients per 1000 receiving general anesthesia experience intraoperative awareness.[98] Accordingly, all operating room personnel should assume that anesthetized patients may be aware and should behave appropriately at all times in their presence.

Prevention

Prevention of awareness depends on steps to ensure that adequate levels of anesthesia are achieved, and that the anesthesia plan incorporates necessary levels of redundancy.

Maintaining anesthesia with low doses of multiple anesthetics instead of a single agent is an example of redundancy. TIVA with propofol offers a visual cue that the agent is reaching the patient, because the vehicle is colored, so that it is visible as it is carried into the circulation by the intravenous infusion.

Recognition

Awareness results from "light" anesthesia that is too light. The signs of light anesthesia (and hence increased risk of awareness) include hypertension, tachycardia, and sweating, as well as movement in those patients who are not paralyzed. These findings are nonspecific, but none of them are "normal" during laparoscopy, and each should prompt consideration of inadequate anesthesia as a cause.

Many anesthesiologists employ or at least consider level-of-consciousness monitoring if a light anesthetic technique is used. Patients actually tend to receive higher doses of anesthetics when level-of-conscious monitors are *not* used, however.[99] Unfortunately, the disposable components of commercially available level-of-consciousness monitors each add 10% to the total pharmacy and supply costs for a typical laparoscopy anesthetic procedure. To counter this, many economically based cost-benefit arguments have been made to justify routine monitoring of level of consciousness. In one study, the lighter anesthesia achieved with level-of-consciousness monitoring translates into a few minutes of operating room time saved per case due to faster emergence.[99] On the other hand, a recent meta-analysis of all controlled trials reporting outcomes in terms of supply costs, anesthetic consumed, and times to discharge from the PACU indicates that the cost of the level-of-consciousness disposable monitor outweighs all of the other savings combined.[100]

Management

Management begins with prevention, and the anesthesia team should be diligent during the case to ensure a reasonable depth of anesthesia and adequate analgesia. Like positioning injuries, awareness usually does not come to the care team's attention until well after the event has occurred. Awareness can be quite distressing and can lead to lasting problems, including debilitating post-traumatic stress disorder. Symptoms are diverse, ranging from overt combativeness and angry remonstrations immediately on emergence to vague sleep disturbances after surgery. Patients with overt recall should possibly receive an anxiolytic immediately and must receive immediate care from a psychiatrist. This goal is to institute therapy to minimize the likelihood of post-traumatic stress disorder.

Before discharge, all patients should be queried specifically about intraoperative recall with semistructured questions such as the following:

- "What is the last thing you remember before surgery?"
- "What is the next thing you remember after that?"
- "Do you recall anything that seemed to happen during surgery?"

Positive responses should prompt referral to a psychiatrist. Patients who report postoperative anxiety or sleep disturbances at follow-up visits also merit attention, because they may be experiencing symptoms of recall.

Arrhythmia

Prevention

Arrhythmias are common during surgery, occurring in 70% of a large population of patients given general anesthesia, 90% of whom would be considered healthy (i.e., American Society of Anesthesiologists [ASA] physical status category I or II).[101,102] In general, such arrhythmias are benign and resolve quickly after anesthesia ends. For example, ventricular extrasystolic beats occur frequently during laparoscopy. These aberrant beats commonly are described as resulting from hypercarbia-induced acidosis, but this may not be the case.[6] Ventricular extra systoles usually are self-limited and of no consequence to the patient. Perioperative arrhythmias recently have been reviewed in depth,[103] and the reader is referred to this work for more details. General preventive measures to avoid arrhythmias during laparoscopy focus on managing hypercarbia and on minimizing the impact of vagotonic stimuli that might otherwise induce severe bradycardia.

Recognition

Arrhythmias are recognized from the electrocardiogram (ECG) displayed continuously on the physiologic monitor. A normal ECG tracing is shown in Figure 2–1. The most common arrhythmia encountered during laparoscopy is bradycardia, occurring in approximately 5% to 20% of procedures,[104,105] regardless of the patient's state of health. This disturbance frequently is attributed to increased endogenous vagal tone from sudden insufflation,[106] omental and mesenteric traction, or cervical manipulation. Other, more rare inciting events, such as uterine injection of vasopressin, have been cited in case reports.[107] Vagally mediated bradycardia is potentially worsened by vagotonic drug combinations such as fentanyl plus vecuronium.

Other arrhythmias such as ventricular tachycardia can occur, although probably at the same rate at which they are observed in the population of all surgical patients. Rare case reports, for example, attributing ventricular fibrillation to electrocautery during laparoscopy[108] have appeared.

Management

Bradycardia during laparoscopy occasionally progresses to asystolic cardiac arrest requiring CPR and advanced cardiac life support (ACLS)-level resuscitation, and it is our practice to abort elective surgery if this occurs. Consultation with a cardiologist is warranted, although causes for asystole (other than anesthesia and laparoscopy) are almost never discovered.

Succinylcholine infusions sometimes are used for skeletal muscle paralysis for short procedures, and symptomatic bradycardia is common (occurring in 1 in 10 cases) among these patients. The brief nature of some laparoscopic procedures, coupled with the need to use operating room time efficiently, ensures that succinylcholine will continue to be used. The drug is given in bolus doses or by continuous infusion using syringe microinfusion pumps. Repeat or continuous succinylcholine administration, especially coupled with pneumoperitoneum, commonly causes rapidly developing severe

bradycardia, and cardiac arrest also can result. Brief laparoscopic procedures have high task demands competing for operating room team members' attention, and heart rate changes induced by succinylcholine can go unnoticed until severe. In many cases, we use glycopyrrolate 0.2 mg given intravenously as prophylaxis before repeat doses of succinylcholine, or for rapid treatment of bradycardia if the heart rate drops below 40 beats per minute.

In general, when a significant arrhythmia occurs, a potential inciting event (e.g., initial insufflation, peritoneal traction) often can be identified and should be immediately reversed. Often the arrhythmia resolves and does not return with more gentle repetition of the previously inciting maneuver. Management of arrhythmias that persist and are hemodynamically significant should follow the relevant ACLS protocols. In such instances, surgery should be terminated as quickly as possible. Patients who are successfully resuscitated need not remain intubated if they are hemodynamically stable and no other contraindication to extubation exists. Consultation with a cardiologist should be obtained, and many (but not all) patients should have this evaluation in an ICU setting.

Increasingly, patients present for laparoscopy with pacemakers and implantable cardioverter-defibrillators (ICDs). The management of patients with these devices must be carefully considered, because electrocautery in the operating room can interfere with their function.[103] Patients with pacemakers may or may not be entirely pacemaker dependent for their cardiac rhythm. Each patient should be carefully evaluated for pacemaker dependence by review of records and consultation with the patient's cardiologist, because inadvertent pacemaker inhibition in a pacemaker-dependent patient during surgery can have catastrophic consequences. All patients with ICDs should be considered device dependent, because ICDs are implanted for the specific purpose of detecting and treating lethal arrhythmias. Patients with pacemakers and ICDs should be evaluated by an anesthesiologist well in advance of surgery, and they should be instructed to bring any documentation related to their device, as well as contact information for their cardiologist, to the preanesthetic evaluation.

In general, pacemakers should be left alone and protected from electrocautery output during surgery.[103,109] Older pacemakers would generally convert to an electrocautery-insensitive VOO mode (see the article by Vijayakumar[103] for details) when a magnet was placed on them. Modern pacemakers are much less sensitive to electrocautery interference and have a much less predictable response to magnets (i.e., they may reprogram, or they may lose output entirely). Therefore, it is now recommended (1) to establish, if possible, the pacemaker manufacturer, the model, and its response to magnets; (2) *not* to apply magnets to pacemakers; (3) to use electrocautery in short (less than 5 seconds) bursts; and (4) to interrogate the pacemaker to confirm normal functioning after surgery.[103,109] The electrocautery dispersion pad should be placed so that current lines run away from pacemaker and ICD generators.[110] The commonly used anterior thigh location for the dispersion pad meets this criterion during abdominal surgery.

Some pacemakers have additional features that can be troublesome or at least disconcerting in the operating room. For example, models that augment the heart rate in response to exercise demand sense the demand by monitoring the respiratory rate. If the anesthesiologist raises the respiratory rate in an attempt to relieve hypercarbia during laparoscopy, the pacemaker may respond by raising the heart rate. Some authors recommend turning off these types of features in pacemakers during surgery,[103,109,111] but our current practice is to learn the settings of such programmable features and to work within that envelope, leaving the pacemaker undisturbed. It is prudent to have the pacemaker interrogated in the PACU to confirm normal function after surgery.

When patients have ICDs, the recommended practice is to suspend arrhythmia detection but *not* to disable therapeutic modes in the operating room. This is the safest practice, because high-frequency discharge by the electrocautery frequently is interpreted as ventricular fibrillation, triggering the ICD to deliver a spurious shock.[103,109,111] Most ICDs suspend detection in response to donut magnet application. When the magnet is removed, arrhythmia detection resumes. If the magnet is removed in response to a true arrhythmia, detection resumes and therapy will be delivered, usually within 10 seconds. Because the patient's ICD will have been "tuned" to deliver the best therapy for that patient's unique arrhythmia, this often is the safest approach—therapy will be precisely tailored and quicker than external defibrillation.

One ICD model, the Guidant-CPI, responds to magnet application by producing an audible tone (audible to an ear placed near the device), after which the device turns off. The device can be turned back on by removing the magnet and reapplying it for 30 seconds. Audible tones should again be heard, confirming that the device is back on.

Most ICDs have a backup pacing mode, either VVI or DDD (see ref. 103 for details of pacemaker nomenclature), that is unaffected by magnet application.

Magnet application is preferable to reprogramming ICDs to turn off arrhythmia detection, because in almost all cases, removing the magnet restores the ICD to normal function, almost instantaneously providing optimal arrhythmia therapy should it be needed. If the ICD is turned off, either as a first choice or by necessity in the case of devices that turn off in response to magnet application, we recommend making provision for external pacing and defibrillation, to the point of actually applying external pacemaker electrodes before induction of anesthesia.

After surgery, ICDs should be interrogated by the hospital's electrophysiology service before the patient is discharged from the hospital, and ideally in the PACU.

Perioperative Myocardial Ischemia

Perioperative myocardial ischemia in at-risk patients during noncardiac surgery remains a problem. Myocardial ischemia is caused by atherosclerotic plaque rupture and acute thrombosis, or when myocardial oxygen demand outstrips supply, as reviewed by Akhtar and Silverman[112] and Roizen.[113] Myocardial ischemia is not among the complications of laparoscopy that first come to mind—but minimally invasive surgery is not minimal surgery. Intraoperative physiologic derangements can be severe, upsetting the myocardial oxygen supply-and-demand balance. Surgery induces an inflammatory and prothrombotic state, increasing the likelihood of atherosclerotic plaque rupture and thrombosis. Both mechanisms have been proposed as the cause of perioperative myocardial ischemia and infarction.[114,115]

Prevention

Prevention of myocardial ischemia and infarction is based on appropriate risk stratification, risk factor modification, and control of the myocardial oxygen supply-and-demand balance during surgery. Perioperative evaluation and perioperative management for patients at risk of cardiac events during noncardiac surgery have been reviewed recently.[116-119] In appropriately selected patients, perioperative beta blockade reduces the incidence of myocardial ischemia[120] and confers a lasting longevity advantage.[121] In high-risk patients, perioperative beta blockade confers dramatic protection from perioperative cardiac events.[122] Recent work shows that alpha-2 agonism with clonidine has a similar effect.[123]

As the patient population ages and minimally invasive surgery becomes pervasive, more patients at elevated risk for perioperative myocardial ischemia will present for laparoscopy and hysteroscopy. Appropriate risk stratification must be conducted and may be initiated in the surgeon's office. This process includes preoperative cardiac testing as appropriate and perioperative medical therapy (including beta blockade) when indicated. Screening should follow the American College of Cardiology and American Heart Association guidelines published in 1997 and updated in 2002.[117]

Giving beta blockers to patients soon to be at risk for clinically significant bradycardia due to surgical maneuvers may seem ill advised, but the long-term salutary effects of beta blockade in patients at risk for perioperative myocardial ischemia are well established.[119] Beta blockade increases the incidence of bradycardia during surgery,[119] but beta blockade was well tolerated in at least one small population of laparoscopy patients.[124] In fact, inappropriate withholding of beta blockade from at-risk patients[125] with consequent failure of protection from perioperative cardiac complications has been reported.[126]

In patients for whom coronary revascularization is contemplated before surgery, it is critical to respect the need to delay surgery by at least 6 weeks,[117] and preferably 3 months after coronary stenting.[127] Even when these guidelines are followed, acute stent thrombosis occurs in the perioperative period and can be fatal.[128]

Recognition

Recognition of myocardial ischemia in the operating room most commonly is accomplished by electrocardiographic monitoring with computerized ST segment analysis, a modality that has become almost universally available. Subendocardial ischemia is the most common type of ischemia in the perioperative setting and is manifested by ST segment depression on the ECG.[129] ECG changes consistent with ischemia are difficult to detect in patients with right bundle branch blocks, left ventricular hypertrophy with a strain pattern, or atrial fibrillation.[130] Ischemia monitoring by ECG is considered to be impossible in patients with left bundle branch block or pacemaker dependency,[130] although in practice, changes in the ECG morphology in these patients should arouse suspicion. Lead V_5 is the single most sensitive lead for detecting intraoperative ischemic changes (75% of episodes were evident in this lead); the sensitivity increases to 80% by monitoring leads II and V_5 together.[131] With a three-lead system (leads II, V_4, and V_5), 96% of ischemic changes were detected.[131] In practice, usually only a single precordial lead is available in the operating room, and recent work suggests that V_4 may be the most useful lead used in concert with lead II.[129] Computerized ST segment trend monitoring (see Fig. 2–1) provides a reliable way to monitor for ischemia: Following the trend for ST segment elevation or depression over time provides high sensitivity to events manifested in the leads observed. To be most useful, however, the ECG leads must be placed before anesthetic induction and should not be moved for the duration of the procedure. Moving the leads artifactually changes the ECG complex morphology, rendering the previous ST segment trend useless as a baseline. Hence, careful initial ECG lead placement is essential so that leads will not need to be moved during preparation for surgery.

Occasionally, laparoscopy patients without ischemia present with a convincing clinical picture of myocardial ischemia. For example, pneumopericardium may mimic myocardial ischemia, manifesting as chest pain and T wave inversions on ECG.[132] These episodes should be investigated vigorously, because some maneuvers common during laparoscopy, such as administration of intrauterine vasopressin to control bleeding, can cause myocardial ischemia.

Management

Intraoperative myocardial ischemia is relatively rare, probably because (1) anesthetics decrease adrenergic tone, (2) most of the determinants of myocardial oxygen supply and demand are under tight control of the anesthesiologist, and (3) intraoperative ischemia monitoring is effective and continuous. When myocardial ischemia occurs intraoperatively, the anesthesiologist will work to improve the oxygen supply-and-demand balance by regulating the depth of anesthesia, controlling the heart rate, and optimizing hemodynamics. These considerations lead to significant interaction with the laparoscopist, because the increased intra-abdominal pressure to create pneumoperitoneum has an unfavorable effect on hemodynamics.[6] Specifically, pneumoperitoneum decreases venous return and increases systemic vascular resistance, adding to myocardial workload. Hence, minimizing insufflation pressure becomes an important goal with respect to optimizing the myocardial oxygen supply-and-demand balance.

When intraoperative myocardial ischemia is recognized, surgery should be completed expeditiously or terminated if possible. In the PACU, aggressive diagnostic and therapeutic management of a presumed acute coronary syndrome should be initiated immediately, with subsequent care guided by a cardiologist.

Myocardial ischemia is most common in the postoperative period, when the patient's medical status is much less tightly controlled. Postoperatively, virtually every determinant of myocardial oxygen supply and demand is altered by factors such as hypothermia, fluid shifts, blood loss, pain, circulating catecholamines, altered coagulability, and ventilatory insufficiency. Control of each of these factors is essential to lower the risk of postoperative ischemia and infarction. It also is important to continue useful medication regimens from the preoperative period. Patients receiving beta blockers chronically before surgery should have these medications continued on the day of surgery and postoperatively. Abrupt discontinuation of beta blockers probably removes their cardioprotective effect and can cause rebound tachycardia and hypertension. Patients begun on beta blockers in the immediate preoperative period should continue to receive them postoperatively until discharge. At hospital discharge, beta blockade may be continued after consultation with the patient's cardiologist or primary care physician.

Hypercarbia

Prevention

Hypercarbia is an almost inevitable consequence of laparoscopy because it is almost always facilitated by CO_2 insufflation. CO_2 is well suited for use as a distending gas for all of its good properties: It is optically clear and does not support combustion. It also is rapidly absorbed from blood, minimizing the impact of emboli. Unfortunately, this rapid absorption causes hypercarbia and acidosis if the anesthesiologist cannot manage the patient's ventilation to compensate for the added CO_2 load. Because CO_2 insufflation is an obligate part of laparoscopic surgery, managing the consequences of CO_2 insufflation becomes a primary anesthesia goal.

Extraperitoneal procedures lead to more CO_2 uptake than that observed in intraperitoneal procedures of similar duration.[133-136] It has been speculated that this difference in uptake is due to the development of extensive subcutaneous emphysema, which provides a larger surface area for absorption and less compression of perfusing vessels, both contributing to a larger ongoing uptake rate.[133] In contrast with intraperitoneal procedures, in which the rate of CO_2 uptake plateaus after 15 to 20 minutes,[6] hypercarbia and acidosis worsen throughout the duration of extraperitoneal laparoscopies, requiring progressively more aggressive ventilation. Occasionally hypercarbia becomes uncontrollable, requiring a break in surgery to ventilate off CO_2 or even conversion to an open technique.

Recognition

The normal arterial P_{CO_2} is 40 mm Hg. In intubated patients, it is possible to measure the P_{CO_2} of the expired breath, giving a value known as end-tidal CO_2 (ET_{CO_2}). The capnogram (CO_2 tracing during ventilation) and the ET_{CO_2} for a typical laparoscopy patient are shown in Figure 2–1. ET_{CO_2} is always lower than arterial P_{CO_2} because of the dead space in the respiratory system. Studies in awake patients undergoing laparoscopy reveal that they increase minute ventilation to defend the P_{CO_2} setpoint, and that they do this by increasing the respiratory rate rather than the tidal volume. During general anesthesia, ET_{CO_2} is used as a surrogate for the arterial P_{CO_2}, with the assumption that the ET_{CO_2} is at most a few points lower than arterial P_{CO_2}.

The ET_{CO_2} may not reflect arterial P_{CO_2}, especially in patients with severe chronic obstructive pulmonary disease (COPD) or bronchospasm. If elevated ET_{CO_2} during laparoscopy is not easily managed by simple ventilatory maneuvers or if the patient has significant evidence of obstruction on capnogram, it is likely that the ET_{CO_2} gives a poor reflection of the arterial P_{CO_2}. Under these circumstances, insertion of an arterial catheter for arterial blood gas analysis should be considered.

Management

During mechanical ventilation, increasing the minute ventilation by 15% to 20%, by increasing either the tidal volume or the respiratory rate, or both, should readily compensate for CO_2 insufflation–induced hypercarbia. Additionally, allowing permissive hypercapnia is safe, so the ventilatory manipulations can be relatively modest.

Anesthesiologists will take pains to minimize the risk of barotrauma (probably actually volutrauma), either by careful attention to airway pressures using the volume control ventilator most commonly found on anesthesia machines, or by using pressure control ventilation (PCV). Pressure control ventilation is not the ideal answer to preventing barotrauma, because tidal volumes (and hence minute ventilation) may drop over time if compliance decreases as a result of pneumoperitoneum or progressively accumulating CO_2 subcutaneous emphysema. If PCV is used, the ventilator's "low minute ventilation" alarm should be set at a threshold that provides early alert to diminishing ventilation.

Eliminating the hypercarbia caused by CO_2 spurred early interest in other distending gases such as helium.[137] These investigations ultimately proved unfruitful: Inert gases do not cause hypercarbia, but their insolubility in blood, coupled with the frequency of embolism under ordinary laparoscopy conditions,[80] made them unacceptable from the standpoint of reducing embolism risk.[138] For example, continuous infusion of 0.1 mL/kg per minute of insoluble gases in an animal model was likely to be fatal, whereas equivalent infusion rates of soluble gases did not cause death.[139] In general, inert gases exert smaller hemodynamic effects than CO_2, and cause minimal acidosis. With inert gas pneumothoraces, however, reabsorption of gas is slow, and inert gas embolism is poorly tolerated, severely limiting the utility of these gases relative to CO_2.[140,141]

Ineffective Muscle Relaxation

Laparoscopy does not require muscle relaxation, but in practice effective relaxation facilitates surgery. Patient straining collapses the pneumoperitoneum, impeding the surgeon's view of the field. When relaxation is inadequate, surgeons may compensate by raising insufflation pressure, thereby enhancing CO_2 uptake (worsening hypercarbia) and increasing the chance of gas embolism, devlopment of pneumothorax, and other problems. Conversely, providing good relaxation allows lower insufflation pressures and facilitates surgery. "Perfect"—that is, complete—muscle relaxation has its own pitfalls, however. Laparoscopic procedures tend to end quickly, with minimal effort (and time) needed for closure. Thus, effective reversal of neuromuscular blockade from deep paralysis can be problematic.

Prevention

Most anesthesiologists use short-acting (e.g., mivacurium) or, for longer cases, intermediate-acting (e.g., rocuronium, vecuronium, atracurium, cisatracurium) nondepolarizing paralytic agents to provide adequate relaxation.

Recognition

Surgeons often recognize inadequate relaxation by the need for higher insufflation pressures to maintain a view of the "operative field" during laparoscopy, by the collapse of the pneumoperitoneum, or by unwanted movement of the diaphragm. Occasionally, overt patient movement is observed.

Anesthesiologists gauge the depth of paralysis using a "twitch monitor," applied most commonly over the ulnar nerve so as to stimulate contractions of adductor pollicis brevis. Strength in this motor nerve–muscle circuit returns later than diaphragmatic strength, so the twitch monitor is not a perfect reflection of paralysis in the surgical field. Often the anesthesiologist will assess the depth of paralysis with this device as a first response to complaints of inadequate paralysis. The purpose is to obtain a "calibration" of how much strength at the monitored site leads to signs of inadequate relaxation in the surgical field.

Management

Inadequate relaxation requiring immediate treatment can be promptly addressed with 20 to 50 mg of propofol, with concomitant administration of additional paralytic agent. Propofol decreases muscle tone indirectly by increasing the depth of anesthesia on a seconds-to-minute time scale. This strategy works to repair inadequate relaxation during the early and middle part of a typical laparoscopic case. Even the shortest-acting nondepolarizing paralytic drug, however, does not provide the ideal characteristics of profound relaxation followed immediately by complete off-set for laparoscopic cases with operative times of 15 to 25 minutes. The alternative is to use succinylcholine, which is the fastest-onset and shortest-lived skeletal muscle paralytic currently available. The drug is given as a bolus of 0.5 to 2.0 mg/kg as an initial dose. Relaxation is prolonged by subsequent doses of 20 to 40 mg or by continuous infusion using syringe microinfusion pumps. Typical infusion rates for succinylcholine of 85 ± 15 µg/kg per minute are satisfactory for laparoscopic surgery.[142,143] This results in a cumulative dose of less than 5 mg/kg, and phase II block does not occur. The neuromuscular monitoring goal for succinylcholine infusion during laparoscopy is reduction of the train-of-four response to a just perceptible level.

Volume Overload

Prevention

Laparoscopic surgery does not entail the large-scale insensible and third space fluid losses seen in equivalent open procedures. Thus, total fluid administration usually does not need to exceed the sum of (1) deficits due to fasting, (2) maintenance fluids, and (3) blood loss. Though rare, volume overload due to overzealous crystalloid administration can occur.

Recognition

Recognition of perioperative volume overload from fluid administration is fairly straightforward and is based on an accounting of fluids administered and lost during the procedure. Fluid overload not leading to physiologic compromise and in the absence of oliguric renal failure does not need to be treated, nor should it delay extubation or discharge from the operating room or PACU, because affected patients will eliminate the excess fluid on their own.

Management

If volume administration leads to pulmonary edema with compromised oxygenation, administration of modest doses of furosemide (e.g., 5 to 10 mg given intravenously) in patients with normal renal function will produce a dramatic diuresis within 20 minutes. In such cases, it probably is wise to keep the patient intubated, appropriately sedated, and supported by a mechanical ventilator until inspired oxygen requirements (i.e., fraction of inspired oxygen [FiO_2]) and work of breathing have diminished to the point that the patient is capable of independent respiration (usually only a few hours). Many clinicians would guide such ventilator management, using serial blood gas determinations, entailing the placement of an arterial catheter. Hence, the consequences of a readily avoidable complication (volume overload) can include otherwise needless procedures, each with its own attendant risks, as well as increased patient discomfort and use of hospital resources.

Postoperative Nausea and Vomiting

Postoperative nausea and vomiting (PONV) has become an increasingly important end point for anesthesiologists as the safety profile of anesthesia with respect to major morbidity and mortality has steadily improved.[144] One third of surgical patients experience PONV.[145] PONV also is an increasingly important consideration to patients as anesthetic techniques leading to earlier recovery from anesthesia and fast-track discharge from postoperative care have become more prominent.[144] These developments have meant that increasing numbers of patients are fully awake while suffering from PONV, and they are being asked to assume more of their own care while coping with a decidedly unpleasant feeling. In fact, many patients rank PONV on a level with pain as an anesthetic outcome they wish to avoid[146,147]—and they are willing to pay out of pocket to do so.[148,149]

Prevention

In theory and in practice, multimodality drug regimens can reduce the incidence of PONV to nearly zero.[145,150] PONV risk factors and treatment recently have been described in detail elsewhere.[145,151,152] The incidence of PONV commonly is thought to be influenced by a variety of factors, including the choice of anesthetic technique and the type of surgery. General anesthesia clearly is more emetogenic than are regional techniques, and most laparoscopic procedures are performed with the patient under general anesthesia. Most nonanesthetic drugs given in the perioperative period are only weakly emetogenic, if at all. For example, neostigmine, a cholinesterase inhibitor used to antagonize nondepolarizing paralytics, is not consistently emetogenic.[153,154] Unfortunately, many anesthetics and all opioid analgesics are emetogenic. PONV in the early postoperative period is strongly influenced

Table 2–1 ▪ Major Risk Factors for Postoperative Nausea and Vomiting (PONV)*
Female gender
History of PONV or motion sickness
Nonsmoker
Use of postoperative opioids

*See text for description of scoring system based on these risk factors.

by *both* exposure to *and* duration of exposure to volatile anesthetics,[155] and this effect was larger than the relative risk of PONV incurred with nitrous oxide exposure.[145,156] Propofol, a ubiquitous anesthetic induction agent, probably has antiemetic properties, however,[157,158] and in fact has been used as a rescue antiemetic after surgery.[158-160] Young age is an independent but weaker predictor of PONV; the type of surgery is less clearly linked to PONV incidence (reviewed by Apfel and Roewer[151]).

Recognition

Recognition of established PONV is not difficult. Preoperative recognition of patient groups most likely to experience PONV also is straightforward, although pinpointing which persons will be affected in advance is still impossible. Four factors clearly increase the likelihood of PONV: (1) female gender, (2) history of previous PONV or motion sickness, (3) nonsmoking status, and (4) postoperative opioids (Table 2–1). These four factors have been developed into a simplified risk scoring system that has been validated across different institutions.[161] The scoring scheme is as follows: For adults undergoing general anesthesia with volatile agents, the presence of 0, 1, 2, 3, or 4 of these risk factors is associated with a 10%, 20%, 40%, 60%, or 80% risk of PONV, respectively. Hence, the chain-smoking octogenarian male tugboat captain presenting for laparoscopic cholecystectomy and the 25-year-old woman complaining of car sickness presenting for complex laparoscopic infertility surgery define opposite ends of the spectrum of risk, and PONV in the latter patient is almost unavoidable. This scoring system has been used to rationally guide antiemetic prophylaxis and anesthetic management,[152] leading to reductions in PONV and duration of PACU stay.

Management

Management of PONV begins before the induction of anesthesia, with risk stratification, appropriate use of prophylactic antiemetics, and prudent choices of anesthetic drugs. Propofol is a logical drug choice for induction of anesthesia in patients at high risk for PONV because it is not emetogenic. Beyond this, the choice of anesthetic drugs for maintenance probably has little effect on the incidence of PONV, with a single exception: Propofol probably should be included as an infused maintenance anesthetic, replacing volatile agents (and perhaps nitrous oxide). Propofol maintenance (as opposed to use of volatile agents) is associated with reduced incidence of PONV. For example, the incidence of PONV in patients who received inhalational anesthesia for tubal sterilization procedures was higher than in a group of patients who received

TIVA using propofol plus alfentanil.[96] Use of propofol for maintenance seems to reduce the risk of PONV by a factor of approximately 2.[155] Propofol maintenance appears to be roughly equivalent to use of a volatile agent in combination with an antiemetic.[162] Shorter-acting opioids during anesthesia also may reduce the incidence of PONV.[163]

Consensus guidelines for prophylaxis against PONV, as well as rescue from PONV when it occurs, have been developed.[164] In general, PONV prophylaxis is not thought to be warranted in any but the highest-risk groups of patients. This is because all antiemetic drugs are relatively ineffective, compromising the cost-effectiveness of prophylactic administration. PONV prophylaxis is indicated in certain patients at high risk for PONV (see Table 2–1). Additionally, some surgical procedures (e.g., airway surgery, antireflux procedures, oral surgery in which the mouth is wired shut postoperatively) necessitate PONV prophylaxis.

Each of the widely available antiemetics is effective in roughly 60% of patients as monotherapy,[145,165-168] but they differ widely in cost and, to some extent, in the incidence and severity of side effects. 5-Hydroxytryptamine-3 (5-HT$_3$) antagonists, butyrophenones such as droperidol and haloperidol, the steroid dexamethasone, and scopolamine administered subcutaneously and transdermally all are widely used at our institution. Each of these agent groups attacks PONV by a different mechanism, which probably explains why their beneficial effects are additive when they are given in combination. Thus, we prefer to prevent and treat PONV by giving drug combinations tailored to the patient's specific risk factors and anticipated postoperative course, rather than persisting with increasing doses of a single agent. For example, the dose-response curve for ondansetron, a common 5-HT$_3$ antagonist, is quite flat, with little improvement in results between doses of 2 mg and 8 mg (i.e., half and twice the manufacturer's recommended unit dose, respectively).[169] Evidence indicating that any one 5-HT$_3$ antagonist is superior to another is lacking.[169] These drugs have few side effects, so they frequently are first-line agents, but their costs are roughly an order of magnitude higher than those of other, equally effective drugs with similar side effect profiles.

We take an aggressive, multimodality approach to PONV preemption in patients for laparoscopy, particularly in those for whom day-of-surgery discharge is anticipated. Because these patients tend to be young female nonsmokers undergoing gynecologic laparoscopy, we use at least two and sometimes three drugs from different classes prophylactically. For example, this patient population receives ondansetron, 4 mg given intravenously immediately after placement of the intravenous line, and dexamethasone, 4 mg given intravenously just before induction. Dexamethasone's efficacy is greatest when it is administered before anesthetic drugs are given,[170] but it occasionally causes a transient but marked perineal burning sensation. Induction of anesthesia almost always is with propofol, although use of this agent probably serves only to avoid the emetogenic effects of other induction agents, rather than providing lasting antiemesis on its own.[171] Additionally, some of these patients receive a scopolamine patch while they are in the preoperative holding area. This approach well exceeds the recommendations of recent guidelines and investigations of PONV prophylaxis[145,164] and incurs additional pharmacy expense but has been associated with a high level of

patient satisfaction.[172] In contrast with ambulatory patients, those who are at risk for PONV and because of other factors are expected to be hospitalized after surgery are more likely to receive an antiemetic with sedating properties (e.g., a butyrophenone such as haloperidol, 1 mg, or promethazine, 12.5 to 25 mg, both given by the intravenous route). If PONV occurs, we treat early with drugs likely to be effective (i.e., those from a class other than those already administered). We frequently use haloperidol, 1 mg given intravenously, for rescue. This drug and other butyrophenones are effective in at least 60% of patients and work with miraculous rapidity. These agents exert their effects in the time to circulate from the arm to the brain, meaning that a retching patient frequently will stop vomiting within seconds of drug administration.

Certain patient populations are at risk for compromise of the surgical result by the injurious effects of retching in the immediate postoperative period. For example, laparoscopic procedures involving the diaphragm, stomach, and esophagus (e.g., Nissen fundoplication) could theoretically be complicated by early failure from excessive retching. A study by Soper and associates retrospectively associated PONV (along with several other factors) with failure of the fundoplication in the early postoperative period.[173] Although this study far from proves the role of PONV in early fundoplication failure, many surgeons doubtless have this study in mind when they request that the anesthesiologist attempt to minimize this side effect of anesthesia and surgery.

Pain

Although once considered a normal physiologic response to surgery, operative pain and postsurgical pain are now widely viewed as triggering events in a multichannel, positive-feedback cascade transmitted by nociceptive neurons whose discharge characteristics are sensitized, amplified, and sustained by the inflammatory and immunologic mediators released with tissue injury. Branch points in this cascade include induced neural plasticity at the spinal cord dorsal horn, contributing to increased wound sensitivity and leading to muscle splinting, decreased pulmonary function, atelectasis, and pneumonia, and sympathetic activation, leading to tachycardia or hypertension with consequent increased oxygen demand and consumption, which directly contribute to coronary ischemia in susceptible patients.[174] Although it is widely recognized that minimization of pain can improve clinical outcomes,[175] an estimated 50% to 75% of postoperative patients still receive inadequate pain relief.[176]

One reason for inadequate control of pain is the operating room and postoperative care teams' concern for opioid side effects. Opioids continue to form the foundation of intra- and postoperative pain control; however, at the doses traditionally required to provide adequate analgesia, they also contribute to respiratory depression, PONV, exacerbation of postoperative gastroparesis, constipation, urinary retention, decreased rapid eye movement sleep,[176] and unanticipated hospitalization of same-day surgical patients. Thus, the prescribing physician is caught on the horns of a dilemma with respect to opioids: Use them sparingly, thus leaving the patient with inadequately treated pain (albeit often at home and hence out of sight), or use them more liberally and run the risk of their very visible side effects. In this context, the last decade has seen an expanded interest in multimodal approaches to analgesia. The use of non-narcotic and sometimes nonpharmacologic means to reduce the need for opioids and thereby limit their side effects lies at the heart of the concepts of balanced or multimodal analgesia and preemptive or preventive analgesia.[176]

Among the options used to provide preventive analgesia are nonsteroidal anti-inflammatory drugs (NSAIDs). These drugs inhibit cyclooxygenase, a protein complex that catalyzes steps in prostaglandin synthesis. Prostaglandin production leads to inflammation and pain. Traditional NSAIDs inhibit both forms of cyclooxygenase, COX-1 and COX-2. COX-1 is a constitutive protein that is constantly expressed as part of normal homeostasis. Inhibition of COX-2 can adversely affect renal function, gastric mucosal integrity, and platelet adhesiveness.[174] This side effect profile has limited the usefulness of NSAIDs in the perioperative period. COX-2 is selectively expressed after tissue injury and augments inflammation. COX-2 inhibitors decrease inflammation and have been shown to reduce postoperative morphine requirements.[177] In addition, the timing of drug administration may be important. One study at least has shown that COX-2 inhibitors given pre-incision had a greater morphine-sparing effect than that observed for the same dose given postoperatively.[178]

N-methyl-D-aspartic acid (NMDA) receptor antagonists—ketamine, dextromethorphan—are other potential agents for providing preventive analgesia. Activation of the NMDA receptor has been implicated in the induction and maintenance of central sensitization to pain.[179,180] In addition to possibly blocking central sensitization, NMDA receptor antagonists also may reduce opioid tolerance, thereby making smaller doses of opioids more effective.[181] Although large doses of ketamine (greater than 2 mg/kg) are associated with hallucinations, hypersalivation, and cardiac stimulation, smaller doses (0.15 mg/kg) given before skin incision have been shown to decrease postoperative pain and to reduce morphine consumption in patients undergoing laparoscopic gynecologic procedures without producing the side effects as described.[179]

Current tactics in operative and postoperative pain management attempt not only to block pain transmission (narcotics, local anesthetics) but also to inhibit the positive feedback mechanisms responsible for pain amplification and prolongation (COX-2 inhibitors, NMDA receptor antagonists) and to use old therapies in new ways (local anesthetics instilled into the peritoneum during laparoscopy or applied directly to the fallopian tubes during laparoscopic tubal ligation).[182-184] Nonpharmacologic modalities that have shown a pain-reducing (and therefore morphine-sparing) effect include soothing music played during the perioperative period.[185-190]

MINIMIZATION OF RISKS DURING SURGERY

Error suppression in medicine is a laudable goal, but one that can never be fully realized. Paradoxically, as modern surgery asymptotically approaches the best performance that can be achieved by gradual refinement of the techniques currently in use, the concern arises whether it has become harder to recognize and respond appropriately in the rare event of a true

complication. This conundrum was expressed by Cooper and co-authors[191] as follows:

Perhaps the most insidious hazard of anesthesia is its relative safety. The individual anesthetist rarely, on average, will be responsible for a serious iatrogenic complication. It is our impression from the process of collecting incidents, that most seemingly minor errors are not taken seriously and that risk management depends almost solely on the anesthetist's ability to react instinctively and flawlessly every time a problem arises.

Minimally invasive surgery *usually* is minimally invasive. Therefore, anesthesiologists' supportive interventions have decreased. Immediately recognizing that a complication has occurred is only part of the challenge. An effective laparoscopic team will immediately and decisively ramp up the level of support to meet the new needs of the patient. Thus, it is important to focus on two goals at once: (1) error *suppression*, to further reduce the incidence of complications, and (2) error *management*, that is, neutralizing or mitigating the effects of errors that do occur and proactively training to correctly diagnose and manage rare catastrophic complications. The remainder of this section describes common approaches to suppressing or minimizing the incidence of complications; the following section describes simple interventions to improve error detection and early management.

Patient Selection

Preoperative evaluation should determine the presence of conditions that would adversely affect the course and outcome of laparoscopic surgery. Absolute contraindications to necessary laparoscopy have been narrowed to uncorrected coagulopathy and the inability to tolerate laparotomy. It is now routine practice, for example, to perform laparoscopic cholecystectomy in patients with severe myocardial dysfunction[192] or, in cases of acute cholecystitis, just a few days before valvuloplasty for critical aortic stenosis. Relative contraindications include previous abdominal surgery, peritonitis, obesity, pregnancy, umbilical abnormalities, and severe pulmonary disease.

Preanesthetic Evaluation

The past decade has brought a shift from managing presurgical patients as inpatients to an outpatient based model. Most hospitals now have a presurgical clinic where patients are evaluated for surgical and anesthetic risk, with appropriate interventions made a few days before surgery. Increasing demand for anesthesia services[193] has contributed to a further shift toward deferring some parts of the preanesthetic evaluation until the day of surgery.[194] For example, in our institution, many patients are screened in the preoperative clinic by nurse practitioners, who complete a standardized presurgical and preanesthetic examination. Patients with complicated medical histories or complex current medical problems are then directed to specialist anesthesiologists in the clinic. For uncomplicated patients, the final preanesthetic evaluation, formulation of anesthetic plans, and discussion of options, as well as obtaining informed consent, are all conducted on the day of surgery by the responsible anesthesiologist. This system

Table 2–2 ▪ American Society of Anesthesiologists (ASA) Classification

Physical Status Class	Description	Example(s)
ASA I	Normal, healthy patient, without organic, physiologic, or psychiatric disturbance	Healthy with good exercise tolerance
ASA II	Patient who has a controlled medical condition without significant systemic effects	Controlled HTN; controlled diabetes without systemic effects; cigarette smoking without evidence of COPD; anemia; mild obesity; age <1 yr or >70 yr
ASA III	Patient who has a medical condition with significant systemic effects intermittently associated with significant functional compromise	Controlled CHF; stable angina; old MI; poorly controlled HTN; morbid obesity; bronchospastic disease with intermittent symptoms; chronic renal failure
ASA IV	Patient who has a medical condition that is poorly controlled and associated with significant dysfunction and is a potential threat to life	Unstable angina; symptomatic COPD; symptomatic CHF; hepatorenal failure
ASA V	Patient who has a critical medical condition that is associated with little chance of survival with or without the surgical procedure	Multiorgan failure; sepsis syndrome with hemodynamic instability; hypothermia; poorly controlled coagulopathy
ASA VI	A patient who is brain dead and undergoing anesthesia for the purposes of organ donation	
E	Signifies a procedure that is being performed as an emergency and may be associated with a suboptimal opportunity for risk modification	

CHF, congestive heart failure; COPD, chronic obstructive pulmonary disease; HTN, hypertension; MI, myocardial infarction.

works well for many patients undergoing laparoscopy, who tend to have uncomplicated medical pictures.

Not all patients can be managed using this distributed model of preoperative evaluation. As the population ages, increasing numbers of patients with complex medical problems present for elective or semielective laparoscopic surgery. Our hospital has developed a set of guidelines to assist nonanesthesiologists in deciding who needs a preoperative evaluation by an anesthesiologist (see later on). The decision tool is basically a 4×3 grid based on the ASA physical status classification and the expected severity of the contemplated surgical procedure. The ASA physical status classification, presented in Table 2–2, is well validated and can be reasonably applied by nonanesthesiologists, making it a useful first-pass screening tool. Descriptions and a scoring schema for surgical severity are given in Table 2–3. Laparoscopic procedures inevitably fall into the low- and moderate-risk groups. The surgical severity axis is somewhat more problematic when applied to laparoscopic surgery, as laparoscopic procedures tend to have a better postoperative recovery profile but may be every bit as physiologically challenging to the anesthesiologist and the patient during the perioperative period. Therefore, we recommend erring on the side of caution. The complete grid is given in Table 2–4. The success of this tool in appropriately segregating patients needing extensive preoperative preparation guided by an anesthesiologist from those who need minimal intervention before the day of surgery depends on effective assignment of ASA physical status and surgical severity in the surgeon's office. Basically, poor ASA physical status or increased predicted surgical severity would automatically prompt sending the patient for consultation with an anesthesiologist, as would combinations of moderately impaired ASA physical status in combination with elevated anticipated surgical severity. For the remaining patients, the surgical history and findings on physical examination, as well as the laboratory data called out in Table 2–4, should

almost always provide sufficient framework for a focused and timely preanesthetic assessment and plan on the day of surgery.

As mentioned previously, patients with pacemakers and ICDs should have additional evaluation pertaining specifically to these devices *before* the day of surgery. If such evaluation is to be conducted in the preanesthetic clinic, patients should be instructed to bring any documentation related to their device, as well as contact information for their cardiologist, to the preanesthetic evaluation. Alternatively, such patients may be referred to their cardiologist for perioperative management, but alerting the anesthesia team preoperatively to the presence of such devices is prudent, because this team will be managing these devices on the day of surgery.

One final group of patients must ALWAYS be evaluated by an anesthesiologist before the day of surgery: those with a known or likely difficult airway. In such patients, failure to control the airway during induction of anesthesia is likely to lead to severe injury or death. Some patients with known difficult airways (e.g., those who present with a letter from an anesthesiologist describing difficulty with their airway, or a medical alert bracelet) are easy to identify. Other patients with known difficult airways may be readily identified by history. Therefore, it is important to ask patients being prepared for surgery if they have had any difficulties with anesthesia in the past, and in particular if some difficulty with the anesthetic procedure had been reported. Any positive response should trigger referral to an anesthesiologist well in advance of surgery.

Airway problems can be anticipated by three simple examinations in the office to evaluate the following:

- The ability to open the mouth widely
- The ability to extend the neck
- The distance between the tip of the mandible and the top of the larynx

Table 2–3 ■ Surgical Procedure–Related Risk Categories

Risk Category	Type of Procedure	
	Description	Examples
Low	Procedures associated with minor blood loss (less than 200 mL) and minimal physical insult	Diagnostic laparoscopy Tubal ligation Hernia repair (laparoscopic/open) Incisional hernia repair
Moderate	Procedures associated with some degree of fluid shift, blood loss potential of up to 1000 mL, or moderate procedure-related morbidity/mortality	Laparoscopic cholecystectomy Colectomies (laparoscopic/open) Uterine myomectomy (laparoscopic/open) Laparoscopic-assisted vaginal hysterectomy Vaginal hysterectomy Lysis of adhesions (laparoscopic/open) Laparoscopic Heller myotomy Laparoscopic Nissen fundoplication Prostatectomy (laparoscopic/open)
High	Procedures in upper abdominal, thoracic, or intracranial locations associated with: Potential blood loss greater than 1000 mL Potential for major fluid shifts Potential need for postoperative cardiopulmonary support and monitoring Significant procedure-related morbidity/mortality	Open cholecystectomy Open Nissen fundoplication Liver resection Lung resection Esophagectomy Whipple's procedure Craniotomy

Table 2–4 ■ Anesthesiology Consultation Decision Tool

ASA Class	Indicated Laboratory Tests/Consultation		
	Low Risk	Moderate Risk	High Risk
I	ECG in M >45 yr or F >55 yr, BUN/Cr/Gluc in M/F >65 yr	ECG in M >45 yr or F >55 yr, CBC, BUN/Cr/Gluc in M/F >65 yr	**Anesthesiology consultation** ECG, chest film, CBC, BBS, BUN/Cr/Gluc in M/F >65 yr
II	ECG in M >45 yr or F >55 yr, chest film,* BUN/Cr/Gluc in M/F >65 yr	ECG in M >45 yr or F >55 yr, CBC, chest film,* BUN/Cr/Gluc in M/F >65 yr	**Anesthesiology consultation** ECG, chest film, CBC, BBS, BUN/Cr/Gluc in M/F >65 yr
III	**Anesthesiology consultation** ECG, chest film,* CBC, electrolytes, BUN/Cr/Gluc	**Anesthesiology consultation** ECG, chest film,* CBC, electrolytes, BBS, BUN/Cr/Gluc	**Anesthesiology consultation** Laboratory tests as dictated by underlying condition
IV	**Anesthesiology consultation** Laboratory tests as dictated by underlying condition	**Anesthesiology consultation** Laboratory tests as dictated by underlying condition	**Anesthesiology consultation** Laboratory tests as dictated by underlying condition

*Chest radiograph should be obtained in patients older than 70 years of age or in those with a history of goiter or malignancy.

ASA, American Society of Anesthesiologists; BBS, blood bank sample for typing and antibody screen; BUN, blood urea nitrogen; CBC, complete blood count; Cr, [serum] creatinine; ECG, electrocardiogram; F, female patient; Gluc, glucose; M, male patient.

These three examinations are readily performed in the surgeon's office and should be conducted and documented in the record, particularly if the patient otherwise meets criteria to bypass preanesthetic evaluation. The entire evaluation requires approximately 30 seconds and should be conducted with the patient sitting up. Mouth opening is scored using the Mallampati classification (Fig. 2–3), a four-point classification scale indicating how widely the patient can open the mouth and how much free space is available in the back of the mouth when it is fully open. Higher scores are associated with increased difficulty in visualizing laryngeal structures during intubation attempts. Neck extension is assessed by having the patient tip the head as far back as possible while sitting upright. *Normal* neck extension should allow the patient to look directly at the ceiling while sitting erect; any less would be considered *limited*. The distance between the tip of the mandible and the top of the larynx (formally known as the *thyromental distance*) should be roughly three fingerbreadths. This is readily assessed by placing three fingers between the patient's Adam's apple and the chin; if the examiner's fingers protrude beyond the chin, the thyromental distance is considered to be *short*.

Patients with good mouth opening (low Mallampati scores), normal neck extension, and normal thyromental dis-

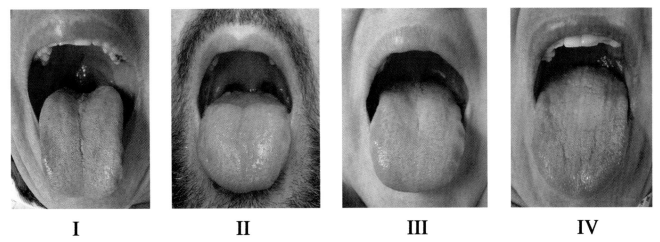

I   **II**   **III**   **IV**

Figure 2–3 ▪ **Mallampati classification of the airway.** The airway is described as class I if the tonsillar pillars and all of the uvula are visible when the patient maximally opens the mouth. In a class II airway, more than the base of the uvula can be seen, but not the tonsillar pillars. In a patient with a class III airway, only the base of the uvula is visible. In a patient with a class IV airway, neither the uvula nor the tonsillar pillars are visible.

tances are unlikely to have airway problems. Similarly, patients with poor mouth opening (high Mallampati scores), limited neck extension, and short thyromental distance are unlikely to suffer airway catastrophes because anesthesiologists anticipate difficulty and prepare effectively. Patients with more subtle indications of difficulty (i.e., only one or two difficult airway predictors) are at greatest risk for problems because the possibility of such problems can easily escape preoperative attention. The value of the airway examination in such patients is clear: Patients at risk should be identified early so that appropriate preparations can be made.

Evidence is beginning to accumulate that medical management choices made in the immediate perioperative period have long-term consequences. For example, perioperative beta blockade in patients at risk for cardiac complications during noncardiac surgery confers a long-term survival advantage over those not receiving beta blockade. Because increasing numbers of such patients are presenting for laparoscopic surgery, it is important to take a more holistic view of the patient well in advance of the surgery. As a rule of thumb, any patient whose medical condition cannot be comfortably managed by the surgical team alone without assistance from consultants in the preoperative period probably should be evaluated by an anesthesiologist before the day of surgery.

Early Recognition of Developing Problems in the Operating Room

All members of the operating room team should be alert to the possibility of complications at any time. To the extent that members of the team can absorb, either by design or incidentally, the knowledge and skills of other members of the team, a redundant system can be created. Thus, "situational" awareness by all members of the team, coupled with cross-training redundancy, enhances the likelihood that a developing complication will be caught early.

Surgeons recognize intraoperative complications using their senses of touch, vision, and, to some extent, hearing,

either by direct contact with the patient or through the laparoscopic view. Anesthesiologists recognize intraoperative complications most frequently by means of indirect patient contact, mediated by the physiologic monitor. Physiologic monitors are arguably the most important piece of equipment in the operating room for the early diagnosis of intraoperative complications, particularly during key parts of laparoscopic procedures, such as blind insufflation of CO_2 through a Veress needle.

Monitoring configurations vary between institutions, and even between operating rooms in a single institution, but each physiologic monitoring package includes certain basic functions that are of critical diagnostic value during the early development of the most catastrophic intraoperative complications of laparoscopic surgery. Each person in the operating room should be sufficiently familiar with these functions to sense immediately that something is going wrong when readings deviate rapidly from nominal values. Figure 2–1 shows a typical physiologic monitor with key trends displayed for a 6-minute period. The most important information on the monitor changes during the course of the procedure. For example, during the initial establishment of pneumoperitoneum, the SpO_2, $ETCO_2$, and heart rate are the key information; rapid diminution of these waveforms as CO_2 is being insufflated into the abdomen should prompt immediate cessation of insufflation and arouse suspicion of CO_2 embolism. Similarly, dramatic slowing of the heart rate (or occasionally asystole) during insufflation also should prompt rapid release of pressure.

All members of the operating room team should have at least passing familiarity with the most basic physiologic constellations indicating intraoperative complications for which these monitors are useful in diagnosis. At the most basic level, the unannounced disappearance of the pulse oximeter's audible tones (implying in the worst case a sudden loss of circulation) should create immediate and compelling anxiety among all members of the operating room team until resolved.

Optimized Work Environment

Human factors design is a relatively new consideration in medicine.[195] In other industries such as air transportation and nuclear power, it is widely recognized that poor ergonomics contributes to bad outcomes by diverting people's attention and cognitive resources away from the ultimate goal and toward making the system go.[195] Conversely, good ergonomics and clear display of useful data enhance the likelihood of good outcomes. We recently completed the design and implementation of a large ergonomics optimization project focused on laparoscopic operating rooms, with the goal of creating an environment that is as near to the ideal as could be supported by current technology.

To achieve this redesign, we took a multidisciplinary approach to reorganizing perioperative patient flow, work processes, and surgical, nursing, and anesthesia ergonomics for maximum operating room effectiveness. This "Operating Room of the Future" (ORF) Implementation Project required (1) application of advanced technology, (2) changes to operating room architecture, and (3) reengineering of work processes to enhance operating room working conditions. The ORF Project was designed for optimal support of advanced minimally invasive surgery and its associated anesthesia and nursing practices.

A multidisciplinary team surveyed other "best-of-breed" operating rooms in the United States and Europe and used the accumulated experience to inform the initial designs of the ORF. After several rounds of design refinement, including full-scale mockups and modeling of patient flow in the space, a multispace design was chosen. We constructed an operating suite with a functioning induction room and a space for early recovery, both attached to the operating room in a fashion sometimes found in European facilities. As shown in Figure 2–4, patients enter the ORF from the main operating room area (*red arrow* in the figure). Movements within the ORF suite, such as from the induction area to the operating room to the emergence area, are denoted by the *yellow arrow*. Egress to the main PACU is denoted by the *green arrow*. Construction of a self-contained three-room suite created an additional 100 square feet of patient care space compared with a typical operating room at our institution.

Equipment in the ORF was chosen to facilitate throughput and good ergonomics. The operating room table is a transporter–operating room table-top–fixed column system (Fig. 2–5, *left*) that eliminates surface-to-surface transfers. Monitoring is continuous (without cable swapping) (see Fig. 2–5, *right*). Postoperatively, patients can be transferred fully monitored, on the operating room table-top, directly to patient care units. The ORF quickly exceeded its throughput

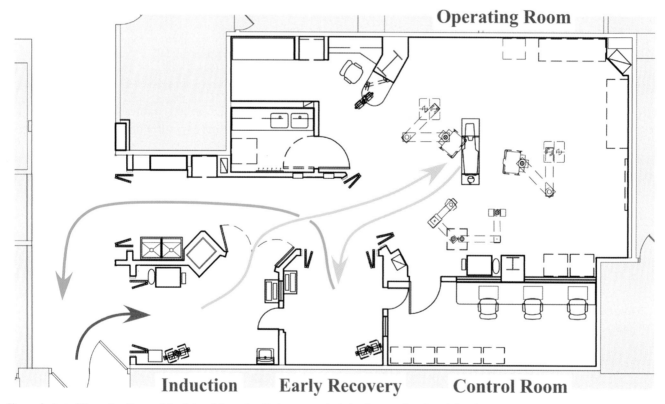

Operating Room

Induction   Early Recovery   Control Room

Figure 2–4 ■ **"Operating Room of the Future" floor plan.** Patients enter the induction area from hospital perioperative areas and are admitted to the unit by the perioperative nurse. Anesthesia is induced in the induction area while operating room setup proceeds. At the end of the procedure, the perioperative nurse receives a report of the case events. At the conclusion of the procedure, the patient is either extubated in the operating room or moved to the early recovery (emergence) area and extubated, after which the perioperative nurse resumes care. The anesthesia team then promptly anesthetizes the next patient in the induction area as the operating room team proceeds with room setup. At the end of setup, the anesthetized (subsequent) patient is transported to the operaing room, and the work flows join. During turnover, the surgeons work (e.g., dictating operative notes, looking up results, writing orders on the hospital information system, teleconferencing with patient's family) in the control room.

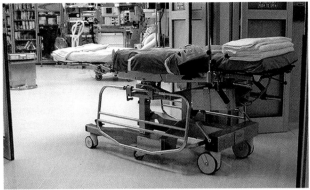
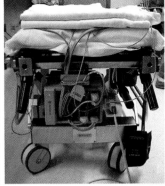

Figure 2–5 ▪ **Mobile operating room table-top, transporter, and fixed column. Left panel,** The fixed column can be seen on the *left.* When the operating room table-top is on the transporter *(foreground),* it is easily moved between operating suite spaces by a single person while it is occupied by a patient. **Right panel,** The physiologic monitor data acquisition unit is mounted to the underside of the head of the operating room table-top. Once monitors are applied, they are not removed as the patient moves between spaces in the operating suite and through induction, maintenance, and emergence from anesthesia.

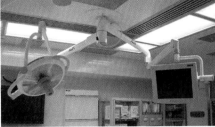

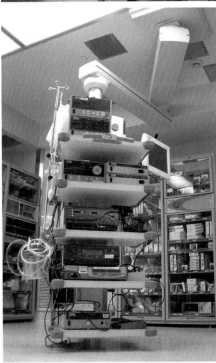

Figure 2–6 ▪ **Integrated endosurgical system. Upper panel,** Flat-panel liquid crystal display (LCD) devices used for surgery share space with operating room field lights and video camera (in light handle). When not in use, the display can simply be pushed up out of the way. **Lower panel,** Complete endosurgery equipment package on ceiling-mounted boom in the operating suite. No interconnect cabling is required, and the equipment is permanently deployed, minimizing setup time.

goals, but the improved ergonomics of the facility is the key element for the following discussion.

The ORF itself contains a dedicated, integrated endosurgical equipment package that is pendant mounted to facilitate room turnover between cases (Fig. 2–6, *top*).[196] More important, the endosurgical equipment is permanently deployed in the ORF (see Fig. 2–6, *bottom*), effectively eliminating cabling and configuration errors. This ensures that the equipment is more likely to be properly configured and will perform as expected when needed. Lightweight flat-panel displays can be readily positioned for optimal surgical viewing, minimizing fatigue for the surgical team.

The ORF anesthesia workspace is designed as an ergonomic "cockpit" (Fig. 2–7). Everything needed for patient care is within reach of the anesthesiologist standing at the head of the bed, without any need to move.

The final piece of technology deployed in the ORF is aimed at enhancing situational awareness of the operating room team. To accomplish this, a plasma screen video display keeps everyone in the operating room registered with the surgical process (Fig. 2–8). Continuous display of live images from laparoscopes or light-mounted cameras in the operating room is standard practice whenever surgery is being performed. This allows team members not directly in the surgical field to "self-update" to surgical events. It also minimizes interruptions of the surgical team's work by reducing other team members' need to ask for progress updates. Finally, a continuous visual display of the operation allows the rest of the team to see most of what the surgeons see when a surgical complication develops. In this way, the plasma display gives the same visibility to surgical events that the physiologic monitor display gives to anesthesia events.

Creation of the ergonomic anesthesia workspace and the provision of the large-format plasma video display serve to keep the members of the anesthesia and the surgical teams integrated and in proximity, effectively removing the psychologic separation that can inadvertently be created by the physical presence of drapes separating these team members.

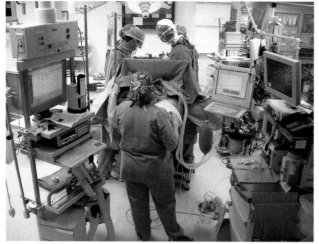

Figure 2–7 ▪ **Ergonomic "cockpit" for the anesthesia team in the operating suite.** On the *right*, an anesthesia machine, physiologic and level-of-consciousness monitors, and an automated anesthesia information management system (AIMS) with vital signs trend display are deployed. The anesthetist can address the AIMS *(second screen from right)* when standing facing the patient's head and the surgical field. The physiologic monitor display (see Fig. 2–2 for detail) and the displays on the anesthesia machine are optimally positioned at the anesthesia team's right side and are readily visible to the surgical team. Additionally, dedicated task lighting, telephones, ample electric power, and local area network (LAN) connections are available for future expansion. To the *rear* is an anesthesia supply workstation, as well as waste and sharps containers. On the *left*, an auxiliary boom organizes infusion pumps, as well as intravenous fluid and forced-air patient warming devices. The auxiliary boom also provides extra electric power and LAN connectivity. Also included on the *left* side of the anesthesia cockpit is a computer to access patient medical data and for computerized order entry *(left screen)*. The computer also connects to hospital knowledge bases, the university library system, and the National Library of Medicine, providing a valuable resource for information searching at the patient's bedside.

PROSPECTIVE MANAGEMENT OF COMPLICATIONS: PRACTICING RECOGNITION AND MANAGEMENT OF ADVERSE EVENTS

With laparoscopic surgery, there is no substitute for experience. Where studied, the complication rates for individual surgeons have shown an inverse correlation with the number of procedures performed.[25,197–200] This finding is at least partly explained by the challenge of visualizing a three-dimensional operation on a two-dimensional video display.[201] An additional mechanism for reduced complication rates as a function of experience is the opportunity to experience, manage, and learn from complications throughout the practitioner's career. An approach that affords this opportunity is simulation—practicing the avoidance, diagnosis, and management of complications. Technologies for simulation allow surgeons, anesthesiologists, and other members of the care team to gain relevant experience in a safe environment and without involving patients.

Part-Task Simulation

In view of the initial steepness of the learning curve for mastering laparoscopic surgical skills and techniques, a reliable way to teach these skills without putting patients at risk is eminently desirable. Traditionally this has been done with mechanical box trainers (also known as part-task simulators) and animal models.

More recently, computer-based virtual reality (VR) simulators are being used to teach and develop laparoscopic skills. Specifically, graduate students (without previous surgical experience) who were given structured intracorporeal knot

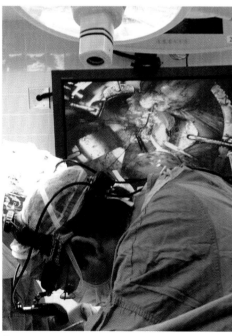

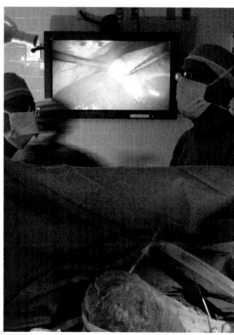

Figure 2–8 ▪ Plasma video display in the operating suite during open (**A**) and laparoscopic (**B**) surgery. In **A**, the video feed to the display is from a camera in the light handle at the top of the image. In **B**, the view on the plasma display is from the laparoscopic camera. In both instances, the entire operating room team sees what the surgeon is viewing.

A

B

tying training on simulators mastered the task more quickly than those who received unstructured training.[202] The value of this approach was further demonstrated in a prospective, randomized, blinded study of teaching laparoscopic cholecystectomy to surgical residents. In this study, eight surgical residents were assigned to VR training on a laparoscopic diathermy task until they achieved expert performance, defined as meeting criteria established by expert laparoscopists. Eight additional residents received no simulator training. Next, each resident performed laparoscopic cholecystectomy in the operating room with an attending surgeon unaware of the resident's VR training exposure. Videotapes of gallbladder dissection were reviewed independently by two surgeons blinded to resident identity and VR training status, and the number of each of eight predefined errors was scored every minute. VR-trained residents "made fewer errors, were less likely to injure the gallbladder and burn non-target tissue, and were more likely to make steady progress throughout the procedure" than were non–VR-trained residents. The investigators observed that it may soon be possible to "train out the learning curve for technical skills on a simulator, rather than on patients."[203] This study is an example of the successful transfer of skills learned in a VR simulation environment to the operating room.

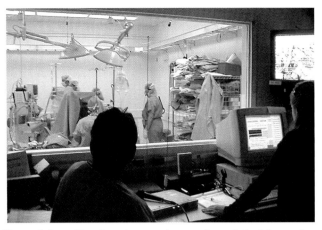

Figure 2–9 ▪ View from the control room of a realistic, full-operating-room simulator during execution of a scenario. The computer to the *right* is used to control the response of the simulated patient to interventions by the care team in the operating suite. Video monitors, direct viewing through the one-way mirror (here transparent), and voice feeds from simulator personnel in the operating room allow the care team's actions to be recorded and translated into appropriate patient responses. Members of the surgical team usually are simulator confederates but need not be so.

Anesthesia Crisis Resource Management Training

Full-operating-room simulation, also known as anesthesia crisis resource management (ACRM), was developed to educate anesthesia teams by allowing them to rehearse the diagnosis and management of adverse events.[204] ACRM is a development of crew resource management, a success story from the airline industry.[204] Full-operating-room simulation allows anesthesiologists to experience, with great realism, events that are only rarely encountered, if ever, during a career but could have disastrous consequences if not recognized and effectively managed. Relevant to anesthesia, these have included oxygen source failure, cardiac arrest, malignant hyperthermia, tension pneumothorax, and complete power failure. More broadly, scenarios featuring almost any perioperative catastrophe can be constructed. Figure 2–9 shows the view from the control room of a realistic, full-operating-room simulator. From the control room, operators can manipulate the mannequin's responses and simulated vital signs as a crisis develops and change the mannequin's condition in response to the actions taken by the care team.

Simulation has been used to investigate how well anesthesiologists respond to crises. As might be expected, clinicians accustomed to the smooth perioperative course so often associated with minimally invasive surgery and modern anesthetic techniques do not readily perceive and respond to the early evidence foretelling the development of rare critical events. For example, ACRM has been used to demonstrate that anesthesia teams do not readily detect or respond appropriately to anaphylactic shock during anesthesia,[205,206] and that they do not respond in a consistent manner to more common critical events.[207] Furthermore, relatively inexperienced providers do not effectively seek help in a crisis.[208]

In addition to pointing out inconsistent performance, full-operating-room simulation is a powerful educational tool. Prospective evidence indicates that even brief exposure (i.e., a single day at the simulator with two simulated critical events) improves performance in responding to a crisis.[209] Review of videotape between simulation sessions, a common component of simulator training, speeds improvement in performance.[210] Moreover, simulation of rare events may lead to improved performance when these events are resimulated at a later date.[211] For example, after simulation training anesthesiologists and residents dealt more effectively with malignant hyperthermia, a vanishingly rare but lethal complication of anesthesia.[211] In this study, 28 participants were divided into two groups and exposed to a prescripted, simulated "control" scenario of anaphylactic shock in a realistic, full-operating-room simulator. The sessions were videotaped and the performances of individual participants were evaluated using a standardized scoring scheme. Performance scores on this first scenario were used to eliminate the effects of interindividual variability (i.e., level of training, experience) on subsequent performance scores. Approximately 2 weeks later, participants from one group repeated simulator training in the management of anaphylactic shock, while the other group trained in simulated malignant hyperthermia. Four months later, each participant returned to the simulator for a "test" scenario of malignant hyperthermia. Participants were not aware in advance of what scenario would be presented. These sessions were again evaluated using the same scoring scheme. The participants previously exposed to the malignant hyperthermia simulation responded more quickly and provided better treatment than those not previously exposed to this simulation.

Unfortunately, this and many other studies of the efficacy of simulation suffer from various methodologic flaws that compromise their dispositive value. In the case of the study cited previously, performance was assessed by a single unblinded evaluator using an unvalidated scoring scheme. Other writers have drawn attention to the general lack of rigor in this area.[212] These criticisms are leveled at the methodologic quality of assessments of simulation, rather than the value of simulation itself. Indeed, the study involving simulated malignant hyperthermia reviewed earlier suggests that simulation of rare events improves performance (i.e., "time to first response" is a fairly objective measure), and even brief simulation exposure to rare events leads to lasting performance improvement.

Indirect evidence suggests that simulation can be used even to improve the performance of routine systems, as evidenced by the following example: We have implemented a model for perioperative patient flow in the operating room that is new to our institution as illustrated in Figures 2–4 and 2–5. These changes amounted to the creation of a completely novel environment and workflow relative to our typical perioperative patient workflow, and we hypothesized that learning would occur (evidenced by improvement in performance) as the team began to use the space. As a measure of familiarity with the new workflow, we studied the times required to complete key steps in the perioperative process. Redesigned-operating-room time data for the nonoperative interval (when the new workflow would have the greatest impact) were compared with time data from conventional operating rooms for the same surgeon doing the same procedure (laparoscopic cholecystectomy) in the two environments (Fig. 2–10). Nonoperative times were significantly reduced in the new operating room, indicating the success of the throughput intervention. An expected finding would be evidence of a learning curve—that is, a rapid reduction in nonoperative time over a period of days or weeks as the team acclimated to the new system. Instead, a minimal learning effect on nonoperative time was observed (in Fig. 2–10, neither slope is significantly different from 0). This finding was unexpected in view of the magnitude of the work process reorganization. The early learning effect for the new system, however, may have been minimized by a form of simulation—the entire team, including surgeons, anesthesiologists, and nurses simulated the perioperative workflow with mock patients during formal rehearsals before the ORF was opened.

Although the most experience with full-operating-room simulation has been accumulated with anesthesiologists, simulation has been effectively used to train physicians and nurses from other specialties.[209,213,214] Simulation allows team members to see how they will perform under pressure (through facilitated review of videotapes of the just-completed simulation) and allows intervention by skilled simulation instructors to correct bad habits, teach effective leadership, and facilitate communication and development of role clarity under extreme duress.[209] We propose that the value of simulation can be extended to full-team, full-operating-room simulations of the rare, devastating complications of laparoscopic surgery, particularly massive venous embolism and cardiac arrest.

FINAL THOUGHTS

Complications inevitably will occur during laparoscopic surgery. Most complications that occur in the operating room can be remediated in the operating room (if they are recognized at the time) and do not necessarily require special postoperative care such as admission to the ICU. If the patient has not been returned to a state of hemodynamic and metabolic stability by the conclusion of the procedure, however, then remedial care necessarily continues into the postoperative period. Postoperative efforts to optimize recovery from a complication should be directed at reversing the problem. In this respect, postoperative care after a complication of laparoscopic surgery does not differ from the management of all surgical patients after a complication. The anesthesiologist and the surgeon should work together to identify what other resources, including ICU admission and appropriate subspecialty consultations, are needed to ensure the best outcome. This discussion should begin when a complication is recognized and continue with frequent updates as the situation unfolds in the operating room. When necessary, intraoperative consultation may contribute to the discussion between the anesthesia team and the surgeon about what resources available within their particular hospital are needed to ensure the best outcome.

Laparoscopic surgery promises patients less discomfort and a speedier recovery than have been possible with open surgery. The operating room team should resist the temptation to be lulled by this promise into a false sense of security. The safety systems surrounding surgery are indeed fallible. The public is now aware that even with today's extraordinary technologic potentials, surgery is at its heart a dangerous undertaking. Modern surgery has exploded into an incredibly complex system, and the risk of failure is embedded within it. These sources of vulnerabilities have been identified by intrinsic attributes of the system: that (1) it has grown beyond the capacity of humans to fully control it and (2) the possibilities for errors are much more expansive than was previously realized.[215]

If, in fact, the basis for error lies innately within the system, then more strategic, technologic advancements (i.e., system-level changes) need to be made for true improvement to occur. The perioperative environment is a particularly

Non-operative Time as a Function of Days Since Room Opening

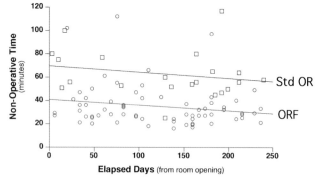

Figure 2–10 ▪ Nonoperative time in the "Operating Room of the Future" (ORF) *(circles)* and standard operating rooms *(squares)* as a function of the number of days since ORF opening. For the same surgical procedure, the nonoperative interval is shorter in the ORF than in the standard operating room at any point in time. The slight negative slopes of the regression lines, suggesting gradual improvement over time, are not significant. If the learning curve for the new patient flow in the ORF were significant, a correspondingly significant reduction in nonoperative time in the ORF during the first days or weeks after room opening would be expected. Inspection of the *left* side of the figure reveals no evidence for such a learning curve.

complex area plagued by fragmented and incomplete systems.[216] The complexity of operating room work is unrelentingly high, yet it is frequently interrupted by such mundane events as missing or nonfunctional equipment. Significant energy is diverted from patient care simply to gather all of the needed elements for modern surgery in the operating room and to make this equipment function. Even the best equipment properly maintained often is saddled with counterintuitive setup procedures. Mundane interruptions occur frequently and in clusters, causing unpredictable responses and high stress levels and diverting the operating room team's attention from patient care. Balky, inefficient, and unreliable perioperative systems have limited the benefits of new surgical techniques and high-level technology, in addition to their impact on patient safety. Nor has the expense of such inefficiency brought added safety. To the contrary, today's increasingly complex perioperative processes are still prone to spectacular failures, despite herculean efforts by practitioners to construct human-based systems to prevent mishaps. Humans cannot be relied on to intercept human error; such a practice only compounds the probability of errors occurring in complex systems.[215]

Even with the acknowledgment that inherent risk exists, many approaches to operating room safety focus on changes in personnel behavior, rather than on approaches that improve safety by fundamentally strengthening the error interception and suppression process. The interventions that have been emphasized as focal points for improved safety are rules and procedures, training, strategic redundancies, teamwork development, and mitigating decision making. In fact, almost all of the recommendations in this chapter have emphasized these approaches. Again, the focus is on the human elements of knowledge, motivation, and skill.[4] More powerful strategies for error interception such as automation and force function have not made it to the operating room.

The complicated undertakings in surgery have until now been carried out solely by humans, with automation for assistance only. In other fields of endeavor, the actual execution and, more important, the monitoring for early signs of trouble have been automated, with human operators moving into planning and global, higher-level monitoring roles.[217] Thus far, perceptions of medicine as a highly specialized field in which art, expertise, and intuition play large roles have limited the penetration of automated safeguards into clinical practice.[215,218] Computer and sensor technologies are increasingly robust, however, and the burgeoning complexity in high-risk medical environments now necessitates an automatic computer-based system to provide feedback, verifications, and safeguards to augment human vigilance for errors during surgical care. Thus, it is now possible to integrate the information stemming from operating room equipment to (1) suppress and eliminate mundane interruptions due to malfunctioning, misconnected, or missing equipment; (2) provide "augmented vigilance" for early and reliable detection of developing problems that manifest themselves at least in part as altered output on a monitor; and (3) provide decision support to suggest likely causes.

Such a technologic solution will not prevent procedural errors such as accidental dural or carotid puncture by anesthesiologists, nor will it prevent inadvertent gas embolization or bowel, vascular, or urinary tract injuries by laparoscopic surgeons. By reducing distractions due to more mundane failures, however, it will allow the entire operating room team to concentrate on its core mission: the care of the patient.

References

1. Institute of Medicine. To err is human: Building a safer healthcare system. Washington, DC: National Academy Press, 1999.
2. Cooper JB, Newbower RS, Long CD, McPeek B. Preventable anesthesia mishaps: A study of human factors. Anesthesiology 1978;49:399.
3. Pierce EC Jr. Looking back on the anesthesia critical incident studies and their role in catalysing patient safety. Qual Saf Health Care 2002;11:282.
4. Turnbull JE. Process management and systems thinking for patient safety. In: Smith LR, ed. The Business of Healthcare: A Journal of Innovative Management Collection. Salem, NH: GOAL/QPC, 2001; 140.
5. Bates DW, Leape LL, Cullen DJ, et al. Effect of computerized physician order entry and a team intervention on prevention of serious medication errors. JAMA 1998;280:1311.
6. Joris JL. Anesthesia for laparoscopic surgery. In: Miller RD, ed. Anesthesia, 5th ed. Philadelphia: Churchill Livingstone, 2000;2003.
7. Danelli G, Berti M, Perotti V, et al. Temperature control and recovery of bowel function after laparoscopic or laparotomic colorectal surgery in patients receiving combined epidural/general anesthesia and postoperative epidural analgesia. Anesth Analg 2002;95:467.
8. Wullstein C, Barkhausen S, Gross E. Results of laparoscopic vs. conventional appendectomy in complicated appendicitis. Dis Colon Rectum 2001;44:1700.
9. Rose DK, Cohen MM, Soutter DI. Laparoscopic cholecystectomy: The anaesthetist's point of view. Can J Anaesth 1992;39:809.
10. Grace PA, Quereshi A, Coleman J, et al. Reduced postoperative hospitalization after laparoscopic cholecystectomy. Br J Surg 1991;78:160.
11. Winfield HN, Hamilton BD, Bravo EL, Novick AC. Laparoscopic adrenalectomy: The preferred choice? A comparison to open adrenalectomy. J Urol 1998;160:325.
12. Baldwin DD, Dunbar JA, Parekh DJ, et al. Single-center comparison of purely laparoscopic, hand-assisted laparoscopic, and open radical nephrectomy in patients at high anesthetic risk. J Endourol 2003;17: 161.
13. Harkki-Siren P, Sjoberg J, Toivonen J, Tiitinen A. Clinical outcome and tissue trauma after laparoscopic and abdominal hysterectomy: A randomized controlled study. Acta Obstet Gynecol Scand 2000;79:866.
14. Eden CG, Haigh AC, Carter PG, Coptcoat MJ. Laparoscopic nephrectomy results in better postoperative pulmonary function. J Endourol 1994;8:419.
15. Frazee RC, Roberts JW, Okeson GC, et al. Open versus laparoscopic cholecystectomy. A comparison of postoperative pulmonary function. Ann Surg 1991;213:651.
16. Joris J, Cigarini I, Legrand M, et al. Metabolic and respiratory changes after cholecystectomy performed via laparotomy or laparoscopy. Br J Anaesth 1992;69:341.
17. Putensen-Himmer G, Putensen C, Lammer H, et al. Comparison of postoperative respiratory function after laparoscopy or open laparotomy for cholecystectomy. Anesthesiology 1992;77:675.
18. Schauer PR, Luna J, Ghiatas AA, et al. Pulmonary function after laparoscopic cholecystectomy. Surgery 1993;114:389.
19. Fahlenkamp D, Rassweiler J, Fornara P, et al. Complications of laparoscopic procedures in urology: Experience with 2,407 procedures at 4 German centers. J Urol 1999;162:765.
20. Soulie M, Seguin P, Richeux L, et al. Urological complications of laparoscopic surgery: Experience with 350 procedures at a single center. J Urol 2001;165:1960.
21. Mirhashemi R, Harlow BL, Ginsberg E, et al. Predicting risk of complications with gynecological laparoscopic surgery. Obstet Gynecol 1998;92:327.
22. Harkki-Siren P, Kurki T. A nationwide analysis of laparoscopic complications. Obstet Gynecol 1997;89:108.
23. Hulka J, Peterson HB, Phillips JM, Surrey MW. Operative laparoscopy: American Association of Gynecologic Laparoscopists' 1993 membership survey. J Am Assoc Gynecol Laparosc 1995;2:133.
24. Sutton C. Operative laparoscopy. Curr Opin Obstet Gynecol 1992;4: 430.

25. Harkki-Siren P, Sjoberg J, Kurki T. Major complications of laparoscopy: A follow-up Finnish study. Obstet Gynecol 1999;94:94.
26. Magrina JF. Complications of laparoscopic surgery. Clin Obstet Gynecol 2002;45:469.
27. Chapron C, Pierre F, Harchaoui Y, et al. Gastrointestinal injuries during gynaecological laparoscopy. Hum Reprod 1999;14:333.
28. Hashizume M, Sugimachi K. Needle and trocar injury during laparoscopic surgery in Japan. Surg Endosc 1997;11:1198.
29. Hasson HM, Rotman C, Rana N, Kumari NA. Open laparoscopy: 29-year experience. Obstet Gynecol 2000;96:763.
30. Bonjer HJ, Hazebroek EJ, Kazemier G, et al. Open versus closed establishment of pneumoperitoneum in laparoscopic surgery. Br J Surg 1997;84:599.
31. Bateman BG, Kolp LA, Hoeger K. Complications of laparoscopy—operative and diagnostic. Fertil Steril 1996;66:30.
32. Philosophe R. Avoiding complications of laparoscopic surgery. Fertil Steril 2003;80(Suppl 4):30.
33. Bishoff JT, Allaf ME, Kirkels W, et al. Laparoscopic bowel injury: Incidence and clinical presentation. J Urol 1999;161:887.
34. Saye WB, Miller W, Hertzmann P. Electrosurgery thermal injury. Myth or misconception? Surg Laparosc Endosc 1991;1:223.
35. Cadeddu JA, Regan F, Kavoussi LR, Moore RG. The role of computerized tomography in the evaluation of complications after laparoscopic urological surgery. J Urol 1997;158:1349.
36. Crist DW, Gadacz TR. Complications of laparoscopic surgery. Surg Clin North Am 1993;73:265.
37. Peterson HB, DeStefano F, Rubin GL, et al. Deaths attributable to tubal sterilization in the United States, 1977 to 1981. Am J Obstet Gynecol 1983;146:131.
38. Peterson HB, Hulka JF, Phillips JM. American Association of Gynecologic Laparoscopists' 1988 membership survey on operative laparoscopy. J Reprod Med 1990;35:587.
39. Cruickshank AM, Fraser WD, Burns HJ, et al. Response of serum interleukin-6 in patients undergoing elective surgery of varying severity. Clin Sci (Lond) 1990;79:161.
40. Nezhat C, Nezhat F, Ambroze W, Pennington E. Laparoscopic repair of small bowel and colon. A report of 26 cases. Surg Endosc 1993;7:88.
41. Reich H. Laparoscopic bowel injury. Surg Laparosc Endosc 1992;2:74.
42. Harris WJ, Daniell JF. Early complications of laparoscopic hysterectomy. Obstet Gynecol Surv 1996;51:559.
43. Chapron CM, Pierre F, Lacroix S, et al. Major vascular injuries during gynecologic laparoscopy. J Am Coll Surg 1997;185:461.
44. Champault G, Cazacu F, Taffinder N. Serious trocar accidents in laparoscopic surgery: A French survey of 103,852 operations. Surg Laparosc Endosc 1996;6:367.
45. Riedel HH, Lehmann-Willenbrock E, Conrad P, Semm K. German pelviscopic statistics for the years 1978-1982. Endoscopy 1986;18:219.
46. Mintz M. Risks and prophylaxis in laparoscopy: A survey of 100,000 cases. J Reprod Med 1977;18:269.
47. Yuzpe AA. Pneumoperitoneum needle and trocar injuries in laparoscopy. A survey on possible contributing factors and prevention. J Reprod Med 1990;35:485.
48. Nordestgaard AG, Bodily KC, Osborne RW Jr, Buttorff JD. Major vascular injuries during laparoscopic procedures. Am J Surg 1995;169:543.
49. Thiel R, Adams JB, Schulam PG, et al. Venous dissection injuries during laparoscopic urological surgery. J Urol 1996;155:1874.
50. Saidi MH, Sadler RK, Vancaillie TG, et al. Diagnosis and management of serious urinary complications after major operative laparoscopy. Obstet Gynecol 1996;87:272.
51. Daly JW, Higgins KA. Injury to the ureter during gynecologic surgical procedures. Surg Gynecol Obstet 1988;167:19.
52. Goodno JA Jr, Powers TW, Harris VD. Ureteral injury in gynecologic surgery: A ten-year review in a community hospital. Am J Obstet Gynecol 1995;172:1817.
53. Hasson HM, Parker WH. Prevention and management of urinary tract injury in laparoscopic surgery. J Am Assoc Gynecol Laparosc 1998;5:99.
54. Nezhat CH, Seidman DS, Nezhat F, et al. Laparoscopic management of intentional and unintentional cystotomy. J Urol 1996;156:1400.
55. Font GE, Brill AI, Stuhldreher PV, Rosenzweig BA. Endoscopic management of incidental cystotomy during operative laparoscopy. J Urol 1993;149:1130.
56. Hulka JF, Peterson HB, Phillips JM. American Association of Gynecologic Laparoscopists' 1988 membership survey on laparoscopic sterilization. J Reprod Med 1990;35:584.
57. Joris JL, Chiche JD, Lamy ML. Pneumothorax during laparoscopic fundoplication: Diagnosis and treatment with positive end-expiratory pressure. Anesth Analg 1995;81:993.
58. Loffer FD, Pent D. Indications, contraindications and complications of laparoscopy. Obstet Gynecol Surv 1975;30:407.
59. Prystowsky JB, Jericho BG, Epstein HM. Spontaneous bilateral pneumothorax—complication of laparoscopic cholecystectomy. Surgery 1993;114:988.
60. Batra MS, Driscoll JJ, Coburn WA, Marks WM. Evanescent nitrous oxide pneumothorax after laparoscopy. Anesth Analg 1983;62:1121.
61. Doctor NH, Hussain Z. Bilateral pneumothorax associated with laparoscopy. A case report of a rare hazard and review of literature. Anaesthesia 1973;28:75.
62. Gabbott DA, Dunkley AB, Roberts FL. Carbon dioxide pneumothorax occurring during laparoscopic cholecystectomy. Anaesthesia 1992;47:587.
63. Ronsse G, Stalport J, Burnon D. [Bilateral pneumothorax; a rare complication of gynecological laparoscopy (author's transl).] Acta Chir Belg 1980;79:345.
64. Whiston RJ, Eggers KA, Morris RW, Stamatakis JD. Tension pneumothorax during laparoscopic cholecystectomy. Br J Surg 1991;78:1325.
65. Woolner DF, Johnson DM. Bilateral pneumothorax and surgical emphysema associated with laparoscopic cholecystectomy. Anaesth Intensive Care 1993;21:108.
66. Reid DB, Winning T, Bell G. Pneumothorax during laparoscopic dissection of the diaphragmatic hiatus. Br J Surg 1993;80:670.
67. Joris J. Anesthetic management of laparoscopy. In: Miller RD, ed. Anesthesia. New York, Churchill Livingstone, 1992;2011.
68. Shanberg AM, Zagnoev M, Clougherty TP. Tension pneumothorax caused by the argon beam coagulator during laparoscopic partial nephrectomy. J Urol 2002;168:2162.
69. Biswas TK, Smith JA. Laparoscopic total fundoplication: Anaesthesia and complications. Anaesth Intensive Care 1993;21:127.
70. Leong LM, Ali A. Carbon dioxide pneumothorax during laparoscopic fundoplication. Anaesthesia 2003;58:97.
71. Khan AU, Pandya K, Clifton MA. Near fatal gas embolism during laparoscopic cholecystectomy. Ann R Coll Surg Engl 1995;77:67.
72. Bongard F, Dubecz S, Klein S. Complications of therapeutic laparoscopy. Curr Probl Surg 1994;31:857.
73. Cottin V, Delafosse B, Viale JP. Gas embolism during laparoscopy: A report of seven cases in patients with previous abdominal surgical history. Surg Endosc 1996;10:166.
74. Croce E, Azzola M, Russo R, et al. Laparoscopic liver tumour resection with the argon beam. Endosc Surg Allied Technol 1994;2:186.
75. Kono M, Yahagi N, Kitahara M, et al. Cardiac arrest associated with use of an argon beam coagulator during laparoscopic cholecystectomy. Br J Anaesth 2001;87:644.
76. Fatal gas embolism caused by overpressurization during laparoscopic use of argon enhanced coagulation. Health Devices 1994;23:257.
77. Root B, Levy MN, Pollack S, et al. Gas embolism death after laparoscopy delayed by "trapping" in portal circulation. Anesth Analg 1978;57:232.
78. Capuzzo M, Buccoliero C, Verri M, et al. Presumptive delayed gas embolism after laparoscopic cholecystectomy. Minerva Anestesiol 2000;66:63.
79. Couture P, Boudreault D, Derouin M, et al. Venous carbon dioxide embolism in pigs: An evaluation of end-tidal carbon dioxide, transesophageal echocardiography, pulmonary artery pressure, and precordial auscultation as monitoring modalities. Anesth Analg 1994;79:867.
80. Derouin M, Couture P, Boudreault D, et al. Detection of gas embolism by transesophageal echocardiography during laparoscopic cholecystectomy. Anesth Analg 1996;82:119.
81. Fahy BG, Hasnain JU, Flowers JL, et al. Transesophageal echocardiographic detection of gas embolism and cardiac valvular dysfunction during laparoscopic nephrectomy. Anesth Analg 1999;88:500.
82. Diakun TA. Carbon dioxide embolism: Successful resuscitation with cardiopulmonary bypass. Anesthesiology 1991;74:1151.
83. Bloomstone J, Chow CM, Isselbacher E, et al. A pilot study examining the frequency and quantity of gas embolization during operative hysteroscopy using a monopolar resectoscope. J Am Assoc Gynecol Laparosc 2002;9:9.
84. Graff TD, Arbgast NR, Phillips OC. Gas embolism: A comparative study of air and carbon dioxide as embolic agents in the systemic venous circulation. Am J Obstet Gynecol 1959;78:259.

85. Kalhan SB, Reaney JA, Collins RL. Pneumomediastinum and sub-cutaneous emphysema during laparoscopy. Cleve Clin J Med 1990;57: 639.

86. Catheline JM, Capelluto E, Gaillard JL, et al. Thromboembolism pro-phylaxis and incidence of thromboembolic complications after laparo-scopic surgery. Int J Surg Invest 2000;2:41.

87. Boike GM, Miller CE, Spirtos NM, et al. Incisional bowel herniations after operative laparoscopy: A series of nineteen cases and review of the literature. Am J Obstet Gynecol 1995;172:1726.

88. Leung TY, Yuen PM. Small bowel herniation through subumbilical port site following laparoscopic surgery at the time of reversal of anesthesia. Gynecol Obstet Invest 2000;49:209.

89. Luck AJ, Moyes D, Maddern GJ, Hewett PJ. Core temperature changes during open and laparoscopic colorectal surgery. Surg Endosc 1999;13: 480.

90. Makinen MT. Comparison of body temperature changes during laparo-scopic and open cholecystectomy. Acta Anaesthesiol Scand 1997;41:736.

91. Nguyen NT, Fleming NW, Singh A, et al. Evaluation of core temperature during laparoscopic and open gastric bypass. Obes Surg 2001;11:570.

92. Camus Y, Delva E, Sessler DI, Lienhart A. Pre-induction skin-surface warming minimizes intraoperative core hypothermia. J Clin Anesth 1995;7:384.

93. Moore SS, Green CR, Wang FL, et al. The role of irrigation in the devel-opment of hypothermia during laparoscopic surgery. Am J Obstet Gynecol 1997;176:598.

94. Nguyen NT, Furdui G, Fleming NW, et al. Effect of heated and humid-ified carbon dioxide gas on core temperature and postoperative pain: A randomized trial. Surg Endosc 2002;16:1050.

95. Nelskyla K, Yli-Hankala A, Sjoberg J, et al. Warming of insufflation gas during laparoscopic hysterectomy: Effect on body temperature and the autonomic nervous system. Acta Anaesthesiol Scand 1999;43:974.

96. Collins SJ, Robinson AL, Holland HF. A comparison between total intra-venous anaesthesia using a propofol/alfentanil mixture and an inhala-tional technique for laparoscopic gynaecological sterilization. Eur J Anaesthesiol 1996;13:33.

97. Tong D, Chung F. Recall after total intravenous anaesthesia due to an equipment misuse. Can J Anaesth 1997;44:73.

98. Sebel PS, Bowdle TA, Ghoneim MM, et al. The incidence of awareness during anesthesia: A multicenter United States study. Anesth Analg 2004;99:833.

99. White PF, Ma H, Tang J, et al. Does the use of electroencephalographic bispectral index or auditory evoked potential index monitoring facili-tate recovery after desflurane anesthesia in the ambulatory setting? Anesthesiology 2004;100:811.

100. Liu SS. Effects of bispectral index monitoring on ambulatory anesthe-sia: A meta-analysis of randomized controlled trials and a cost analysis. Anesthesiology 2004;101:311.

101. Forrest JB, Cahalan MK, Rehder K, et al. Multicenter study of general anesthesia. II. Results. Anesthesiology 1990;72:262.

102. Forrest JB, Rehder K, Cahalan MK, Goldsmith CH. Multicenter study of general anesthesia. III. Predictors of severe perioperative adverse out-comes. Anesthesiology 1992;76:3.

103. Vijayakumar E. Anesthetic considerations in patients with cardiac arrhythmias, pacemakers, and AICDs. Int Anesthesiol Clin 2001;39:21.

104. Ambrose C, Buggy D, Farragher R, et al. Pre-emptive glycopyrrolate 0.2 mg and bradycardia during gynaecological laparoscopy with miva-curium. Eur J Anaesthesiol 1998;15:710.

105. Reed DN Jr, Duff JL. Persistent occurrence of bradycardia during laparo-scopic cholecystectomies in low-risk patients. Dig Surg 2000;17:513.

106. Lehmann LJ, Lewis MC, Goldman H, Marshall JR. Cardiopulmonary complications during laparoscopy: Two case reports. South Med J 1995; 88:1072.

107. Tulandi T, Beique F, Kimia M. Pulmonary edema: A complication of local injection of vasopressin at laparoscopy. Fertil Steril 1996;66:478.

108. Klop WM, Lohuis PJ, Strating RP, Mulder W. Ventricular fibrillation caused by electrocoagulation during laparoscopic surgery. Surg Endosc 2002;16:362.

109. Senthuran S, Toff WD, Vuylsteke A, et al. Implanted cardiac pace-makers and defibrillators in anaesthetic practice. Br J Anaesth 2002;88: 627.

110. Joe RR, Diaz LK. Anesthesia in the cardiac cath lab: Catheter and EPS, therapeutic procedures for pediatrics and adults. ASA Newsletter 2003;67.

111. Bourke ME. The patient with a pacemaker or related device. Can J Anaesth 1996;43:R24.

112. Akhtar S, Silverman DG. Assessment and management of patients with ischemic heart disease. Crit Care Med 2004;32:S126.

113. Roizen MF. Anesthetic implications of concurrent diseases. In: Miller RD, ed. Anesthesia, 5th ed. Philadelphia: Churchill Livingstone, 2000;903.

114. Dawood MM, Gutpa DK, Southern J, et al. Pathology of fatal perioper-ative myocardial infarction: Implications regarding pathophysiology and prevention. Int J Cardiol 1996;57:37.

115. Landesberg G. The pathophysiology of perioperative myocardial infarction: Facts and perspectives. J Cardiothorac Vasc Anesth 2003;17: 90.

116. Auerbach AD, Goldman L. Beta-blockers and reduction of cardiac events in noncardiac surgery: Scientific review. JAMA 2002;287:1435.

117. Eagle KA, Berger PB, Calkins H, et al. ACC/AHA Guideline Update for Perioperative Cardiovascular Evaluation for Noncardiac Surgery—Executive Summary. A report of the American College of Cardiology/American Heart Association Task Force on Practice Guide-lines (Committee to Update the 1996 Guidelines on Perioperative Cardiovascular Evaluation for Noncardiac Surgery). Anesth Analg 2002;94:1052.

118. Fleisher LA. Preoperative cardiac evaluation. Anesthesiol Clin North America 2004;22:59.

119. Stevens RD, Burri H, Tramer MR. Pharmacologic myocardial protection in patients undergoing noncardiac surgery: A quantitative systematic review. Anesth Analg 2003;97:623.

120. Wallace A, Layug B, Tateo I, et al. Prophylactic atenolol reduces post-operative myocardial ischemia. McSPI Research Group. Anesthesiology 1998;88:7.

121. Mangano DT, Layug EL, Wallace A, Tateo I. Effect of atenolol on mor-tality and cardiovascular morbidity after noncardiac surgery. Multi-center Study of Perioperative Ischemia Research Group. N Engl J Med 1996;335:1713.

122. Poldermans D, Boersma E, Bax JJ, et al. The effect of bisoprolol on peri-operative mortality and myocardial infarction in high-risk patients undergoing vascular surgery. Dutch Echocardiographic Cardiac Risk Evaluation Applying Stress Echocardiography Study Group. N Engl J Med 1999;341:1789.

123. Wallace AW, Galindez D, Salahieh A, et al. Effect of clonidine on cardiovascular morbidity and mortality after noncardiac surgery. Anesthesiology 2004;101:284.

124. Burns JM, Hart DM, Hughes RL, et al. Effects of nadolol on arrhyth-mias during laparoscopy performed under general anaesthesia. Br J Anaesth 1988;61:345.

125. VanDenKerkhof EG, Milne B, Parlow JL. Knowledge and practice regarding prophylactic perioperative beta blockade in patients under-going noncardiac surgery: A survey of Canadian anesthesiologists. Anesth Analg 2003;96:1558.

126. Taylor RC, Pagliarello G. Prophylactic beta-blockade to prevent myocar-dial infarction perioperatively in high-risk patients who undergo general surgical procedures. Can J Surg 2003;46:216.

127. Chassot PG, Delabays A, Spahn DR. Preoperative evaluation of patients with, or at risk of, coronary artery disease undergoing non-cardiac surgery. Br J Anaesth 2002;89:747.

128. Marcucci C, Chassot PG, Gardaz JP, et al. Fatal myocardial infarction after lung resection in a patient with prophylactic preoperative coronary stenting. Br J Anaesth 2004;92:743.

129. Landesberg G, Mosseri M, Wolf Y, et al. Perioperative myocardial ischemia and infarction: Identification by continuous 12-lead electro-cardiogram with online ST-segment monitoring. Anesthesiology 2002; 96:264.

130. Norris EJ, Frank SM. Anesthesia for vascular surgery. In: Miller RD, ed. Anesthesia, 5th ed. Philadelphia: Churchill Livingstone, 2000;1849.

131. London MJ, Hollenberg M, Wong MG, et al. Intraoperative myocardial ischemia: Localization by continuous 12-lead electrocardiography. Anesthesiology 1988;69:232.

132. Beaver J, Safran D. Pneumopericardium mimicking acute myocardial ischemia after laparoscopic cholecystectomy. South Med J 1999;92:1002.

133. Glascock JM, Winfield HN, Lund GO, et al. Carbon dioxide homeosta-sis during transperitoneal or extraperitoneal laparoscopic pelvic lymphadenectomy: A real-time intraoperative comparison. J Endourol 1996;10:319.

134. Meininger D, Byhahn C, Wolfram M, et al. Prolonged intraperitoneal versus extraperitoneal insufflation of carbon dioxide in patients under-going totally endoscopic robot-assisted radical prostatectomy. Surg Endosc 2004;18:829.

135. Mullett CE, Viale JP, Sagnard PE, et al. Pulmonary CO_2 elimination during surgical procedures using intra- or extraperitoneal CO_2 insufflation. Anesth Analg 1993;76:622.
136. Wolf JS Jr, Monk TG, McDougall EM, et al. The extraperitoneal approach and subcutaneous emphysema are associated with greater absorption of carbon dioxide during laparoscopic renal surgery. J Urol 1995;154:959.
137. Bongard FS, Pianim NA, Leighton TA, et al. Helium insufflation for laparoscopic operation. Surg Gynecol Obstet 1993;177:140.
138. Mann C, Boccara G, Grevy V, et al. Argon pneumoperitoneum is more dangerous than CO_2 pneumoperitoneum during venous gas embolism. Anesth Analg 1997;85:1367.
139. Roberts MW, Mathiesen KA, Ho HS, Wolfe BM. Cardiopulmonary responses to intravenous infusion of soluble and relatively insoluble gases. Surg Endosc 1997;11:341.
140. Menes T, Spivak H. Laparoscopy: Searching for the proper insufflation gas. Surg Endosc 2000;14:1050.
141. Neuhaus SJ, Gupta A, Watson DI. Helium and other alternative insufflation gases for laparoscopy. Surg Endosc 2001;15:553.
142. DeCook TH, Goudsouzian NG. Tachyphylaxis and phase II block development during infusion of succinylcholine in children. Anesth Analg 1980;59:639.
143. Ramsey FM, Lebowitz PW, Savarese JJ, Ali HH. Clinical characteristics of long-term succinylcholine neuromuscular blockade during balanced anesthesia. Anesth Analg 1980;59:110.
144. Scuderi PE, Conlay LA. Postoperative nausea and vomiting and outcome. Int Anesthesiol Clin 2003;41:165.
145. Apfel CC, Korttila K, Abdalla M, et al. A factorial trial of six interventions for the prevention of postoperative nausea and vomiting. N Engl J Med 2004;350:2441.
146. Macario A, Weinger M, Carney S, Kim A. Which clinical anesthesia outcomes are important to avoid? The perspective of patients. Anesth Analg 1999;89:652.
147. Rashiq S, Bray P. Relative value to surgical patients and anesthesia providers of selected anesthesia related outcomes. BMC Med Inform Decis Mak 2003;3:3.
148. Gan T, Sloan F, Dear Gde L, et al. How much are patients willing to pay to avoid postoperative nausea and vomiting? Anesth Analg 2001;92:393.
149. Tang J, Wang B, White PF, et al. The effect of timing of ondansetron administration on its efficacy, cost-effectiveness, and cost-benefit as a prophylactic antiemetic in the ambulatory setting. Anesth Analg 1998;86:274.
150. Hammas B, Thorn SE, Wattwil M. Superior prolonged antiemetic prophylaxis with a four-drug multimodal regimen—comparison with propofol or placebo. Acta Anaesthesiol Scand 2002;46:232.
151. Apfel CC, Roewer N. Risk assessment of postoperative nausea and vomiting. Int Anesthesiol Clin 2003;41:13.
152. Pierre S, Corno G, Benais H, Apfel CC. A risk score–dependent antiemetic approach effectively reduces postoperative nausea and vomiting—a continuous quality improvement initiative. Can J Anaesth 2004;51:320.
153. Lovstad RZ, Thagaard KS, Berner NS, Raeder JC. Neostigmine 50 microg kg^{-1} with glycopyrrolate increases postoperative nausea in women after laparoscopic gynaecological surgery. Acta Anaesthesiol Scand 2001;45:495.
154. Nelskyla K, Yli-Hankala A, Soikkeli A, Korttila K. Neostigmine with glycopyrrolate does not increase the incidence or severity of postoperative nausea and vomiting in outpatients undergoing gynaecological laparoscopy. Br J Anaesth 1998;81:757.
155. Apfel CC, Kranke P, Katz MH, et al. Volatile anaesthetics may be the main cause of early but not delayed postoperative vomiting: A randomized controlled trial of factorial design. Br J Anaesth 2002;88:659.
156. Divatia JV, Vaidya JS, Badwe RA, Hawaldar RW. Omission of nitrous oxide during anesthesia reduces the incidence of postoperative nausea and vomiting. A meta-analysis. Anesthesiology 1996;85:1055.
157. DeBalli P. The use of propofol as an antiemetic. Int Anesthesiol Clin 2003;41:67.
158. Gan TJ, El-Molem H, Ray J, Glass PS. Patient-controlled antiemesis: A randomized, double-blind comparison of two doses of propofol versus placebo. Anesthesiology 1999;90:1564.
159. Numazaki M, Fujii Y. Reduction of emetic symptoms during cesarean delivery with antiemetics: Propofol at subhypnotic dose versus traditional antiemetics. J Clin Anesth 2003;15:423.
160. Unlugenc H, Guler T, Gunes Y, Isik G. Comparative study of the antiemetic efficacy of ondansetron, propofol and midazolam in the early postoperative period. Eur J Anaesthesiol 2004;21:60.
161. Apfel CC, Laara E, Koivuranta M, et al. A simplified risk score for predicting postoperative nausea and vomiting: Conclusions from cross-validations between two centers. Anesthesiology 1999;91:693.
162. Tang J, White PF, Wender RH, et al. Fast-track office-based anesthesia: A comparison of propofol versus desflurane with antiemetic prophylaxis in spontaneously breathing patients. Anesth Analg 2001;92:95.
163. Rognas LK, Elkj AP. Anaesthesia in day case laparoscopic female sterilization: A comparison of two anaesthetic methods. Acta Anaesthesiol Scand 2004;48:899.
164. Gan TJ, Meyer T, Apfel CC, et al. Consensus guidelines for managing postoperative nausea and vomiting. Anesth Analg 2003;97:62.
165. Fortney JT, Gan TJ, Graczyk S, et al. A comparison of the efficacy, safety, and patient satisfaction of ondansetron versus droperidol as antiemetics for elective outpatient surgical procedures. S3A-409 and S3A-410 Study Groups. Anesth Analg 1998;86:731.
166. Hill RP, Lubarsky DA, Phillips-Bute B, et al. Cost-effectiveness of prophylactic antiemetic therapy with ondansetron, droperidol, or placebo. Anesthesiology 2000;92:958.
167. Tang J, Chen L, White PF, et al. Recovery profile, costs, and patient satisfaction with propofol and sevoflurane for fast-track office-based anesthesia. Anesthesiology 1999;91:253.
168. Tang J, Watcha MF, White PF. A comparison of costs and efficacy of ondansetron and droperidol as prophylactic antiemetic therapy for elective outpatient gynecologic procedures. Anesth Analg 1996;83:304.
169. Kazemi-Kjellberg F, Henzi I, Tramer MR. Treatment of established postoperative nausea and vomiting: A quantitative systematic review. BMC Anesthesiol 2001;1:2.
170. Wang JJ, Ho ST, Tzeng JI, Tang CS. The effect of timing of dexamethasone administration on its efficacy as a prophylactic antiemetic for postoperative nausea and vomiting. Anesth Analg 2000;91:136.
171. Soppitt AJ, Glass PS, Howell S, et al. The use of propofol for its antiemetic effect: A survey of clinical practice in the United States. J Clin Anesth 2000;12:265.
172. Eberhart LH, Mauch M, Morin AM, et al. Impact of a multimodal antiemetic prophylaxis on patient satisfaction in high-risk patients for postoperative nausea and vomiting. Anaesthesia 2002;57:1022.
173. Soper NJ, Dunnegan D. Anatomic fundoplication failure after laparoscopic antireflux surgery. Ann Surg 1999;229:669.
174. Carr DB, Goudas LC. Acute pain. Lancet 1999;353:2051.
175. Ballantyne JC, Carr DB, deFerranti S, et al. The comparative effects of postoperative analgesic therapies on pulmonary outcome: Cumulative meta-analyses of randomized, controlled trials. Anesth Analg 1998;86:598.
176. Huang N, Cunningham F, Laurito CE, Chen C. Can we do better with postoperative pain management? Am J Surg 2001;182:440.
177. Sinatra RS, Shen QJ, Halaszynski T, et al. Preoperative rofecoxib oral suspension as an analgesic adjunct after lower abdominal surgery: The effects on effort-dependent pain and pulmonary function. Anesth Analg 2004;98:135.
178. Reuben SS, Fingeroth R, Krushell R, Maciolek H. Evaluation of the safety and efficacy of the perioperative administration of rofecoxib for total knee arthroplasty. J Arthroplasty 2002;17:26.
179. Kwok RF, Lim J, Chan MT, et al. Preoperative ketamine improves postoperative analgesia after gynecologic laparoscopic surgery. Anesth Analg 2004;98:1044.
180. Woolf CJ, Thompson SW. The induction and maintenance of central sensitization is dependent on N-methyl-D-aspartic acid receptor activation; implications for the treatment of post-injury pain hypersensitivity states. Pain 1991;44:293.
181. McCartney CJ, Sinha A, Katz J. A qualitative systematic review of the role of N-methyl-D-aspartate receptor antagonists in preventive analgesia. Anesth Analg 2004;98:1385.
182. Loughney AD, Sarma V, Ryall EA. Intraperitoneal bupivacaine for the relief of pain following day case laparoscopy. Br J Obstet Gynaecol 1994;101:449.
183. Shaw IC, Stevens J, Krishnamurthy S. The influence of intraperitoneal bupivacaine on pain following major laparoscopic gynaecological procedures. Anaesthesia 2001;56:1041.
184. Wheatley SA, Millar JM, Jadad AR. Reduction of pain after laparoscopic sterilisation with local bupivacaine: A randomised, parallel, double-blind trial. Br J Obstet Gynaecol 1994;101:443.

185. Good M, Anderson GC, Stanton-Hicks M, et al. Relaxation and music reduce pain after gynecologic surgery. Pain Manag Nurs 2002;3:61.

186. Good M, Stanton-Hicks M, Grass JA, et al. Relaxation and music to reduce postsurgical pain. J Adv Nurs 2001;33:208.

187. Good M, Stanton-Hicks M, Grass JA, et al. Relief of postoperative pain with jaw relaxation, music and their combination. Pain 1999;81:163.

188. Nilsson U, Rawal N, Enqvist B, Unosson M. Analgesia following music and therapeutic suggestions in the PACU in ambulatory surgery: A randomized controlled trial. Acta Anaesthesiol Scand 2003;47:278.

189. Nilsson U, Rawal N, Unestahl LE, et al. Improved recovery after music and therapeutic suggestions during general anaesthesia: A double-blind randomised controlled trial. Acta Anaesthesiol Scand 2001;45:812.

190. Nilsson U, Rawal N, Unosson M. A comparison of intra-operative or postoperative exposure to music—a controlled trial of the effects on postoperative pain. Anaesthesia 2003;58:699.

191. Cooper JB, Newbower RS, Kitz RJ. An analysis of major errors and equipment failures in anesthesia management: Considerations for prevention and detection. Anesthesiology 1984;60:34.

192. Carroll BJ, Chandra M, Phillips EH, Margulies DR. Laparoscopic cholecystectomy in critically ill cardiac patients. Am Surg 1993;59:783.

193. Bierstein K. Creative scheduling for anesthesiologists: Physician retention in a tight market. ASA Newsletter 2003;67.

194. Cunningham AJ. Laparoscopic surgery—anesthetic implications. Surg Endosc 1994;8:1272.

195. Vincente K. The human factor: Revolutionizing the way people live with technology. New York: Routledge, 2004.

196. Kenyon TA, Urbach DR, Speer JB, et al. Dedicated minimally invasive surgery suites increase operating room efficiency. Surg Endosc 2001;15:1140.

197. Capelouto CC, Kavoussi LR. Complications of laparoscopic surgery. Urology 1993;42:2.

198. Gill IS, Kavoussi LR, Clayman RV, et al. Complications of laparoscopic nephrectomy in 185 patients: A multi-institutional review. J Urol 1995;154:479.

199. Guillonneau B, Vallancien G. Laparoscopic radical prostatectomy: The Montsouris technique. J Urol 2000;163:1643.

200. See WA, Cooper CS, Fisher RJ. Predictors of laparoscopic complications after formal training in laparoscopic surgery. JAMA 1993;270:2689.

201. Thomas R, Steele R, Ahuja S. Complications of urological laparoscopy: A standardized 1 institution experience. J Urol 1996;156:469.

202. Pearson AM, Gallagher AG, Rosser JC, Satava RM. Evaluation of structured and quantitative training methods for teaching intracorporeal knot tying. Surg Endosc 2002;16:130.

203. Seymour NE, Gallagher AG, Roman SA, et al. Virtual reality training improves operating room performance: Results of a randomized, double-blinded study. Ann Surg 2002;236:458.

204. Gaba D. Human work environment and simulators. In: Miller RD, ed. Anesthesia, 5th ed. Philadelphia: Churchill Livingstone, 2000;2613.

205. Byrne AJ, Jones JG. Responses to simulated anaesthetic emergencies by anaesthetists with different durations of clinical experience. Br J Anaesth 1997;78:553.

206. Jacobsen J, Lindekaer AL, Ostergaard HT, et al. Management of anaphylactic shock evaluated using a full-scale anaesthesia simulator. Acta Anaesthesiol Scand 2001;45:315.

207. Lindekaer AL, Jacobsen J, Andersen G, et al. Treatment of ventricular fibrillation during anaesthesia in an anaesthesia simulator. Acta Anaesthesiol Scand 1997;41:1280.

208. Hammond J, Bermann M, Chen B, Kushins L. Incorporation of a computerized human patient simulator in critical care training: A preliminary report. J Trauma 2002;53:1064.

209. Sica GT, Barron DM, Blum R, et al. Computerized realistic simulation: A teaching module for crisis management in radiology. AJR Am J Roentgenol 1999;172:301.

210. Byrne AJ, Sellen AJ, Jones JG, et al. Effect of videotape feedback on anaesthetists' performance while managing simulated anaesthetic crises: A multicentre study. Anaesthesia 2002;57:176.

211. Chopra V, Gesink BJ, de Jong J, et al. Does training on an anaesthesia simulator lead to improvement in performance? Br J Anaesth 1994;73:293.

212. Byrne AJ, Greaves JD. Assessment instruments used during anaesthetic simulation: Review of published studies. Br J Anaesth 2001;86:445.

213. Marshall RL, Smith JS, Gorman PJ, et al. Use of a human patient simulator in the development of resident trauma management skills. J Trauma 2001;51:17.

214. Reznek M, Smith-Coggins R, Howard S, et al. Emergency medicine crisis resource management (EMCRM): Pilot study of a simulation-based crisis management course for emergency medicine. Acad Emerg Med 2003;10:386.

215. Merry MD, Brown JP. From a culture of safety to a culture of excellence: Quality science, human factors and the future of healthcare quality. In: Smith LR, ed. The Business of Healthcare: A Journal of Innovative Management Collection. Salem, NH: GOAL/QPC, 2002;122.

216. Sandberg WS, Ganous TJ, Steiner C. Setting a research agenda for perioperative systems design. Semin Laparosc Surg 2003;10:57.

217. Barach P, Small SD. Reporting and preventing medical mishaps: Lessons from non-medical near miss reporting systems. BMJ 2000;320:759.

218. Krizek TJ. Surgical error: Ethical issues of adverse events. Arch Surg 2000;135:1359.

Preventing Complications before the Operation

3

Stephen M. Cohen and Andrea J. Singer

Learn from the mistakes of others . . .
You can't possibly live long enough to make them all yourself!
GEORGE W. MORLEY, MD
University of Michigan

The possibility of a potential adverse outcome is always present whenever an operation is performed. Some complications are unavoidable, but the experienced surgeon can reduce the likelihood of their occurrence. The surgeon should possess a thorough knowledge of the anatomy and a complete understanding of the disease process. Oftentimes, many different surgical approaches can be used to treat the same condition. A comprehensive awareness of these various operations will allow the surgeon to choose the procedure that will be the safest. Thorough assessment of the presenting condition, followed by design of a unique treatment plan, is essential, because no two cases are ever exactly alike. Most important, the surgeon will need to anticipate potential complications and develop a strategy that will minimize the likelihood of their occurrence. This chapter presents methods to avoid complications even before the incision is placed, thereby eliminating the possibility of such complications from the outset.

ANTIBIOTICS

Preoperative antibiotics are used in gynecology for the prevention of postoperative intra-abdominal infections and for prophylaxis of subacute bacterial endocarditis (SBE). During the last decade, studies supporting the use of antibiotics in surgery have allowed the development of recommendations that are based on sound scientific evidence, rather than on theory. Very specific guidelines for the use of antibiotics in both surgical site infection (wound infection) prevention and SBE prophylaxis are now available.

Prophylaxis of Subacute Bacterial Endocarditis

In the 1970s, all patients who were discovered to have mitral valve prolapse were prescribed antibiotics for SBE prophylaxis. During the next decade, Doppler ultrasound techniques allowed more accurate study of valve prolapse. The recommendation for the use of antibiotics in surgery was changed, so that antibiotic coverage was no longer recommended in those patients who had mitral valve prolapse without regurgitation.

In the latest advisory from the American Heart Association (AHA), the recommendations for prophylaxis have changed again, leaving even fewer surgical patients in need of SBE antibiotic coverage.[1] Patients have now been divided into three groups based on their risk of developing SBE (Table 3–1).

Low-risk patients have no greater risk than in the normal population for the development of SBE. These are the patients most commonly encountered in clinical practice and include those without a regurgitant mitral valve, those with repaired atrial septal defects or ventricular septal defects, or with implanted pacemakers or defibrillators, and those who have undergone coronary artery bypass grafting. These patients need no antibiotics.

Moderate-risk patients are those patients who have mitral valve prolapse with a regurgitant flow and those with acquired structural abnormalities of valves or congenital cardiac malformations. SBE antibiotic prophylaxis is not required for gynecologic operations in these patients. Cystoscopy and urethral dilation, however, do carry some risk of bacteremia. Thus, patients who will have either of these two procedures performed in addition to their primary minimal-access gynecologic procedure should receive antibiotic prophylaxis.

All *high-risk patients*—those with prosthetic valves of any type or those with a history of SBE—probably should receive prophylaxis, even though the risk of bacteremia is very low after gynecologic procedures.

These recommendations pertain only to patients who are known not to be infected. All moderate- and high-risk patients should receive prophylactic antibiotics if the operation will involve any infected tissue.

Moderate-risk patients who will undergo cystoscopy or urethral dilation should receive 2 g of amoxicillin orally 1 hour before the procedure or ampicillin 2 g administered intramuscularly or intravenously 30 minutes before the procedure. These moderate-risk patients do not need gentamicin. Amoxicillin- or ampicillin-allergic patients should receive

Table 3–1 ▪ Recommendations for Prophylaxis of Subacute Bacterial Endocarditis			
	Need for Prophylaxis with Endocarditis Risk		
Procedure	**High Risk**	**Moderate Risk**	**Low Risk**
Minimal-access procedures	Recommended	None	None
Cystoscopy; urethral dilation	Recommended	Recommended	None
Infected procedures	Recommended	Recommended	None

Adapted from Dajani AS, Taubert KA, Wilson W, et al. Prevention of bacterial endocarditis: Recommendations by the American Heart Association. JAMA 2003;227:1794.

Table 3–2 ▪ Antibiotics for Prophylaxis of Subacute Bacterial Endocarditis				
	Patient Characteristics			
Antibiotic(s)	**High Risk**	**High Risk, Ampicillin Allergic**	**Moderate Risk**	**Moderate Risk, Ampicillin Allergic**
Ampicillin or amoxicillin			X	
Vancomycin				X
Ampicillin or amoxicillin *plus* gentamicin	X			
Vancomycin *plus* gentamicin		X		

Adapted from Dajani AS, Taubert KA, Wilson W, et al. Prevention of bacterial endocarditis: Recommendations by the American Heart Association. JAMA 2003;227:1794.

vancomycin 1 g intravenously infused over 1 hour, completed within 30 minutes of the start of the procedure.

High-risk patients should receive ampicillin 2 g intramuscularly or intravenously plus gentamicin 1.5 mg/kg intramuscularly or intravenously (up to 120 mg) within 30 minutes of the procedure start, followed by ampicillin 1 g intramuscularly or intravenously or amoxicillin 1 g orally 6 hours later. In ampicillin- or amoxicillin-allergic patients, one preoperative dose of vancomycin 1 g intravenously infused over 1 hour should be substituted for the ampicillin or amoxicillin. No subsequent postoperative dose of vancomycin is necessary (Table 3–2).

Surgical Site Prophylaxis

Preoperative antibiotic use has become the standard of care for patients undergoing certain specific procedures for which the literature has shown a statistically significant reduction in postoperative surgical site infections with such prophylaxis. Unfortunately, the use of antibiotics for preoperative prophylaxis has been extended arbitrarily by many gynecologists to include almost all operations that are performed in the pelvis. Data supporting the use of antibiotics in this random fashion are lacking, and antibiotics should not be used in this setting. Even when antibiotics are used in the appropriate cases, they often are inappropriately administered, thereby diminishing their effectiveness.

General guidelines for the administration of prophylactic antibiotics are as follows:

- Antibiotics need to be given within 1 hour of the surgical procedure. (Vancomycin can be given between 1 and 2 hours before incision time.)

- An antibiotic that has been shown to be effective must be used.
- If an operation takes more than 3 to 4 hours, then a second dose of antibiotics should be given. Thus, most patients should receive only one dose.
- The preoperative infusion does not have to be completed before the incision is made.

The only gynecologic procedure for which surgical site prophylaxis has been shown to be beneficial is hysterectomy. The evidence-based data are supportive for both vaginal and abdominal hysterectomy. The data for laparoscopic hysterectomy are scant; nevertheless, we recommend that prophylactic antibiotics be used in this procedure because of its similarity to both vaginal and abdominal hysterectomy.

The antibiotics of choice for gynecologic prophylaxis are the second-generation cephalosporins, including cefazolin, cefotetan, and cefoxitin.[2] A dose of 2 g of one of these drugs should be administered intravenously within 1 hour of surgery. If the operation takes longer than 3 to 4 hours, the patient should receive a second dose. In the penicillin-allergic patient, metronidazole, doxycycline, clindamycin, or one of the quinolones can be substituted.[3]

VENOUS THROMBOEMBOLISM

Venous thromboembolism (VTE), which includes both deep venous thrombosis and pulmonary embolism, is a potential complication of surgery. The mean incidence of deep venous thrombosis (DVT) after gynecologic surgery is approximately 16% (range, 4% to 38%).[4] Fatal pulmonary embolism has been reported in 0.4% of such procedures.[4] The use of thromboprophylaxis has reduced the risk of fatal pulmonary embolism by 75%, from 0.4% to 0.1%.[4] Recognition of surgical patients at heightened risk for VTE presents an opportunity for intervention with effective prophylactic modalities. Unfortunately, actual use of recommended prophylactic measures is variable, with only a minority of patients at increased risk receiving prophylaxis.

Clinical conditions that promote thrombosis by causing venous stasis, venous intimal damage, or increased coagulation, thereby placing patients at risk for VTE, have been described (Table 3–3). Age alone is a risk factor. The potential for postoperative DVT increases linearly from age 40 years. In many surgical patients, multiple risk factors may be present, leading to an even greater cumulative risk for VTE. Patient risk factors have been stratified into low-, moderate-, and high-risk categories on the basis of the reported incidences of DVT and pulmonary embolism (Table 3–4). Recommendations for prophylactic regimens are based on risk category.

Early mobilization of patients has been associated with a decreased relative risk of developing VTE postoperatively, because this strategy helps to reduce the likelihood of venous stasis. One of the significant advantages of minimal-access surgery is the fact that all patients are able to ambulate earlier following surgery. Therefore, immobilization is essentially eliminated as a contributing factor for VTE.

In addition to early ambulation, modalities for the prevention of VTE consist of either mechanical strategies (application of elastic stockings or intermittent pneumatic compression devices) or anticoagulation (with heparin). Mechanical strategies are widely used and very safe. As previously mentioned, early ambulation should be part of routine care for all postsurgical patients. If properly fitted, elastic stockings have essentially no adverse effects and may be appropriate for almost all patients until full ambulation is achieved. Intermittent pneumatic compression devices (IPCs) may be used as the primary method of VTE prophylaxis in selected patients. IPCs appear to have an additive effect when used in combination with anticoagulants.

The decision to institute thromboprophylaxis with anticoagulants must always balance the benefits of VTE prevention against the risk of intraoperative and postoperative bleeding. Furthermore, the characteristics of the individual anticoagu-

lant must be considered in choosing which agent to use. Low-dose unfractionated heparin (LDUH) is a very effective prophylactic agent that clearly reduces the incidence of fatal postoperative pulmonary embolism. In addition, the strongest evidence that thromboprophylaxis is of benefit in gynecologic surgery has been provided for LDUH.[6] Risks associated with use of LDUH include excess bleeding and heparin-induced thrombocytopenia. In comparison, low-molecular-weight heparin (LMWH) preparations have greater activity against activated factor X (Xa), as well as greater bioavailability, longer half-life, more predictable anticoagulant response, and no greater risk of bleeding than with LDUH. These characteristics allow subcutaneous administration once or twice daily without the need for laboratory monitoring. In addition, LMWH is less likely to cause heparin-induced thrombocytopenia and thrombosis than are standard heparin preparations. Aspirin and other antiplatelet agents are ineffective in preventing VTE and are therefore not recommended for surgical prophylaxis.

Table 3–3 ▪ Risk Factors for Venous Thromboembolic Disease

Age older than 40 years
Major surgery, especially abdominal, pelvic, lower extremity
Duration of immobilization (longer than 4 days of bed rest)
Paralysis
Previous venous thromboembolism
Varicosities, venous stasis changes, lower extremity edema
Malignancy
Obesity
Pregnancy/postpartum period
Estrogen therapy
Underlying medical conditions, including inflammatory bowel disease, nephrotic syndrome, systemic lupus erythematosus, acute myocardial infarction, acute stroke
Hypercoagulable states
Activated protein C resistance (factor V Leiden)
Protein C deficiency
Protein S deficiency
Antithrombin III deficiency
Antiphospholipid antibodies (lupus anticoagulant, anticardiolipin antibody)
Hyperhomocystinemia

Table 3–4 ▪ Risk Categories for Venous Thromboembolism

Category	Description	Postoperative Management
Low risk	Minor surgery in patients younger than 40 years of age; no additional risk factors	Early ambulation
Moderate risk	Minor surgery in patients 40 to 60 years of age; no additional risk factors Major surgery in patients younger than 40 years of age; no additional risk factors Minor surgery in patients with additional risk factors	Early ambulation *and* IPC
High risk	Minor surgery in patients older than 60 years of age; no additional risk factors Major surgery in patients older than 40 years of age or with additional risk factors Medical patients with additional risk factors	Early ambulation *and* IPC LDUH *or* LMWH optional
Highest risk	Major surgery in patients older than 40 years of age with multiple risk factors or previous VTE, hypercoagulability, or malignancy	Early ambulation *and* IPC *and* LDUH *or* LMWH pre- and postoperatively

LDUH, low-dose unfractionated heparin; LMWH, low-molecular-weight heparin; IPC, intermittent pneumatic compression device; VTE, venous thromboembolism.
Modified from Geerts WH, Heit JA, Clagett GP, et al. Prevention of venous thromboembolism. Chest 2001;119:132S; and Kaboli P, Henderson MC, White RH. DVT prophylaxis and anticoagulation in the surgical patient. Med Clin North Am 2003;87:77.

Optimal timing for the commencement of VTE prophylaxis is based on when the risk of developing thrombosis begins. For elective surgery, this usually is as soon as the patient is taken to the operating room. Application of elastic stockings and IPC devices should be accomplished preoperatively. LDUH usually is initiated 1 to 2 hours before surgery. Experience with general surgery patients suggests that no adverse consequences are associated with giving the first dose of LMWH (less than 3400 IU) up to 2 hours before operation, with the possible additional benefit of preventing DVT from developing during surgery and in the immediate postoperative period. When higher doses of LMWH are used in high-risk general surgery patients, treatment should be commenced 10 to 12 hours before the operation to avoid excessive intraoperative bleeding.

The ideal duration of thromboprophylaxis is unknown. The only procedure for which strong evidence in favor of extended prophylaxis is available is total hip arthroplasty.[5] Because of safety and cost concerns, it would be appropriate to risk-stratify patients and recommend extended prophylaxis for only the highest-risk patients. The most important risk factors are confinement to bed or wheelchair, history of a previous VTE, presence of a hypercoagulable state, and malignancy.

In conclusion, the incidence of VTE and pulmonary embolism in gynecologic minimal-access surgery appears to be very low, but the data have been extrapolated from case reports and surveys. The incidence of VTE in gynecologic laparoscopy from these studies was 0.0001%[6]; in laparoscopic cholecystectomy, however, the incidence of VTE is reported to be 0.03%.[7] This latter incidence probably more closely resembles that in patients undergoing laparoscopic hysterectomy. It is difficult to give specific recommendations regarding prophylaxis in these patients. The lowest-risk patients (those younger than 40 with no risk factors) need no prophylaxis. Without doubt, the highest-risk patients should receive anticoagulation that should be continued beyond discharge. Moderate- to high-risk patients need IPC and probably will benefit from anticoagulation, but the potential for increased bleeding must be considered in these patients. Thus, the surgeon should individualize the plan for each operation. As laparoscopic procedures become more common in older populations, as well as in the setting of malignancy, VTE prophylaxis may become even more important.

Perioperative Management of Patients on Long-Term Oral Anticoagulation

The most common indications for long-term oral anticoagulation therapy (OAT) include primary and secondary prevention of VTE and prevention of systemic embolization in patients with atrial fibrillation or prosthetic heart valves. When such patients need to undergo surgery, the risks of stopping anticoagulation with the accompanying chance for venous or arterial thromboembolism must be weighed against the risk of continuing anticoagulation and the chance of perioperative hemorrhage. Options for perioperative anticoagulation include the following: (1) continue OAT and perform surgery with the patient anticoagulated; (2) discontinue OAT preoperatively and reinstitute OAT postoperatively as soon as possible, and give prophylactic subcutaneous LDUH or LMWH if clinically indicated; or (3) discontinue OAT preoperatively and administer "bridging therapy" with full-dose intravenous heparin or subcutaneous LMWH while the INR is in the subtherapeutic range. Consensus is lacking on how best to manage anticoagulation in the surgical patient. The following recommendations should be used in conjunction with the physician's clinical judgment in order to individualize therapy for each patient.

Because of the *high risk for bleeding with OAT*, anticoagulants should be withheld before laparoscopic surgery. Surgery generally is safe from major hemorrhagic complications when the INR is less than 1.5. OAT should be discontinued 4 to 5 days preoperatively, to allow the INR to reach 1.5 or less by the time of the surgical procedure.

For patients with a *history of VTE*, elective surgery should be avoided during the first month after the thromboembolic episode because of the high risk of recurrent VTE without anticoagulation.[5,8] If the patient must have surgery, bridging therapy with full-dose intravenous heparin or LMWH should be initiated when the INR falls below 2.0.[5,8] Intravenous heparin should be stopped 6 hours before surgery. If LMWH is being used, the last dose should be given 24 hours before surgery. If no contraindication exists from a surgical standpoint, intravenous heparin should be restarted 12 hours postoperatively with no bolus. Intravenous heparin is preferred over LMWH during the first 24 hours postoperatively because it is more easily reversed should bleeding occur. If the likelihood of postoperative bleeding is low or the patient is to be discharged on the same day, LMWH can be started between 12 and 24 hours postoperatively. OAT usually should resume on the first postoperative day. Bridging therapy is continued until the INR is in the therapeutic range (greater than 2.0) for 2 consecutive days.

For patients with *previous VTE* who are 2 to 3 months from their thromboembolic episode, no need exists for preoperative intravenous heparin or LMWH after the OAT has been stopped preoperatively.[9] Postoperatively, intravenous heparin or LMWH should be used in full doses until the INR is in the therapeutic range, because the risk of postoperative VTE is high.[8]

For patients with *recurrent VTE* with the last episode of thrombosis occurring more than 3 months before surgery, no preoperative or postoperative intravenous heparin is needed.[5,8] These patients should receive postoperative subcutaneous LDUH or LMWH, as described in Table 3–5.

For patients with *mitral or multiple valve prostheses, prosthetic heart valves in combination with atrial fibrillation, or atrial fibrillation with a history of transient ischemic attacks or stroke*, bridging therapy should be used as detailed previously. For patients with aortic valve prosthesis alone or atrial fibrillation alone, bridging therapy is not required. Prophylactic subcutaneous LDUH or LMWH should be given perioperatively, as described in Table 3–5.

PERIOPERATIVE CARDIOVASCULAR EVALUATION

Preoperative evaluation of the surgical patient generally focuses on the cardiovascular system, because cardiac events are the primary cause of death after surgical procedures.

Table 3–5 ▪ Recommended Heparin Prophylactic Regimens*

Low-dose unfractionated heparin (LDUH)
  5000 U every 8 to 12 hours
Low-molecular-weight heparin (LMWH)
  Dalteparin
  General: 2500 IU 2 hours before surgery, then 2500 IU daily
    for 5-10 days postoperatively
  High risk: 5000 IU the evening before surgery, then 5000 IU
    daily for 5-10 days postoperatively
  Malignancy: 2500 IU 2 hours before surgery, then 2500 IU 12
    hours later, then 5000 IU daily for 5-10 days postoperatively
  Enoxaparin
  40 mg 2 hours before surgery, then daily for 5-10 days
    postoperatively

*All regimens to be administered subcutaneously.

Table 3–6 ▪ Clinical Predictors of Increased Perioperative Cardiovascular Risk

Major Risk

Unstable coronary syndromes
  Unstable or severe angina
  Recent myocardial infarction (within 7-30 days)
Significant arrhythmias
  High-grade atrioventricular block
  Symptomatic ventricular arrhythmias with heart disease
  Supraventricular tachycardia with uncontrolled ventricular rate
Decompensated CHF
Severe valvular disease

Intermediate Risk

Class I or II angina
Previous myocardial infarction
Compensated or previous CHF
Diabetes mellitus
Renal insufficiency (serum creatinine greater than 2.0 mg/dL)

Minor Risk

Advanced age
Abnormalities on ECG (left bundle branch block, ST-T
  abnormalities, left ventricular hypertrophy)
Heart rhythm other than sinus
Uncontrolled hypertension
History of stroke

CHF, congestive heart failure; ECG, electrocardiogram.
Adapted from ACC/AHA Guidelines.
Modified from Eagle KA, Berger PB, Calkins H, et al. ACC/AHA guideline update for perioperative cardiovascular evaluation for noncardiac surgery: A report of the American College of Cardiology/American Heart Association Task Force on Practice Guidelines (Committee to Update the 1996 Guidelines on Perioperative Cardiovascular Evaluation for Noncardiac Surgery). J Am Coll Cardiol 2002;39:542.

Furthermore, if the potential for such complications is recognized, many problems are preventable. To minimize such complications, thorough assessment for occult cardiac disease and optimization of existing coronary disease are of the utmost importance. Myocardial ischemia remains the major cardiac risk in gynecologic surgery, with a reported incidence of perioperative infarction of approximately 0.15% to 2%.[9]

Over the past 25 years, numerous studies have examined potential risk factors, and various risk indices, guidelines, and algorithms have been proposed for cardiac risk stratification. The abundance of and inconsistency in parameters available for preoperative evaluation led the American College of Cardiology (ACC) and the AHA to develop consensus guidelines to facilitate preoperative cardiovascular risk assessment. The ACC/AHA guidelines employ a strategy using the urgency of the surgery, history of previous coronary evaluation or revascularization, clinical predictors, level of functional capacity, and surgery-specific risks in a stepwise manner to help determine whether to proceed directly to surgery or to order further testing, consultation, or therapy. In emergent cases, lack of time precludes formal risk assessment, and the urgency of the surgery will take precedence.

Stepwise Approach to Cardiac Assessment in Elective Surgery

A stepwise approach to perioperative cardiac assessment in elective surgery is helpful to identify risk factors and the need for further testing or treatment (Fig. 3–1).

First, a careful history will reveal whether the patient has undergone coronary revascularization within the past 5 years. If the patient has had coronary artery bypass grafting within the previous 5 years or angioplasty within the previous 6 months to 5 years, and if clinical status has remained stable without the recurrence of signs or symptoms of ischemia, the risk of perioperative cardiac complications is low. Further cardiac testing generally is not necessary, and the patient can proceed to surgery.

Second, the assessment should determine whether the patient has had a coronary evaluation in the past 2 years. Favorable findings on either invasive or noninvasive evaluation in this time frame are associated with low surgical risk if

no new signs or symptoms of ischemia have developed. The patient can proceed to surgery.

In the patient who has had no previous cardiac assessment, the clinician needs to examine three variables that will help determine risk for a perioperative cardiac complication: (1) clinical predictors, such as congestive heart failure or diabetes, that are individually specific and categorize patients into major-, intermediate-, and minor-risk groups (Table 3–6); (2) level of functional capacity, which corresponds to activities of daily living (Table 3–7); and (3) the specific type of operation (Table 3–8).

All patients with major clinical predictors of cardiac risk, such as unstable coronary disease, significant arrhythmias, decompensated congestive heart failure, or severe valvular disease, as well as patients with poor functional capacity, need to be referred for further evaluation and treatment.

For patients with predictors of intermediate clinical risk, further decision making depends on the patient's functional capacity and level of surgery-specific risk. Patients with moderate to excellent functional capacity usually can undergo intermediate-risk procedures with little likelihood of cardiac death or myocardial infarction. Such procedures include all laparoscopic procedures of less than 4 hours' duration. Patients with only moderate functional capacity undergoing higher-risk operations should be referred for further noninvasive testing.

Finally, if the patient has minor or no clinical predictors of cardiac risk and moderate to excellent functional capacity,

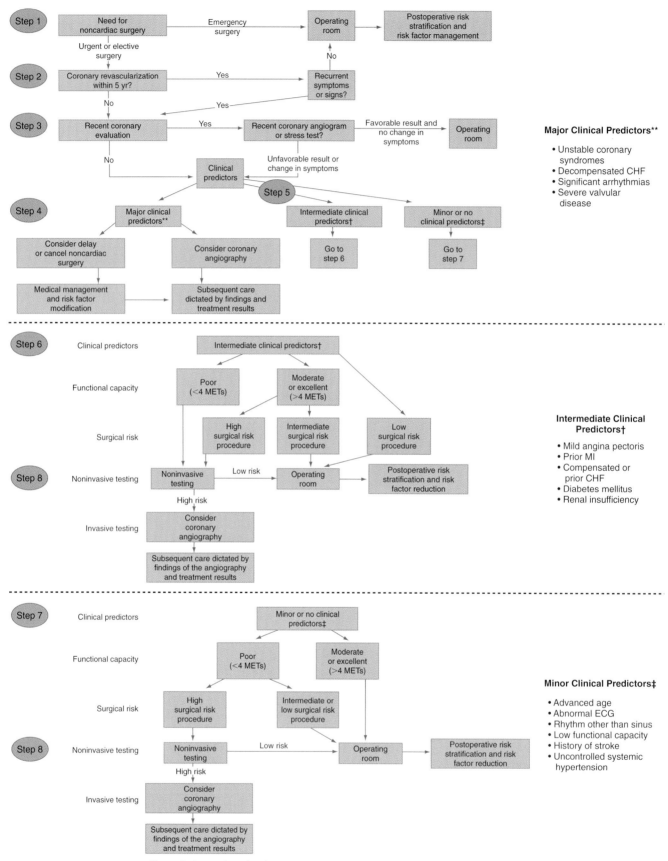

Figure 3–1   ▪   Algorithm for stepwise approach to perioperative cardiac risk assessment.

surgery generally is safe regardless of type of procedure, and no further cardiac evaluation is required.

Perioperative Medical Therapy

The perioperative use of beta blockers has been shown to decrease cardiovascular events and mortality in high-risk patients undergoing surgery.[10] Criteria for beta blocker use include high-risk surgical procedures, ischemic heart disease, cerebrovascular disease (history of transient ischemic attack or cerebrovascular accident), diabetes mellitus requiring insulin, chronic renal insufficiency with a serum creatinine level greater than 2.0 mg/dL, and presence of two or more of the following: age older than 65 years, hypertension, current smoking, total cholesterol greater than 240 mg/dL, or diabetes not requiring insulin.[11] When possible, beta blockers should be started 1 to 2 weeks before surgery, with the dose titrated to lower the heart rate to less than 65 beats per minute. If beta blockers are not going to be continued indefinitely for a chronic indication, they should be continued for a minimum of 1 month postoperatively and then the dose gradually reduced (Table 3–9). Potential contraindications to beta blocker therapy include chronic obstructive pulmonary disease and asthma, bradycardia with heart rate less than 55, second- or third-degree heart block, hypotension with systolic blood pressure less than 100 mm Hg, and acute congestive heart failure or pulmonary edema.

Table 3–7 ■ Estimated Energy Requirements for Various Activities

MET(s) Expended	Self-Reported Activity
1	Self-care activities: Eat, dress, or use the toilet Walk indoors around the house Walk a block or two on level ground at 2 to 3 mph (3.2 to 4.8 km/h)
4	Do light work around the house such as dusting or washing dishes Climb a flight of stairs or walk up a hill Walk on level ground at 4 mph (6.4 km/h) Run a short distance Do heavy work around the house, such as scrubbing floors or lifting or moving heavy furniture Participate in moderate recreational activities such as golf, bowling, dancing, doubles tennis, or throwing a baseball or football noncompetitively
Greater than 10	Participate in strenuous sports such as swimming, singles tennis, football, basketball, or skiing

MET, metabolic energy equivalent.
Adapted from the Duke Activity Status Index and AHA Exercise Standards.
Modified from Eagle KA, Berger PB, Calkins H, et al. ACC/AHA guideline update for perioperative cardiovascular evaluation for noncardiac surgery: A report of the American College of Cardiology/American Heart Association Task Force on Practice Guidelines (Committee to Update the 1996 Guidelines on Perioperative Cardiovascular Evaluation for Noncardiac Surgery). J Am Coll Cardiol 2002;39:542.

Table 3–8 ■ Assessing Surgery-Specific Risk

Risk Category	Cardiac Risk	Procedure
High	>5%	Emergency surgery* Aortic or other major vascular surgery Peripheral vascular surgery Prolonged procedures (longer than 4 hours) Large fluid shifts and/or blood loss
Intermediate	1-5%	Carotid endarterectomy Head and neck surgery Intrathoracic procedures Intraperitoneal procedures, including laparoscopy* Orthopedic surgery Prostate surgery
Low	<1%	Endoscopy Breast surgery Cataract surgery Plastic surgery Extremity procedures Dilation and curettage (D&C)

*Procedures with well-defined risk.
Adapted from ACC/AHA Guidelines.
From Eagle KA, Berger PB, Calkins H, et al: ACC/AHA guideline update for perioperative cardiovascular evaluation for noncardiac surgery: A report of the American College of Cardiology/American Heart Association Task Force on Practice Guidelines (Committee to Update the 1996 Guidelines on Perioperative Cardiovascular Evaluation for Noncardiac Surgery). J Am Coll Cardiol 2002;39:542.

Table 3–9 ■ Beta Blocker Treatment Protocol

Preoperative
Continue outpatient therapy if patient was previously on beta blocker (beta$_1$-selective agent), OR give atenolol 50-100 mg PO daily. Titrate dose to maintain heart rate below 65 beats/min.
If patient is on NPO status, give atenolol or metoprolol 2.5-10 mg IV until target heart rate is achieved.

Immediately Postoperative
Use atenolol or metoprolol 5-10 mg IV until target heart rate is achieved.

Postoperative
Return to the preoperative oral regimen when the patient is able to resume oral intake.
Continue beta blocker therapy for at least 1 month.

NPO, *nil per os* [nothing by mouth].
Adapted from Auerbach AD, Goldman L. Beta-blockers and reduction of cardiac events in non cardiac surgery. JAMA 2002;287:1435.

DIABETES

Patients with diabetes mellitus who undergo surgery have an increased risk of perioperative complications, especially infectious, metabolic, renal, and cardiac complications during and after surgery. To increase the likelihood of a safe and effective surgical outcome without complications, a thorough preoperative evaluation and establishment of plans for managing diabetes during surgery and for postoperative diabetic care are necessary. In general, the perioperative management of the patient with diabetes mellitus should be based on the type of diabetes, the specific diabetes medications the patient has been taking, the status of preoperative diabetic control, and the type and extent of the surgery planned. The goals of management are to prevent hypoglycemia, ketosis, and dehydration.

Patients with diabetes are at risk for both hyperglycemia and hypoglycemia in the perioperative period. Metabolic changes that occur with the onset of anesthesia and surgery can cause insulin resistance and decreases in insulin secretion, both of which can contribute to hyperglycemia during and after surgery. In addition, the stresses of anesthesia and surgery also cause an increase in glucose production and can contribute to poor control of glucose levels, ketosis, and acidosis. Impaired wound healing is one of the most important potential consequences of perioperative hyperglycemia, especially because it contributes to the greater frequency of postoperative wound infections. The cells and processes involved in healing are adversely affected by glucose levels greater than 200 to 250 mg/dL; therefore, target plasma glucose should be less than this level.[12] By contrast, hypoglycemia can result from prolonged fasting, medications, inadequate nutritional therapy, sedation, and postoperative gastrointestinal problems. Many of these factors may be less of an issue in the patient undergoing laparoscopic surgery who usually is able to tolerate an oral diet on same-day discharge.

Diabetic patients are at increased risk for cardiovascular disease, and cardiac complications are common in the perioperative period. In all diabetics, preoperative assessment should include an evaluation of cardiac status as well as an electrocardiogram, determination of overall diabetes control, and any other testing deemed necessary by findings on the history and physical examination. In addition, a chemistry panel to evaluate electrolytes, blood glucose, and renal function should be obtained before surgery. If the hemoglobin A_{1c} concentration is greater than 10% or fasting blood glucose level is greater than 200 mg/dL, special care is essential to avoid dehydration and electrolyte imbalances in the perioperative period.

The management of diabetes during the perioperative period depends on the type of the surgical procedure, the degree of overall glycemic control, and whether the patient is being managed with diet alone, with oral hypoglycemic agents, or with insulin. Diabetic patients whose disease is controlled by diet alone can be monitored with daily fasting glucose levels and given insulin if unacceptable elevations in glucose occur.

The management of patients taking oral hypoglycemic agents varies because they represent a fairly heterogeneous group. In general, all oral hypoglycemic agents should be held on the morning of surgery. For those agents with a half-life longer than 24 hours, such as chlorpropamide, medications should be stopped 2 days before surgery. Metformin should be stopped 48 hours before surgery. Patients whose diabetes is controlled with oral agents only usually do not need insulin during the procedure. Patients with poorly controlled diabetes on oral agents should receive an insulin infusion during surgery. Oral medications generally can be restarted when patients are able to resume their usual diet. Metformin should not be restarted (except following minor procedures) until 48 hours after surgery, until the patient is stable and eating, and, for major procedures, until a postoperative serum creatinine has been measured and demonstrated to be normal, so as to avoid any increased risk for lactic acidosis.

In patients who take insulin, the dose should be modified before minimal-access surgery. They should receive half of their usual dose of morning insulin and an intravenous infusion of 5% dextrose in water and $\frac{1}{2}$ normal saline solution ($D_5W/\frac{1}{2}NS$) during surgery. Patients usually can restart their preoperative insulin regimen once they resume their usual diet.

Patients undergoing major surgery who take insulin should not be given their usual insulin on the morning of surgery but should receive a continuous infusion of regular insulin starting at 1.0 unit per hour.[12] In addition, patients should receive a glucose infusion of $D_5W/0.45NS$ with 20 mEq of potassium chloride in each 1000-mL bag, to run at 100 mL per hour.[13] Blood glucose should be checked every 1 to 2 hours before surgery and every hour during surgery, and the insulin infusion rate adjusted in increments of 0.5 unit per hour to maintain a glucose level of 100 to 200 mg/dL.[12] Intravenous insulin infusion controls diabetes better than subcutaneous insulin, because the absorption of the latter can be erratic and variable during surgery.

Most patients undergoing minimal-access surgery will be able to tolerate their normal diet soon after completion of the procedure. As noted previously, once the patient has resumed this diet, she also can resume her preoperative diabetic medications.

PERIOPERATIVE MEDICATION MANAGEMENT

The management of a patient's medications in the perioperative period can present many challenges for the physician. Among the issues faced are the patient's response to the stresses of surgery, any underlying diseases, and the degree of control afforded by ongoing treatment, as well as the likelihood that oral administration of medication will not be an option at some period during the procedure. In addition, because few controlled trials regarding perioperative medication discontinuation and resumption have been conducted, many decisions about management are based on either the manufacturer's guidelines, consensus opinion, or anecdotal experience.

It is important to obtain a complete medication list from the patient, including over-the-counter medications, herbal preparations, and dietary supplements, because some medications have recognized effects on surgical risk or surgical decision making (Table 3–10). Such medications include antiplatelet agents, anticoagulants, hormonal agents, and

Table 3–10 ▪ Perioperative Medication Considerations

Category	Specific Recommendations	Other Considerations
Cardiac drugs	Beta blockers used for treatment of cardiovascular disease should not be stopped abruptly before surgery. Consider perioperative beta blockers in selected patients to reduce perioperative cardiovascular risk.	If patients cannot resume oral intake soon after surgery, parenteral preparations such as propranolol or esmolol can be used. If possible, continue most medications through surgery.
Agents to control hypertension	Consider decreasing or holding diuretic dose to avoid volume depletion. Abrupt discontinuation of clonidine has been associated with rebound hypertension.	Mild elevations in blood pressure may be acceptable in the perioperative period and are preferable to causing autonomic instability or volume depletion in an effort to maximize blood pressure control. Consider clonidine patch or other alternative parenteral agents to avoid acute hypertension.
Agents to manage pulmonary disease (asthma, COPD)	Inhalers (beta agonists, steroids, and anticholinergic agents) can be used throughout the perioperative period. Leukotriene antagonists and 5-lipoxygenase inhibitors can be continued.	If bronchospasm develops before patient can resume use of inhaler, nebulized or parenteral beta agonists can be used. Because abdominal surgery reduces lung function, consider use of nebulizers over metered-dose inhalers in immediate postoperative period. Encourage incentive spirometry, early ambulation.
Agents for endocrine disease management Diabetes	No oral hypoglycemics are given on day of surgery. For oral agents with half-life of more than 24 hours, stop 2 days before surgery. Metformin should be discontinued 2 days before surgery and restarted after 2-3 days when renal function has been shown to be normal or when patient goes home. *Insulin*: Give half the usual dose of long-acting insulin on the morning of procedure with dextrose in IV fluids; use sliding scale insulin as needed to control periprocedure glucose levels.	Resume oral agents when patient is eating again. Use sliding scale insulin coverage as needed.
Thyroid disease	Continue thyroid supplementation.	
Adrenal disease	Use stress doses of steroids if patient has used steroids regularly or for more than several short courses within the preceding year. Hydrocortisone 100 mg IV every 8 hours, starting immediately before the surgery. For minor procedures, one dose of 50-100 mg immediately before surgery may suffice, with another dose given 6-8 hours postoperatively.	Consider the degree of stress of the procedure itself—major surgery or general anesthesia is more stressful than minor procedures or local anesthesia. The dose can usually be tapered by 50% per day and discontinued by the fourth day.
Antiplatelet agents	*Aspirin* (irreversible platelet dysfunction): Stop 7 days before surgery. *NSAIDs* (reversible platelet dysfunction): Stop 3 days preoperatively. *COX-2 inhibitors* (little or no platelet effects): Can continue until day before surgery. *Clopidogrel* (Plavix) (irreversible platelet aggregation inhibition): Stop 7 days before surgery.	
Antiseizure drugs	Continue seizure medications.	
Psychiatric medications	Continue selective serotonin reuptake inhibitors (SSRIs) in the perioperative period. Continue lithium perioperatively. Continue benzodiazepines in modest doses perioperatively.	Stopping SSRIs abruptly can result in a withdrawal syndrome that can start as soon as 1 day after discontinuation of the drug and can include dizziness, agitation, lethargy, nausea, myalgias, shortness of breath, gait instability, and decreased short-term memory. Consider checking serum lithium levels perioperatively to ensure that they are not in the toxic range. Abrupt cessation following chronic use can cause a significant withdrawal syndrome. Patients who take benzodiazepines chronically may have higher requirements for postoperative opiates. Patients who take significant amounts of benzodiazepines require less medication for anesthesia induction and maintenance.

Table continued on following page

Category	Specific Recommendations	Other Considerations
Herbal supplements	In general, patients should stop taking herbal preparations 1 to 2 weeks before surgery; many potential drug interactions and perioperative effects of herbs are still unknown.	
	Garlic, ginkgo biloba, and ginseng should be stopped 7 days before surgery.	All of these have been found to inhibit platelet aggregation and therefore can cause problems with postoperative bleeding.
	Kava can accentuate the sedative effects of anesthetics and has been associated with severe liver injury. Valerian can affect anesthetic requirements.	

Table 3–10 ▪ **Perioperative Medication Considerations** (Continued)

COPD, chronic obstructive pulmonary disease; COX-2, cyclooxygenase-2; NSAIDs, nonsteroidal anti-inflammatory drugs.
Adapted from Mercado DL, Petty BG. Perioperative medication management. Med Clin North Am 2003;87:41.

herbal preparations. Most medications, however, are well tolerated throughout the surgical period and do not interfere with anesthesia and therefore should be continued through the morning of surgery unless contraindicated. In general, antihypertensive medications, anticonvulsants, and psychiatric medications should be administered unless specifically contraindicated. Medications that cause a withdrawal or rebound phenomenon when abruptly stopped should be continued throughout the perioperative period with as little interruption as possible.

In conclusion, except as noted in Table 3–10, most medications can be continued pre- and postoperatively. The gynecologist must take a detailed drug history, to include medication, over-the-counter products, and health and herbal supplements, so as not to miss any potential perioperative interactions.

NEUROLOGIC INJURY

The laparoscopic approach to gynecologic surgery usually requires the patient to be placed in the lithotomy position. Modern advanced laparoscopic surgery often necessitates placing the patient in this relatively unnatural static position for long periods of time. One must be extremely careful in positioning the anesthetized patient, as she obviously will not be able to alert the surgeon to any discomfort.

Many cases of neurologic injury following laparoscopic surgery have now been reported in the literature. The two most common etiologic factors in nerve injury associated with gynecologic operations are use of abdominal retractors and limb positioning. Because no retractors are used for laparoscopic procedures, most nerve injuries incurred during minimal-access surgery are the consequence of limb placement before the operation. Most of these injuries are preventable with a proper understanding of the neuroanatomy and attention to detail.

Neurologic Injury to the Pelvis and Leg

The mechanism of lower extremity nerve injury usually involves either stretch or vascular compromise of the nerves that supply the leg. Only rarely are they injured from direct surgical trauma. These nerves are fixed in their position, with little accommodation for extremes of adduction or flexion.

The leg is supplied by nerves originating from the lumbar and sacral plexus. The sensory nerves—iliohypogastric, ilioinguinal, genitofemoral, and lateral femoral—arise from T12 to L3. The pudendal nerve originates from S2 to S4. All of the motor nerves—obturator, cutaneous femoral, common peroneal, and tibial—arise from L2 to S4. With the exception of the obturator nerve, all of these motor nerves also have a sensory component. During laparoscopic surgery, both motor and sensory nerves can be injured. The ability to test for both motor and sensory deficits helps in the diagnosis of a nerve injury. Trauma to the sensory nerves is more annoying than disabling. Motor nerve injury can result in severe permanent disability.

The occurrence of a neuropathy after vaginal surgery was first reported in 1905. In 1968, Hopper and Baker theorized that the mechanism of postoperative neuropathy involved ischemia to the femoral nerve.[13] If a woman is placed in a lithotomy position that causes excessive hip flexion, abduction, or external rotation (Fig. 3–2), the femoral nerve will be placed at an extreme angle beneath and against the inguinal ligament. Compromise of the blood supply to the femoral nerve may result in a severe injury.

The obturator and sciatic nerves are injured less frequently than the femoral nerve. When an injury does occur, it most commonly results from either direct trauma or suturing during the dissection, rather than from stretch or ischemia. The sciatic nerve is relatively fixed in the pelvis and cannot lengthen as the leg is put into extremes of position. This nerve can be injured either with excessive external rotation of the thigh or with extreme flexion at the hip. In addition, the sciatic nerve also can be injured when the knees are fully extended, such as can occur with the "candy cane" stirrups.

The common peroneal nerve is very superficial in location as it crosses the lateral lower leg over the head of the fibula just below the knee. This nerve most often is injured by direct compression against the stirrup.

If a patient complains of loss of sensation, paresthesia, numbness, or weakness in her leg after laparoscopy, a neurologic examination should be performed. The examination findings usually will reveal which nerve has been injured. Femoral nerve injury may manifest as inability to walk, climb stairs, perform a straight-leg raise, or extend the lower leg. Other possible manifestations of injury include numbness over the medial thigh and loss of the knee jerk reflex. Occasionally, multiple nerve injuries may make the injury more

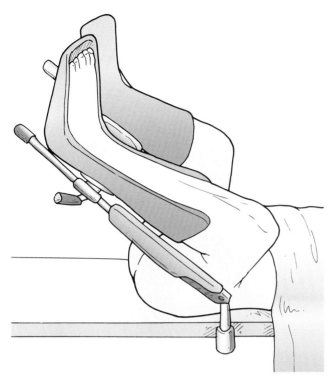

Figure 3–2 ▪ **Common mechanism for lower extremity neurologic injury.** Extreme hip flexion in lithotomy position, as shown, can cause damage to the femoral nerve.

difficult to identify. It has been shown that nerve injuries occur more commonly when the lithotomy position is maintained for longer than 4 hours.

Neurologic Injuries to the Arm

Upper extremity injuries are much less common than those of the lower extremity in laparoscopic surgery. These injuries usually are caused by stretching of the brachial or cervical plexus or by direct compression of the ulnar nerve. Brachial plexus injuries are almost always caused by positioning of the arm board at an angle greater than 90 degrees from the long axis of the patient's body (Fig. 3–3A–C). These injuries usually result in wrist drop and decreased sensation over the dorsum of the radial side of the hand. Cervical plexus injuries incurred during laparoscopy usually are caused by the use of shoulder brackets during steep Trendelenburg positioning, which allows the torso to slide cranially while the shoulders remain fixed. This situation creates a stretch injury of the cervical plexus.

A less common arm injury is that involving the ulnar nerve. This injury is caused by ischemia secondary to compression at the elbow. When this superficial nerve, which is located medial to the epicondyle of the humerus, is allowed to rest against the operating room table or a rigid arm board, a compression injury can result, leading to paresthesia and weakness of the fourth and fifth fingers.

Compartment Syndrome

Compartment syndrome occurs when pressure is increased in a confined space, such as the fascial compartments of the leg,

compromising blood flow and damaging nerve and muscle in that area. A vicious circle ensues as edema in this area reduces blood flow further. Compartment syndrome is well known to occur frequently after traumatic injuries to the extremities. Complications from compartment syndrome following surgery are rare. Most case reports of the syndrome in this setting involve operations in which the patient remains in the lithotomy position for long periods. Symptoms include pain or tense swelling of an isolated area of the leg; pulses may remain intact. Orthopedic consultation must be obtained. A fasciotomy may be necessary to relieve the pressure and restore perfusion to the lower extremity. Care must be taken in positioning and padding the leg so as to avoid excessive pressure over an isolated area.

Prevention of Neurologic Injuries

The prevention of neurologic complications resulting from compression or stretch of the nerves is relatively easy if the mechanisms of injury just described are kept in mind.

Lower extremity nerve injuries usually can be prevented by always keeping the knee flexed and never placing the hip in extremes of flexion, external rotation, or abduction during long operative laparoscopic procedures (Fig. 3–4). If procedures are likely to last longer than 4 hours, the surgeon should decide whether frequent vaginal and rectal access will be necessary. Uterine manipulation can be accomplished using modern uterine manipulators with the patient in the recumbent position. If the need for frequent vaginal or rectal probing is not anticipated, the surgeon should consider performing laparoscopy with the patient in the recumbent position with legs minimally separated.

The incidence of peroneal nerve injury and compartment syndrome can be reduced by paying attention to the positioning and padding of the lower leg. The calf should be placed centrally in the middle of the modern supporting leg holder, to prevent the peroneal nerve from being compressed against the side of the stirrup. Stirrups without padding should not be used. If care is taken, peroneal injuries and compartment syndromes should be rare.

Upper extremity nerve injury can be reduced by never placing the arm at an angle greater than 90 degrees from the longitudinal axis of the body (Fig. 3–5). To reduce the incidence of ulnar nerve injury, the arm should be placed palm down if kept by the patient's side, and palm up if positioned on an arm board. The incidence of cervical plexus injury can be minimized by either eliminating the use of shoulder brackets if possible or, when necessary, positioning the brackets over the acromioclavicular joint.

CONCLUSIONS

The process of avoiding complications in surgery begins long before the operation begins. The surgeon must obtain a comprehensive history from the patient, to identify all of her medical problems, allergies, and prescribed and over-the-counter medications. The surgeon must then decide which preventive preoperative therapies will help reduce perioperative complications in each case. Potential cardiac,

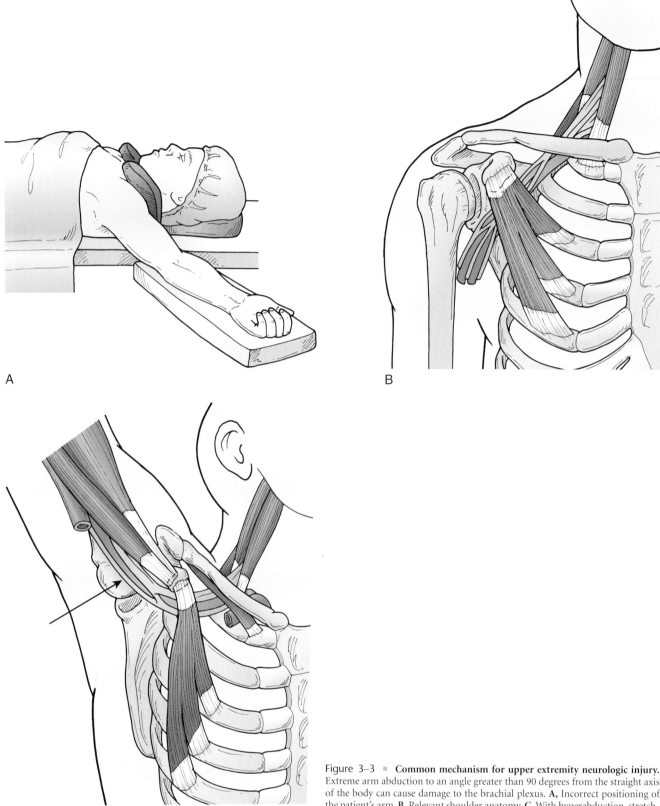

A

B

C

Figure 3–3 ▪ **Common mechanism for upper extremity neurologic injury.** Extreme arm abduction to an angle greater than 90 degrees from the straight axis of the body can cause damage to the brachial plexus. **A,** Incorrect positioning of the patient's arm. **B,** Relevant shoulder anatomy. **C,** With hyperabduction, stretching of the brachial plexus *(arrow)* may occur, with resultant injury.

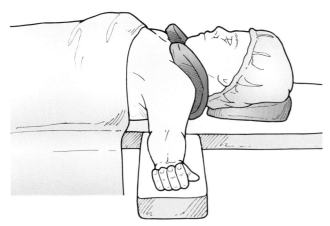

Figure 3–4 ▪ Upper extremity nerve injury may be prevented by correct positioning of the patient's arm, as shown.

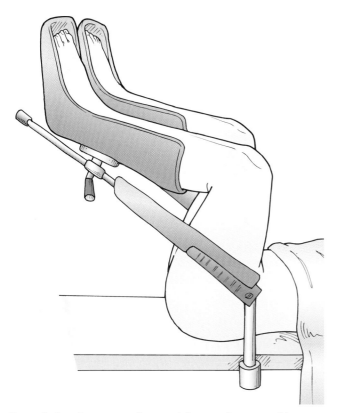

Figure 3–5 ▪ Lower extremity nerve injury may be prevented by correct positioning of the legs for gynecologic procedures, as shown.

thrombotic, and infectious complications can be significantly reduced with careful preoperative planning and attention to detail.

References

1. Dajani AS, Taubert KA, Wilson W, et al. Prevention of bacterial endocarditis: Recommendations by the American Heart Association. JAMA 2003;227:1794.
2. Bratzler DW, Hook PM. Antimicrobial prophylaxis for surgery: An advisory statement from the National Surgical Infection Prevention Project. Clin Infect Dis 2004;38:1706.
3. Soper M. Antibiotic prophylaxis for gynecologic procedures. ACOG Pract Bull 2001;23:1.
4. Geerts WH, Heit JA, Clagett GP, et al. Prevention of venous thromboembolism. Chest 2001;119:132S.
5. Kaboli P, Henderson MC, White R. DVT prophylaxis and anticoagulation in the surgical patient. Med Clin North Am 2003;87:77.
6. Connolly TP, Jachtorowycz MJ, Knaus JV. Incidence of thromboembolic complications after gynecologic laparoscopy: A review of the literature. J Pelv Med Surg 2001;7:350.
7. Lindberg F, Bergquist D, Rasmussen I. Incidence of thromboembolic complications after laparoscopic cholecystectomy: review of literature. Surg Laparos Endosc 1997;7:324.
8. Kearon C, Hirsh J. Management of anticoagulation before and after elective surgery. N Engl J Med 1997;336:1506.
9. Shaw HA, Shaw JA. Perioperative management of the female patient. Emedicine 2004;3290 (emedicine.com/med/topic3290.htm).
10. Mangano DT, Layug EL, Wallace A, Tateo I. Effect of atenolol on mortality and cardiovascular morbidity after noncardiac surgery. Multicenter Study of Perioperative Ischemia Research Group. N Engl J Med 1996; 335:1713.
11. Auerbach AD, Goldman L. Beta-blockers and reduction of cardiac events in non cardiac surgery. JAMA 2002;287:1435.
12. Schiff RL, Welsh GA. Perioperative evaluation and management of the patient with endocrine dysfunction. Med Clin North Am 2003;87:175.
13. Hopper CL, Baker JB. Bilateral femoral neuropathy complicating vaginal hysterectomy: Analysis of contributing factors in 3 patients. Obstet Gynecol 1968;32:543.

Complications of Laparoscopic Access

4

Malcolm G. Munro

Complications of peritoneal access that may confer significant morbidity include bleeding from the abdominal wall, injury to the great vessels of the pelvis, and damage to intraperitoneal viscera, including the bowel and urinary tract. Other complications that have been recognized as being related to port insertion are subcutaneous emphysema, metastatic seeding from malignant neoplasms, and the development of other wound complications such as dehiscence and hernia. Reducing the risk of laparoscopic access complications is based on a combination of surgical judgment, proper instrumentation, and appropriate technique. In gynecologic surgery, insertion of laparoscopic cannulas most commonly has been accomplished with sharp-tipped obturators called *trocars*—instruments that can cause potentially life-threatening injuries to abdominal viscera and major blood vessels. Modifications and innovations in device design and the use of new or rediscovered strategies and techniques for port insertion are potentially important factors that may reduce the incidence of access-related morbidity and mortality.

INSTRUMENTATION FOR LAPAROSCOPIC ACCESS

Instrumentation used for laparoscopic peritoneal access serves one or a combination of purposes, including insufflation of gas for achieving or maintaining a pneumoperitoneum, and allowing the insertion of instruments, usually while maintaining the integrity of the already established pneumoperitoneum. A noncombustible gas, generally CO_2, is provided by an insufflator that can be adjusted to control and maintain both the flow rate and the intraperitoneal pressure. Laparoscopic peritoneal access systems generally comprise an outer cannula or port and an internal obturator that is removed after the cannula is positioned in the peritoneal cavity, or other cavity as appropriate, thereby allowing insertion of the endoscope or hand instrument. When preinsufflation of the peritoneal cavity is performed, an insufflation needle is used before positioning of the access cannula.

Gasless laparoscopy is a technique that eliminates the need for a pneumoperitoneum by suspending the anterior abdominal wall with an external mechanical lifting device. Although gasless laparoscopy has clearly recognized limitations,[1] which in turn have limited its adoption, the need for access ports designed for the purpose of maintaining a pneumoperitoneum is obviated with this technique. Consequently, standard or laparoscopic instruments may be placed through small abdominal wall incisions. In addition, the lack of increased intraperitoneal pressure removes one intraoperative variable that may have significant hemodynamic impact on patients with cardiovascular compromise.[2] The gasless technique may therefore have clinical value at least in selected cases.

Insufflation Needles

The needles used for insufflation of the peritoneal cavity have generally been designed based on the device introduced by Veress in the 1930s (Fig. 4–1). For laparoscopy, a 2-mm-diameter (i.e., outer diameter [OD]) (approximately) sharp-tipped hollow needle is attached to a Luer interface proximally and fitted with a sprung obturator within the hollow of the cannula. This obturator retracts when it engages firm abdominal wall structures such as the fascia, thereby allowing the sharp distal tip of the needle to penetrate the various layers. When the device completes its journey through the abdominal wall, with the tip entering the peritoneal cavity, the obturator is free to rapidly redeploy. This process creates a limited degree of protection for intraperitoneal vessels and viscera; however, bowel adherent to the anterior abdominal wall is at risk without application of additional force from the surgeon, and moreover, should the needle encounter, for example, retroperitoneal vessels such as the aorta or vena cava, they may be damaged. Consequently, insufflation needles should not be considered to be devices that are free of risk.

LAPAROSCOPIC TROCAR-CANNULA SYSTEMS

The hollow access cannula allows insertion of a laparoscope or hand instrument into the peritoneal cavity, while establishing a seal that maintains the pneumoperitoneum. Laparoscopic access systems designed for penetrating the abdominal wall generally have a narrow-tipped obturator, usually called a *trocar*, that fits within the cannula and is used to create and

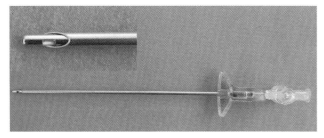

Figure 4–1 ▪ **Insufflation needle.** This disposable insufflation needle is approximately 2 mm in outside diameter and has an inner sprung obturator that retracts when a firm surface is encountered, thereby exposing the blade. When resistance is lost, such as when entering the peritoneal cavity, the obturator snaps back into place.

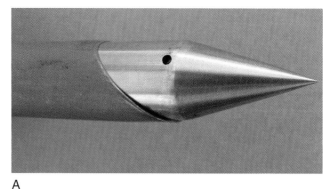

A

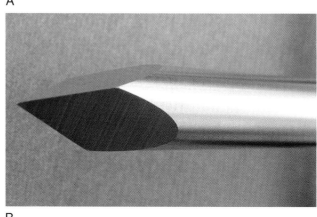

B

Figure 4–3 ▪ **Reusable conical and pyramidal trocars.** Blunt conical (**A**) and pyramidal (**B**) trocars. The knife-like edge of the pyramidal trocar makes insertion through the abdominal wall easier, but causes more tissue damage around the point of entry.

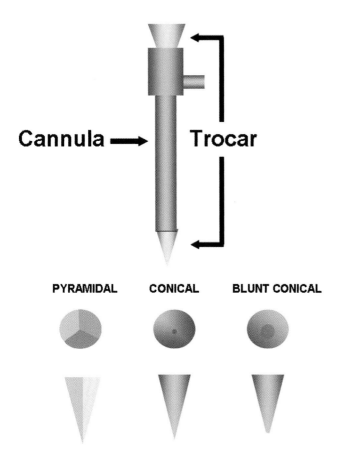

Figure 4–2 ▪ **Trocar-cannula system.** These systems comprise an outer cannula, which is left in the abdominal wall, and an inner trocar, which is used to penetrate the abdominal wall, thereby positioning the cannula. Trocar tips have traditionally been pyramidal or conical, but blunt conical devices also can be used to penetrate the abdominal wall, with slightly greater force but resulting in a smaller wound. Such devices also may be less likely to penetrate blood vessels or other viscera when passed into the peritoneal cavity.

Trocars were traditionally created with a sharp tip based on either a conical or a pyramidal design (Fig. 4–3). Historically, pyramidal trocars (see Fig. 4–3B) have been the most commonly employed devices, largely because they require the smallest entry force owing to the three knife-like edges that can relatively easily slice open the encountered tissue.[3] Conical trocars (see Fig. 4–3A) do not have such sharp edges and instead dilate the fascial and muscular tissue after a small opening is made with the pointed tip. Reusable trocars have been available for many decades and are rather simple devices. In the mid- to late 1980s, with the explosion in laparoscopic surgery, came disposable systems that were fitted with retractable blades or deployable sheaths, purported to provide a degree of protection against injury to intraperitoneal structures. Such "safety shields," however, are known not to be protective for the patient[4]—indeed, the U.S. Food and Drug Administration (FDA) forbids using the term in marketing these devices.

The last 10 years have seen the introduction of a number of other laparoscopic access system designs, including "optical" trocars, blunt dilating tips, and hybrid systems. The optical trocars have a clear tip of variable design that has been purported to allow visualization of entry by placing a laparoscope in its hollow center (Fig. 4–4). The value of this approach is questionable, however, and the evidence suggests that such instrumentation may not reduce the incidence of

then expand an abdominal wall defect. Collectively, these access devices can be called trocar-cannula systems (T-CSs) (Fig. 4–2). The inside diameter (ID) of the most commonly used systems ranges from 5 to 12 mm, but the full range of IDs for all such devices is from 2.7 mm to 15 mm; the usual length of the devices ranges from 120 to 150 mm, although both shorter and longer lengths are available.

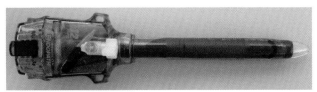

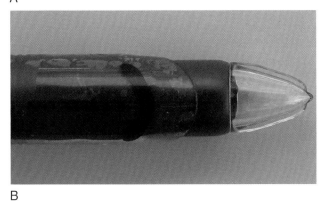

Figure 4–4 ▪ **Visual access device. A,** This device is portrayed as a blunt conical trocar and seems to cause abdominal wounds similar to those produced by other blunt devices. **B,** The rather sharp tip, however, distinguishes it from other blunt devices and may carry an increased risk for damage of internal structures.

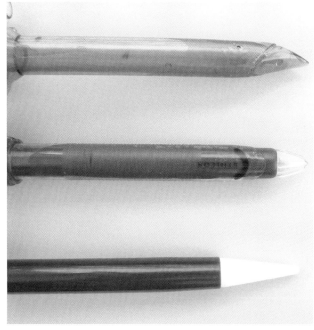

Figure 4–5 ▪ **Access systems with dilating obturators.** Each of these devices has the same impact with respect to creating abdominal wounds, and all are smaller than those of pyramidal devices. The ADAPT device (Taut Medical Inc., Geneva, Illinois) *(top)* and the STEP device (United States Surgical Corp., Norwalk, Connecticut) *(middle)* both are blunt devices, whereas the Optiview device (Ethicon Endosurgery Inc., Cincinnati, Ohio) *(bottom)* has a sharper tip.

vascular and bowel complications.[5] Blunt tips require more force for insertion[6] but have been shown to result in a smaller incisional diameter[3,7] and, because of their tip, *may* provide a greater measure of safety with respect to bowel and vascular injury (Fig. 4–5).[8] Most of these devices have a very simple design, with no moving parts; however, the "Step" system (Autosuture Division of the United States Surgical Corp., Norwalk, Connecticut) comprises four parts: the insufflation needle, the dilating sheath, the cannula, and the obturator. The principal difference between this device and other blunt-tipped cannulas is the dilating sheath. The wounds resulting from this device, however, are similar to those produced with all of the other blunt-tipped devices that we have tested in our laboratory. Consequently, the added value of the dilating sheath is questionable at least, and this feature is at most an unnecessary additional component serving only to add to the cost of the device.

In an attempt to reduce entry force, but to achieve wound dimensions similar to those produced by blunt conical devices, hybrid devices have been introduced (Fig. 4–6). These generally comprise a blunt obturator with a small blade at the tip that deploys, usually transiently, when a force compatible with fascia is encountered. Alternatively, such devices can be manufactured with a pyramidal tip that is then shaped to transform to a blunt dilating instrument (Fig. 4–7). Although reported objective evaluations of these devices are relatively few, our study showed no advantages of one such design over the traditional pyramidal systems with respect to wound area. In addition, I have repeatedly observed the deployable tip remaining exposed following entry into the peritoneal cavity, thereby presenting risk of injury to vessels and viscera (Fig. 4–8).

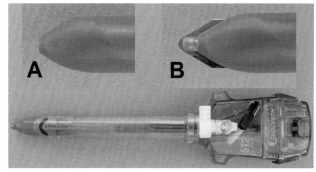

Figure 4–6 ▪ **Hybrid trocar-cannula system.** This hybrid device, the Endopath (Ethicon Endosurgery Inc., Cincinnati, Ohio), is similar to those of a number of other manufacturers. It is a blunt dilating obturator (A) that retracts (B) while traversing the abdominal wall, thereby exposing the sharp tip. The tip frequently remains deployed shortly after the peritoneum is breached, leaving an opportunity for damage to internal structures.

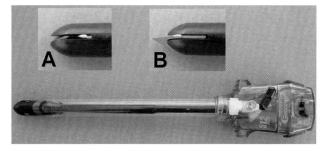

Figure 4–7 ▪ **Pyramidal tip with retractable obturator.** A blunt obturator (A) with a deployable pyramidal tip (B) is shown. This device is conceptually similar to that shown in Figure 4–6, but with a pyramidal design.

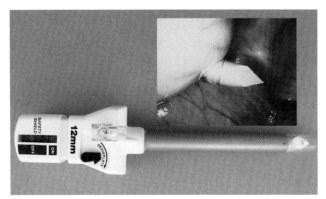

Figure 4–8 ▪ **Failure of sheath deployment.** Sheath redeployment may be delayed with any of the shielded devices. With the device shown (from United States Surgical Corp., Norwalk, Connecticut), deployment of the "Safety Shield" is delayed enough to place the patient at risk for injury if proper insertion technique is not followed.

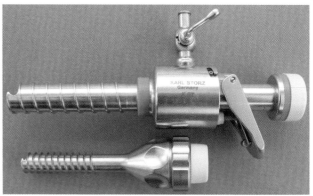

A

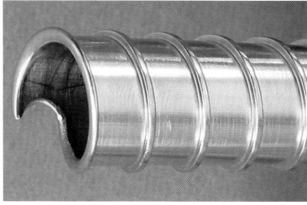

B

Figure 4–9 ▪ **Threaded, trocarless access cannulas.** The EndoTIP (Karl Storz Endoscopy America, Culver City, California) threaded, trocarless cannula (**A**) is twisted into the peritoneal cavity. An endoscope may be passed through the lumen (seen to best advantage in **B**) to visualize passage through the layers of the abdominal wall. Although the manufacturer originally required that a fascial incision be made, this step usually is not necessary. Wound parameters are similar to those for the blunt trocar-cannula system.

Another relatively new design is a threaded cannula designed to be inserted without a trocar (Fig. 4–9). This hollow device allows the surgeon to position a laparoscope within its canal, thereby allowing visualization of the layer-by-layer entry into the peritoneal cavity (Endoscopic Threaded Imaging Port [EndoTIP], from Karl Storz Endoscopy America, Culver City, California). This device has a number of potential benefits.[9,10] Because no trocar is used, the risk of visceral and, in particular, major blood vessel injury would seem to be limited. More important, this device virtually eliminates the need for the surgeon to direct force internally, instead requiring the application of a rotational force that is exerted in effect parallel to the skin surface. The external threads of the cannula cause the layers of the abdominal wall to be lifted up rather than being pushed down toward the viscera. Because the cannula is rotated to obtain access, it is suggested that the injuries in the muscle, fascia, and peritoneum are not aligned, thereby reducing the incidence of incisional hernias. We have evaluated this system in our model, both with[11] and without[12] cannula manipulation, and found that wound area and muscle damage were less than those associated with use of a similarly sized pyramidal device, and more similar to those observed with use of a conical T-CS. These findings suggest that the incidence of associated hernia and dehiscence would be similar to that reported for conical systems. Of note, this device probably is much safer than the other so-called optical access devices, for which the reported incidence of major vascular and visceral injury has been high.[5] With these devices, the force is directed toward the peritoneal cavity, as is the case for other trocar-based access systems, leaving the potential for injury. Presumably, although it has not been proved, such threaded cannulas would have little chance of causing visceral or vascular injury because of the rotational nature of the force applied.

Relatively recent advances in fiberoptic instrument design have allowed the introduction of narrow-caliber endoscopes that, in turn, allow the surgeon to use access ports of narrower caliber. For example, some manufacturers have modified the design of the Veress needle to allow the sprung obturator to be removed like a trocar, so that the needle can function as a laparoscopic cannula for small-caliber laparoscopic instru-

mentation (Fig. 4–10). With these devices, the surgeon can confirm intraperitoneal placement using only the very-narrow-caliber device, potentially reducing the extent, if not the frequency, of intraperitoneal injuries.

The so-called open laparoscopy systems designed for positioning after minilaparotomy, and first described by Hasson, are essentially cannulas with blunt obturators and a conical sleeve that serves to establish a seal between the instrument and the skin, to prevent the escape of the peritoneal gas (Fig. 4–11). The seal usually is maintained with sutures secured to both the fascia and the instrument, but other novel devices such as balloon-tipped cannulas also have been introduced for the same purpose.

Abdominal Wall Suturing Devices

Suturing of the abdominal wall is sometimes necessary to close selected fascial wounds or to obtain hemostasis in the event of a trocar-related injury to an abdominal wall blood vessel such as the deep inferior epigastric artery. It is possible to accomplish these tasks with "off-the-shelf" ligatures and needles. Closure of fascial defects in thin persons may be

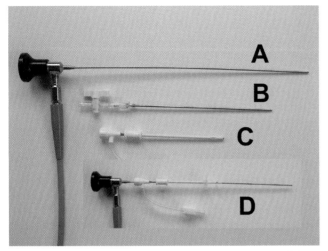

Figure 4–10 ▪ **Small-caliber (2 mm) laparoscope.** The ConMed (Utica, New York) 2-mm access system comprises a 2-mm-fiber laparoscope (A) and an insufflation needle (B) that also serves as the trocar for the cannula or sheath (C). After placement of the trocar-cannula system in the abdominal wall, the laparoscope passed through the sheath, as shown in the *inset* (D).

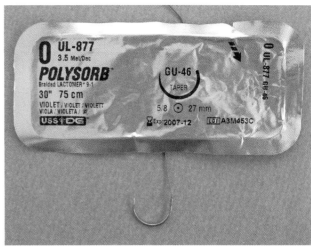

Figure 4–12 ▪ **Urologic needle, three-quarter round.** The most readily available device for fascial closure is a needle that allows positioning in the small confines of the small incisions created for laparoscopy. It is difficult to close the peritoneum with such needles, however, particularly outside the umbilical area. Consequently, Richter's hernia would remain a possible threat.

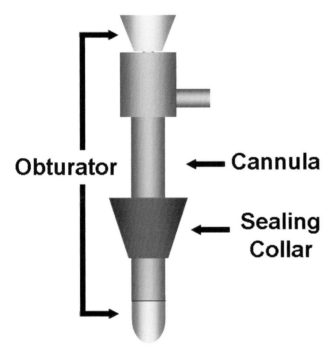

Figure 4–11 ▪ **Hasson system for open laparoscopy.** This cannula is designed to be placed after creation of a minilaparotomy, generally in the sub-umbilical area, and is named after Harreth Hasson, its inventor. The device is retained in the abdominal wall either with two or more sutures or with a balloon positioned at the distal end of the cannula. The obturator is removed to allow insertion of the laparoscope.

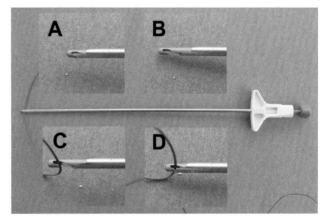

Figure 4–13 ▪ **Endoclose ligature carrier.** The Endoclose (United States Surgical Corp., Norwalk, Connecticut) ligature carrier is modeled after a Veress insufflation needle, with the internal, sprung obturator modified to allow capture and release of a ligature. Closing fascial wounds or securing lacerated deep inferior epigastric vessels must be accomplished under laparoscopic visualization. The unloaded device in the neutral position is shown in *inset* A. Depressing the blue button in the handle opens the obturator (*inset* B) so that it can capture the ligature (*inset* C). Releasing the button secures the ligature (*inset* D) so that the device can be passed through the abdominal wall. Alternatively, capturing the intraperitoneal free end of a ligature previously passed will allow externalization so that a knot might be tied.

accomplished with three-quarter round urologic needles (Fig. 4–12). Particularly in obese patients, however, such devices are not effective at closing the peritoneum, leaving the possibility for bowel to become entrapped below the fascia in the resulting defect—thereby creating a Richter's hernia.[13] Consequently, in such circumstances, specially designed instruments may be both more efficient and more effective.

The devices that seem most useful are called *ligature carriers*, designed to first pass a free tie on one side of a vessel or wound, into the peritoneal cavity. Then, after disengaging the ligature, the ligature carrier is removed, leaving the ligature hanging in the peritoneal cavity. The ligature carrier is then inserted into the peritoneal cavity on the other side of the blood vessel or wound and is used to grasp the intraperitoneal free end of the tie, which is then externalized by removing the ligature carrier. The surgeon then ties and tightens an appropriate series of knots. A number of ligature carrier designs are available, two of which are displayed in Figures 4–13 and 4–14.

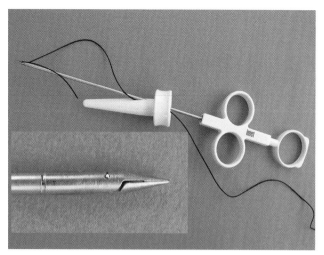

Figure 4–14 ■ **Carter-Tomasson ligature carrier.** Also positioned under laparoscopic direction, the Carter-Tomasson (Inlet Medical, Minneapolis, Minnesota) system includes a stopper that serves both to prevent the egress of distending gas, thereby facilitating laparoscopic visualization, and as a ligature guide allowing proper positioning of the ligature around the wound. *Inset*, The end is an alligator forceps with a notch that allows the jaws to remain completely closed (thereby maintaining the needle-tip profile) while securely holding the ligature.

The disposable Surgineedle (Autosuture Division of United States Surgical Corp.) device resembles an insufflation needle and comprises a sharp-tipped external cannula with an internal sprung obturator. The obturator contains a notch that is used to trap the ligature against the outer sheath of the device for transfer into the peritoneal cavity. Subsequently, the ligature is released by extending the inner obturator after insertion. The now empty device is placed on the other side of the incision and passed into the peritoneal cavity, where it is used to capture and then externalize the ligature to allow formation and tightening of the knots. The Carter-Tomasson (Inlet Medical, Minneapolis, Minnesota) ligature carrier is a single-use sharp-tipped device that achieves the same ends, with the same basic technique as that for the Surgineedle but does so with a different design. The device is actually an alligator forceps grasper that, when closed, creates a sharp needle tip. The Carter-Tomasson ligature carrier is packaged with a needle guide that also serves to occlude the wound, thereby maintaining the pneumoperitoneum.

ACCESS COMPLICATIONS: RECOGNITION AND MANAGEMENT

Interstitial Insufflation

Interstitial insufflation related to access most commonly results from preperitoneal placement of an insufflation needle but may occur as a consequence of leakage of CO_2 around the cannula sites, in the latter case frequently caused by excessive intraperitoneal pressure. Alternatively, gas can be directly injected with an insufflation needle into the retroperitoneal area, the omentum, or the mesentery of the small or large bowel. Although the condition usually is mild, limited, and of

no clinical significance, in some instances it can become extensive, involving the extremities and the neck, when it is referred to as *subcutaneous emphysema*. Should the gas dissect its way to the mediastinum in substantial amounts, cardiovascular collapse could occur.

Recognition. Often the diagnosis of interstitial insufflation will not be a surprise—the surgeon may have had difficulty in positioning the insufflation needle or the primary cannula, or both, within the peritoneal cavity and experienced one or more unsuccessful attempts at insufflation. Subcutaneous emphysema often remains hidden beneath the fascia but if more extensive may be readily identified by the palpation of crepitus in the abdominal wall. If it extends along contiguous fascial planes to the neck, it can be visualized directly. Such a finding can be a reflection of the development of mediastinal emphysema, which, if severe, may lead to pneumothorax and cardiovascular collapse.

Management. If the surgeon finds that the initial insufflation has occurred extraperitoneally, a number of options exist. Although removing the laparoscope followed by reinsufflation is possible, the procedure may be made more difficult because of the new configuration of the anterior peritoneum. Ensuring that the entry point is exactly at the base of the navel, where all layers of the anterior abdominal wall fuse, may allow for successful insufflation. The use of a 2- to 3-mm laparoscope and an accompanying small-caliber insufflation needle or access port may facilitate confirmation of proper placement. Other options include open laparoscopy and the use of an alternate access site such as the left upper quadrant. Another approach is to visually direct insertion of the insufflation needle after leaving the laparoscope in the expanded preperitoneal space.

For mild cases of subcutaneous emphysema, no specific intraoperative or postoperative therapy is required, because the abnormalities, in at least mild cases, quickly resolve following evacuation of the pneumoperitoneum. When the extravasation extends to involve the neck, it usually is preferable to terminate the procedure, because pneumomediastinum, pneumothorax, hypercarbia, and cardiovascular collapse may result. At the end of the operation, it is prudent to obtain a chest film. The patient should be managed expectantly unless a tension pneumothorax develops, in which case immediate evacuation must be performed.

Intravascular Insufflation

The intraperitoneal distention medium can gain access to the systemic circulation by means of direct injection or through breaches in the systemic circulation created during the process of surgical dissection. CO_2 is the most widely used peritoneal distention medium and, because of its high degree of solubility, also is the safest. The vast majority of CO_2 microemboli are absorbed, usually by the splanchnic vascular system, quickly and without incident. Severe cardiorespiratory compromise may result, however, if large amounts of CO_2 gain access to the central venous circulation, such as with inadvertent intravascular placement of an insufflation needle followed by prolonged intravascular insufflation. The use of less soluble distention media such as nitrous oxide generally is discouraged.

Recognition. Clinically insignificant CO_2 emboli are common and can even create the classical "mill-wheel" heart murmur without clinical sequelae. A massive CO_2 embolus may result in sudden cardiovascular collapse with otherwise unexplained cyanosis, hypotension, and cardiac arrhythmia. Other clinical sequelae include an increased end-tidal CO_2, findings consistent with pulmonary edema, and pulmonary hypertension, resulting in right-sided heart failure.

Management. At the first suggestion of cardiovascular compromise secondary to CO_2 embolus, the insufflation apparatus should be immediately turned off and the peritoneal cavity decompressed. The patient should be placed in the Durant or left lateral decubitus position, with head below the level of the right atrium. Immediate establishment of a large-bore central venous line may allow aspiration of gas from the heart. Because the findings are nonspecific, other causes of cardiovascular collapse should be considered in the differential diagnosis.

Vascular Injury

Laparoscopic access may result in injury to vessels in the abdominal wall, to the great vessels located retroperitoneally, or to smaller-caliber vessels directly supplying the structures and viscera of the peritoneal cavity.

GREAT VESSELS

The great vessels include the aorta, the inferior vena cava, and the common, internal, and external iliac arteries and veins. Injury can occur regardless of the method of access, largely because of the often close proximity of these vessels to the abdominal wall, which in thin patients can be as little as 2 cm.[14] Catastrophic hemorrhage may occur if the sharp tip or edge of a laparoscopic trocar or insufflation needle injures one of these vessels. Such injuries usually require conversion to laparotomy and, if bleeding is massive or diagnosis is delayed, constitute a major cause of serious morbidity and mortality associated with laparoscopic technique.[15,16]

The incidence of major vascular injuries has been the subject of a number of surveys and retrospective studies and is estimated to range from 0.04% to 0.5%. This relatively wide range reflects any of a number of factors that include the surgical specialty studied, the training and experience of the surgeon, the difficulty of the case, and the limitations of surveys and other retrospective studies, each of which can be hampered by various types of bias. The initial report of laparoscopic complications from Germany, which comprised minor gynecologic laparoscopic surgical procedures almost entirely, described the complications occurring in approximately 300,000 procedures performed between 1978 and 1982. The incidence of major vascular injury was reported to be 0.07%.[17]

The highest reported incidence of major vascular injury is 0.5%, in a survey of nearly 13,000 major operative procedures performed by Italian general surgeons.[18] In this series, the risk of such injury with "closed" technique was twice that when open technique was used, although a relatively small number of closed approaches were reported. Furthermore, the absence of any comparison of other variables potentially related to outcome, such as surgeon training and patient co-morbidity, makes interpretation of these results difficult. In a French report of a large group of just over 100,000 laparoscopic operations associated with just under 400,000 trocar-cannula insertions, however, the incidence of major vascular injury was much lower, approximately 0.04%.[19] A large Dutch review compared the incidence of vascular injury in 489,335 patients with that in 12,444 in whom open laparoscopy was performed.[20] In this cohort, the incidence of major vascular injury with closed technique was 0.075% and 0% when open laparoscopy was performed.

Some concern has been expressed that publication bias may affect the reporting of complications, particularly when associated with great vessel injury. The medical-legal climate may inhibit clinical investigation into the matter, thereby obfuscating the true incidence of at least some adverse events, and potentially obscuring the mechanisms by which the trauma occurs. It is in some ways fortunate that a few investigators have started to report major vascular injury from the perspective of other sources. One such source is the pooled records of medical-legal litigation cases, whereby, for example, a number of groups of investigators have demonstrated that even open laparoscopy can be associated with catastrophic major vascular injury.[21-23] Another group of investigators reviewed the list of 408 trocar-related major vascular injuries reported to the U.S. Food and Drug Administration (FDA) between 1993 and the end of 1996.[4] Although the incidence of injury cannot be ascertained from the data, the report does provide important information regarding the location of the lesions and the clinical impact of major vascular injury. Of the 408 reported injuries, 26 resulted in death, and 87% occurred despite the use of disposable T-CSs with "safety shields." The most common site of injury was the aorta (23%), followed by the vena cava (15%).

A more recent review of FDA reports focused on two optical access devices (Visiport, from United States Surgical Corp, Norwalk, Connecticut; Optiview, from Ethicon Endo-Surgery Inc., Cincinnati, Ohio) that purported to provide a degree of safety by allowing the operator to insert a clear but sharp trocar with a laparoscope positioned within it.[5] In this report, however, 37 major vascular injuries of the aorta, vena cava, and iliac vessels, are described, with a total of 4 deaths related to vascular injury. Although the incidence of these injuries with these "optical trocars" cannot be calculated from the data, the report does give rise to concern about the technique. These reports also seem to validate the concern that "safety shields," designed to protect vessels and viscera, in fact do not provide such protection, thereby justifying the FDA decision to forbid use of the term in product labeling. Furthermore, such reports, although hampered by the absence of a denominator from which outcome incidence may be calculated, provide some unique insights. For example, it is apparent that even major vascular injury may manifest in delayed fashion, usually involving retroperitoneal bleeding. In such instances, the clinical features of shock may not manifest until the patient is in the recovery room.

Recognition. Most often the problem manifests as profound hypotension, with or without the appearance of a significant volume of blood within the peritoneal cavity. In some instances, the surgeon aspirates blood through the insufflation needle, before introduction of the distending gas medium. Frequently the bleeding may be confined to the retroperitoneal space, a feature that usually delays the diagnosis. Consequently, the development of hypovolemic shock in the recovery room may well be secondary to an otherwise unrecognized laceration to a great vessel. To avoid the specter of late recognition, it is important to evaluate the course of each great vessel before completion of the procedure.

Management. If pure blood is drawn up by the insufflation needle, the needle should be left in place while immediate preparations are made to obtain replacement blood products and to perform laparotomy. If the diagnosis of hemoperitoneum is made on initial visualization of the peritoneal cavity, a grasping instrument may be used, if possible, to temporarily occlude the vessel. Although it is unlikely that significant injury can predictably be repaired by a laparoscopically directed technique, if temporary hemostasis can be obtained, and the laceration visualized, selected localized lesions can be repaired, with suture, under laparoscopic guidance. Such an attempt should not be made by other than experienced and technically adept surgeons. Even if such an instance exists, fine judgment should be used so as not to delay the institution of life-saving open surgical repair.

Most surgeons will be able to gain immediate entry into the peritoneal cavity by laparotomy and immediately compress the aorta and vena cava just below the level of the renal vessels, obtaining at least temporary control of blood loss. At that juncture, the most appropriate course of action, including the need for vascular surgical consultation, will become more apparent.

Abdominal Wall Vessels

Injury to the vessels of the abdominal wall, especially the deep inferior epigastric artery, can result in significant morbidity.[24] These injuries usually are secondary to the positioning of the accessory ports. The injury can occur with the initial insertion of a sharp trocar directly into the vessels, or later in the procedure when the incision is widened to allow passage of a larger cannula or for removal of tissue from the peritoneal cavity. Such injuries frequently are trivial but can account for nuisances such as blood dripping into the operative field. In some instances, however, they may result in postoperative bruising and occasionally significant morbidity from blood loss that often is not appreciated until well after completion of the procedure. Although injury to the deep inferior epigastric vessels generally is considered to be a common complication, information on the incidence of such injuries is lacking, at least in the gynecologic literature.

Recognition. Recognition of vessel injury is by visualization of the blood dripping down the cannula, or by the postoperative appearance of shock, abdominal wall discoloration, or a hematoma located near the incision. In some instances the

blood may track to a more distant site, manifesting as a pararectal or vulvar mass. Delayed diagnosis may be prevented at the end of the operation by laparoscopic evaluation of each peritoneal incision after removal of the cannula.

Management. Superficial inferior epigastric vessel lacerations usually heal with expectant management, and suturing is rarely necessary. Rotation of the cannula to a position at which compression is maximal also may be helpful.

Lacerated deep inferior epigastric vessels should be ligated. The use of a modified, straight ligature carrier such as that described in the section on instrumentation is most useful. After removal of the trocar and cannula, the ligature carrier is used to advance a suture under laparoscopic guidance, directing it laterally and inferiorly, where it is held by a grasping forceps. The ligature carrier is removed and subsequently passed through the incision again, without a suture, but this time medial and inferior to the lacerated vessels. The suture is threaded into the carrier from within the peritoneal cavity and is then externalized and tied. For small incisions, narrower than the diameter of the surgeon's finger, the knot may be tightened with a laparoscopic knot manipulator.

Other, less uniformly successful methods may be used for obtaining hemostasis from a lacerated deep inferior epigastric vessel. The most obvious is the placement of large, through-and-through mattress sutures, usually removed approximately 48 hours later. Electrodesiccation occasionally can be successful, as may temporary compression with the balloon of a Foley catheter that has been passed through the incision into the peritoneal cavity and then secured and tightened externally with a clamp. Although some clinicians suggest that the balloon should be left in place for 24 hours, the delicate channel may be damaged by the clamp, making it impossible to deflate the balloon. For this reason, this option is not recommended.

If the lacerated vessel presents postoperatively as a hematoma, initial management should be with local compression. The temptation to open or aspirate the hematoma should be resisted, because such a maneuver may inhibit the tamponade effect and could increase the risk of abscess formation. If the mass continues to enlarge, however, or if the patient demonstrates signs of hypovolemia, wound exploration is indicated.

Gastrointestinal Injury

Gastrointestinal injury secondary to laparoscopic access may result from the use of insufflation needles, the insertion of sharp trocars, or even the performance of the minilaparotomy required for the positioning of the cannula used in open laparoscopy (Fig. 4–15). Such trauma more frequently is encountered in the setting of previous abdominal surgery or peritonitis that results in fixation of the bowel to other structures, particularly to the anterior abdominal wall.[25] In such instances, the intestines are more susceptible to penetrating trauma from a sharp object, or even a relatively blunt trocar. The incidence of visceral injury has been estimated at 0.06% by Catarci and colleagues,[18] and a group from the Netherlands, using a retrospective comparative study, has reported the incidence of visceral injury to be 0.083% with closed technique and 0.048% in women in whom open laparoscopy is per-

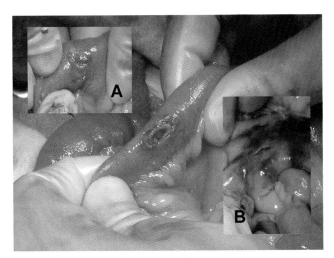

Figure 4–15 ▪ **Trocar injuries to small bowel.** These injuries occurred with the use of a hybrid deployable device similar to that depicted in Figure 4–6. In the *main photograph* and in *inset* A, bowel perforation occurred; in *inset* B, a mesenteric injury that resulted in intraperitoneal bleeding was found. Reexamination of the bowel demonstrated another transmural bowel injury *(not shown)*, emphasizing the need to carefully inspect the entire intestine for breaches in its integrity.

formed.[20] Some evidence suggests that a large proportion, if not a majority, of all bowel injuries incurred at gynecologic laparoscopy are related to laparoscopic access.[26] Many if not most gastrointestinal injuries are not recognized at the time of the index surgery, instead manifesting later in the postoperative course, often with catastrophic outcomes such as peritonitis, abscess, enterocutaneous fistula, or death.[23,26-28]

It is likely that most clinically significant injuries are created during the process of positioning the initial or primary cannula, although insertion of ancillary ports also may result in trauma, particularly to the iliac vessels or to the gastrointestinal tract. Insufflation needle–related injuries of the gastrointestinal tract may be more common than has been reported, for they may occur both unnoticed and without further complication. Nevertheless, the notion that such injuries are limited in caliber to the diameter of the needle should be discarded, because a needle that strikes the bowel in a tangential fashion may indeed function as a knife, rendering a linear lesion of substantial size.

Recognition. Recognition of gastric entry by the insufflation needle may follow identification of any or all of the signs of extraperitoneal entry, including increased filling pressure (to greater than 8 to 10 mm Hg), asymmetrical distention of the peritoneal cavity, and aspiration of gastric particulate matter through the lumen of the needle. The hollow, capacious nature of the stomach, however, may allow the initial insufflation pressure to remain normal. Unfortunately, in many instances, the problem is not identified until the trocar is inserted and the gastric mucosa is identified by direct vision. Recognition of bowel entry usually follows observation of the signs as described for gastric injury, with, in the case of colonic entry, the addition of feculent odor to the list of potential findings.

When a primary port is positioned using a trocar and closed technique, penetration of bowel often is diagnosed when the surgeon visualizes a mucosal lining on insertion of the laparoscope. If large bowel is entered, a feculent odor may be noted after withdrawal of the trocar. Frequently, however, the injury may not immediately be recognized, because the cannula may not stay within the bowel, or it may pass through the lumen and out the other side of the viscus. Such injuries usually occur when a loop of bowel is adherent to the anterior abdominal wall near the entry point, or with the insertion of ancillary cannulas. Such injuries may escape the surgeon's notice until they manifest postoperatively. Early postoperative symptoms can include increasing abdominal pain, abdominal distention, and initial leukopenia.[29,30] Fever generally is absent or low grade, and computed tomography (CT) findings may show an increasing amount of free intraperitoneal gas.[31,32] Unfortunately, later presentation, particularly of colonic perforation, is associated with peritonitis, septic shock, or even death.[30] Consequently, it is important for the surgeon to directly observe the insertion of all ancillary cannulas and, at the end of the procedure to directly view the removal of the primary cannula, either through the device itself or through an ancillary port. Furthermore, it is important to be diligent and responsive in both the institutional and postdischarge phases of care to patients' complaints of increasing abdominal pain.

Management. The management of any trauma to the gastrointestinal tract depends in part on the nature of the injury and in part on the organ(s) involved. In general, insufflation needle punctures that have not resulted in a defect significantly larger than needle diameter may be handled expectantly.[33] Larger defects should be repaired or resected by laparoscopic or laparotomy-based technique, the choice depending on the skill of the operator and the extent of the lesion.

If, after insertion of an insufflation needle, particulate debris is identified, the needle should be left in place and an alternate insertion site identified, such as the left upper quadrant. Alternatively, and if the insufflation needle possesses a removable obturator, a narrow-caliber laparoscope may be passed to evaluate the location of the tip and to aid in later identification of the puncture site. If another access site is selected, immediately after successful entry into the peritoneal cavity, the site of injury is identified. Unless significant injury or bleeding is identified, expectant management is adequate. If unexpected extension of the laceration occurs, it should be managed in a fashion similar to that for a trocar injury.

Trocar injuries to the gastrointestinal tract almost always require repair. If it can be ascertained that the injury is isolated, and if the operator is capable, the lesion may be repaired under laparoscopic guidance using appropriate suture. A number of approaches, many with single-layer closure, are possible; the preferred approach is use of a running 3-0 delayed absorbable suture, followed by placement of an imbricating layer of 2-0 caliber delayed absorbable suture that could be either running or interrupted, depending on the size of the defect and the preference of the surgeon. Surgeons using laparoscopic approaches should have had training and extensive experience in simulated or laboratory conditions to ensure that they are both effective and efficient with this approach. Extensive lacerations may require resection and reanastomosis, which may be performed under laparoscopic direction but in most instances will require laparotomy. If the injury is to sigmoid colon, primary laparoscopic or laparotomic repair may be attempted if the bowel has been mechanically prepared preoperatively. If uncertainty exists regarding the extent of injury, laparotomy is always indicated.

Bladder Injury

In gynecologic procedures, access-related vesical injury can occur during primary port insertion[34] but usually is secondary to trauma from the trocar used to insert an ancillary port entering the previously undrained bladder.

Recognition. The diagnosis of bladder injury is relatively easy if the surgeon recognizes entry into the bladder or when urine is found in the operative field. Hematuria is suggestive of urinary tract injury, and pneumaturia (CO_2 in the indwelling drainage system) is diagnostic of bladder wall entry. The existence of a bladder laceration may be confirmed with the injection of sterile milk or a dilute methylene blue solution through an indwelling catheter. Nevertheless, bladder injury may occur absent visualization of any of these findings and may manifest postoperatively with lower abdominal pain, fever, and sepsis, singly or in combination.[35] CT imaging may demonstrate free fluid within the peritoneal cavity and, if contrast is used, extravasation of dye from the bladder on delayed films.[31] Alternatively, a fluoroscopic or CT urogram can be performed after insertion of an indwelling catheter and injection of suitable contrast medium.

Management. The surgeon should first determine the extent of the damage. Because such injuries may take place without direct visualization, the potential exists that through-and-through damage has occurred.[35,36] Consequently, in some instances, cystoscopy, performed either transurethrally or transfundally, may be necessary.

Small-caliber injuries to the bladder (up to approximately 2 to 3 mm in diameter) will heal spontaneously with prolonged catheterization for 1 to 2 weeks.[34] The duration of such catheterization can be reduced or the need eliminated, however, if repair is undertaken intraoperatively. When a more significant injury to the bladder is identified, it usually can be repaired under laparoscopic guidance if the surgeon has the requisite skill and the location of injury makes repair amenable to use of laparoscopic technique.[37] Further evaluation of the location and extent of the laceration may be provided by direct laparocystoscopic examination of the bladder lumen using a small-caliber endoscope (1.5 to 2 mm in diameter). Should the laceration be near to or involve the trigone, open repair may be preferable.

For relatively small lesions, such as those made with insufflation needles or trocars (up to 1 cm), a single-layer, simple or pursestring closure may be fashioned using any of a number of synthetic absorbable sutures of 2-0 to 3-0 caliber, tying the knot either intra- or extracorporeally. For linear lacerations, the defect preferably is closed in two layers using absorbable suture.

The recommended extent of postoperative catheterization is changing and therefore remains controversial. Appro-

priately repaired intentional cystotomies in nondependent portions of the bladder may require no more than 24 hours of drainage.[38] These types of injury may be considered similar to simple insufflation- or trocar-related injuries. For large-caliber injuries, catheterization with either a urethral or suprapubic catheter of large caliber should be maintained for 5 to 7 days for simple fundal lacerations, and for 2 weeks for injuries closer to the trigone, or the vaginal vault.

Incisional Dehiscence and Hernia

Separation of the incision made for positioning a laparoscopic cannula may occur immediately after completion of the procedure, when it is deemed a *dehiscence*, or at a time more remote from the surgery, when if the peritoneal surface, with or without intraperitoneal content, passes through the defect, the defect is termed a *hernia*. Although originally considered to be rare occurrences, such incisional dehiscence and hernia have proved to be more common than was previously thought. In a survey of members of the American Association of Gynecologic Laparoscopists performed from our center, 933 such complications were reported.[39] Using an extrapolated denominator, we estimated the incidence at approximately 21 in 100,000 cases overall, or approximately 0.02%, with a higher incidence with the use of T-CSs larger than 10 mm ID—results that had been previously suggested by other investigators.[40] We suspect that these complications may be still underreported for a variety of reasons, such as failure to diagnose, delay in diagnosis, patient tolerance of asymptomatic hernia, the increasing number and size of cannulas used, and the resistance to publication of negative or adverse results. Indeed, one study reported an incidence of 1.8% for these complications in a group of patients in whom pyramidal trocars were used.[41] A sinister type of laparoscopy-related hernia is Richter's hernia, which contains only a portion of the intestinal wall in a defect of the peritoneum and, potentially, if present, the posterior fascia (Fig. 4–16). The entrapped portion of the bowel wall is susceptible to localized ischemia and necrosis. In patients so affected, the typical, externally visualized bulge of a hernia is not present, and the diagnosis often is delayed, sometimes with catastrophic results.[13] Diagnosis of this condition is difficult, requiring a high index of suspicion, and may be confirmed with an ultrasound study or a CT scan.[42]

Recognition. The most common defect appears in the immediate postoperative period when bowel or omentum passes through the unrepaired or inadequately repaired incision. The patient may be asymptomatic or can present with pain, fever, periumbilical mass, obvious evisceration, or the symptoms and signs of mechanical bowel obstruction, often within hours and usually within the first postoperative week. Because the patient usually is discharged home shortly after surgery, the clinical manifestations typically appear after hospital discharge, with signs and symptoms reported by telephone. Consequently, the surgeon should take care to assess the patient's complaints in timely fashion to determine whether or not they are consistent with herniation.

Because Richter's hernias contain only a portion of the circumference of the bowel wall in the defect, the diagnosis is

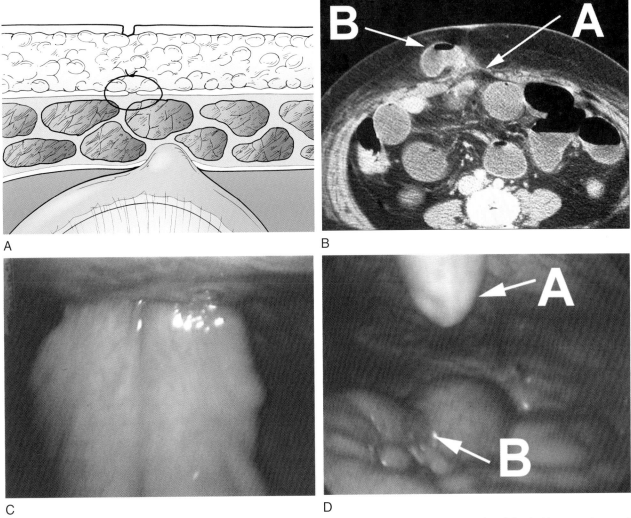

Figure 4–16 ▪ **Richter's hernia that occurred despite fascial closure. A,** Failure to close the peritoneal component of an abdominal laparoscopic wound can result in herniation of bowel that is not apparent clinically. Resulting infarction can result in peritonitis or even death. **B,** CT scan showing facial defect (A) and bowel herniating into subcutaneous tissue (B). **C,** Laparoscopic view of herniated bowel shown in **B. D,** Finger (A) passed through incision, releasing the bowel (B). (Photographs courtesy of Dr. Resad Pasic.)

often delayed.[13] It is likely that such lesions most commonly occur in incisions that are made away from the midline. The initial presenting symptom usually is pain, because the incomplete obstruction still allows the passage of intestinal contents. Fever can develop if incarceration occurs, and peritonitis may result from the subsequent perforation. The diagnosis is difficult to make and requires a high index of suspicion. Ultrasound examination or CT scanning may be useful in confirming the diagnosis.

Although many defects probably remain asymptomatic, late presentation is possible if bowel or omentum becomes trapped. The symptoms and findings are similar to those described for earlier presentations.

Management. Management of laparoscopic incisional defects depends on the timing of the presentation and the presence or absence of entrapped bowel and its condition.

Evisceration will always require surgical intervention. If the diagnosis is made in the recovery room, the patient may be returned to the operating room, the bowel or omentum replaced in the peritoneal cavity (provided that any evidence of necrosis or suture incorporation is absent), and the incision repaired, usually under laparoscopic guidance. If the diagnosis is delayed, however, it is likely that the bowel is incarcerated and at risk for perforation. In such circumstances, resection probably will be necessary, usually by means of laparotomy. Most gynecologic surgeons should request a general surgical consultation.

Wound Infection

Whereas wound infections following laparotomy are relatively common, those occurring after laparoscopic surgery—at least those of clinical significance—appear to be relatively rare. Most are minor skin and subcutaneous tissue infections that can be treated successfully with expectant management, antibiotics, or, in some instances, drainage.[42] The clinician should strive to carefully evaluate localized inflammation and swelling, because such findings may portend a wound dehiscence. Severe necrotizing fasciitis can occur rarely.[43]

Incisional Metastasis

An association of incisional metastases from intraperitoneal malignancy and laparoscopic surgery has been described. Published reports have included both gynecologic malignancies and a number of nongynecologic cancers, most notably adenocarcinoma of the colon. All of the gynecologic malignancies that have been the object of laparoscopic surgical intervention have been involved, including cancers of the cervix,[44-46] endometrium,[47] ovary,[48] and fallopian tube.[49] Additional published literature describes metastatic disease in laparoscopic incisions found in association with gastrointestinal malignancies.

Concern has arisen that incisional metastases may be more common after laparoscopic procedures than after laparotomy, and that the prognosis for the patient may be adversely affected. Experimental animal models evaluating the role of intraperitoneal pressure in the genesis of port site metastasis have produced conflicting results. The results of some of these studies show that increased intraperitoneal pressure increases the risk of incisional metastasis,[50-52] whereas others fail to demonstrate such a difference.[53,54] Some investigators have suggested that the difference in the incidence of seeding of laparoscopic and laparotomic incisions is insignificant. For example, in a randomized controlled trial (RCT) in patients with colonic cancer treated either by laparotomy or by laparoscopic technique, no difference was observed in any clinical outcomes, including the incidence of incisional metastatic disease.[55]

MINIMIZING THE RISK OF ACCESS COMPLICATIONS

Risk reduction requires a discipline of patient preparation, selection of proper instrumentation, and application of technique appropriate to the clinical situation. Simply put, the surgeon is charged with positioning cannulas in the abdominal wall sufficient in number and appropriate in location to allow for expeditious and safe completion of the procedure. The first objective is the positioning of a cannula through which an endoscope can be passed for visualization of the procedure to be performed. Ancillary ports, through which the hand instruments are passed, are inserted under direct laparoscopic guidance after establishment of the pneumoperitoneum.

Insertion of the Primary Cannula

A number of approaches to positioning the initial or primary cannula are possible, including the preinsufflation technique, direct insertion without preinsufflation, and the creation of a minilaparotomy (i.e., open laparoscopy). Each technique for positioning the initial cannula has a number of variations that may provide value depending on the specific clinical situation. Regardless of the technique selected, a number of important steps are necessary before the procedure itself is begun.

PREPROCEDURAL PREPARATION

Informed consent should be obtained well before the patient comes to the operating room. The informed consent process should include some discussion of the potential for access complications. Although such complications are relatively rare, the potentially catastrophic nature of some, such as injury to the great vessels, should be disclosed to and fully discussed with the patient. The possibility that risk may be greater with previous surgery is a factor that should be stressed. Although my patients undergo mechanical bowel preparation for any laparoscopic procedure except routine sterilization, such an approach is strongly recommended for any patient who has had previous abdominal surgery. This measure generally improves exposure of the operative field. Moreover, should large bowel injury occur, adequate mechanical bowel preparation means that repair can be undertaken without resorting to a proximal defunctioning colostomy.

The surgeon should ensure that appropriate access instrumentation is available for each surgical case. For example, obese patients may require longer insufflation needles and access cannulas, and certain types of endoscopes or hand instrumentation may require cannulas of especially narrow or wide caliber. As discussed later on, patients with previous abdominal surgery may be selected for primary access in the left upper quadrant. In such instances, the anesthesiologist should position an orogastric or nasogastric tube after the induction of anesthesia but before the access process is commenced. The surgeon also should be cognizant of difficulties that the anesthesiologist may have had with the intubation. For example, if the esophagus was inadvertently intubated, the stomach could become so distended as to be susceptible to injury from the insufflation needle or trocar tip. In such circumstances, the stomach should be decompressed.

Consistent positioning of patients for laparoscopic access is important to retain the relationships of the intraperitoneal vessels and viscera to the various anatomic landmarks used by the surgeon. This is especially true for the closed or "blind" entry techniques, which generally employ a sharp-tipped instrument of some kind. The patient should be positioned supine on the table, without rotation or tipping into a head-down or modified Trendelenburg position. In such instances, the location of the great vessels may be brought into line with the axis of insertion of the insufflation needle or T-CS. Similarly, rotation of the patient may bring the iliac vessels into the path of the access instrumentation, thereby facilitating injury (Fig. 4–17).

PREINSUFFLATION TECHNIQUE

A narrow-caliber hollow needle is used to inflate the peritoneal cavity before insertion of a larger-caliber access cannula for the laparoscope. The safety of this blind process is

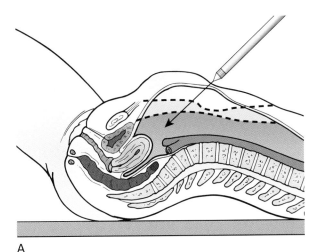

A

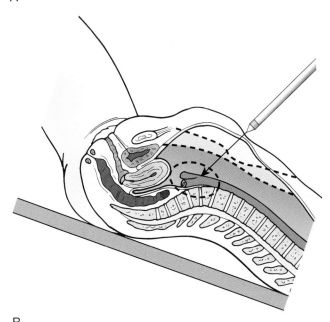

B

Figure 4–17 ▪ **Perils of blind insertion with patient in the Trendelenburg position.** If the same angle of insertion is used in Trendlenburg's position (**A**) as in the supine position (**B**), the trocar may be directed at the great vessels in the midline (*dotted oval* in **B**). Consequently, it is best to position at least the first umbilical trocar-cannula system with the patient supine. Also see Figure 4–22.

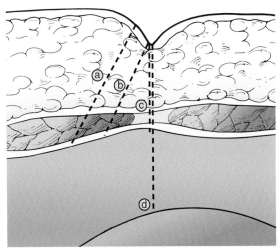

Figure 4–18 ▪ **Abdominal wall thickness and angle of insertion.** With increasing abdominal wall thickness, the distance traversed by insufflation needles or trocar-cannula systems increases disproportionately with distance below the umbilicus and angle of insertion. For example, when a device is inserted through a subumbilical incision and directed at an angle (a), the distance is greater than when the device is passed at the same angle through an intraumbilical incision (b). Although in thin patients this difference may not be of clinical significance, in obese persons it may be the determining factor in success versus failure at correct intraperitoneal placement. In very obese patients, inserting the device through a 90-degree angle (to horizontal) may be necessary (c), but care must be taken to avoid injury to vessels located immediately beneath (d). In most (but not all) obese persons, the umbilicus is below these vessels when the patient is supine.

dependent on the absence of adhesions beneath the insertion site. The presence of surgical scars in the abdomen should provide a warning that underlying adhesions may exist, potentially involving bowel and increasing the risk of gastrointestinal injury. In such instances, alternative approaches to peritoneal entry should be considered.

Positioning the Insufflation Needle in the Umbilical Location

The usual site for insertion of the insufflation needle is deep in the umbilicus, where the abdominal wall is the thinnest. A longitudinal or transverse incision is made at the discretion of the surgeon, generally depending on the anatomy of the umbilicus. If a subumbilical incision is made, the likelihood of preperitoneal placement is greater, especially in obese patients (Fig. 4–18).

The needle should be checked for patency, the sprung obturator for appropriate function, and the integrated Luer-Lok placed in the open position. It is best to lift the abdomen firmly with the nondominant hand to create a space between the peritoneum and the retroperitoneal structures. If it is difficult to grasp and lift adequately, an assistant should be used. Application of Baccus clamps (towel clips) around the umbilicus may further assist in this elevation process, particularly in obese patients. The needle is gently held between the thumb and first two fingers of the dominant hand as close to the distal tip as possible, thereby facilitating proprioception during insertion and limiting the length of the needle that can enter the peritoneal cavity. It is then purposely directed in a midline sagittal plane toward the hollow of the sacrum, where no major vessels are present and where the bowel generally is mobile and capable of moving away if hit by the insertion device. In obese patients, this angle necessarily is steeper, approaching 90 degrees to the horizontal. In general, two "pops" are heard or felt, reflecting breaching of the anterior rectus sheath and then of the peritoneum, but if the location of the incision is at the base of the umbilicus, only one such "pop" may be noted, reflecting the fusion of all layers at this location.

Techniques purported to confirm proper needle placement include saline injection and aspiration to detect blood or stool, the ability to create negative intraperitoneal pressure by lifting the abdominal wall, the early detection of loss of percussed liver dullness with the onset of insufflation, and measurement of an initial intraperitoneal pressure of less than 10 mm Hg. Although such measures may have clinical value, evidence is lacking that any is individually or collectively absolutely predictive of proper positioning.

Despite the putative application of these measures, vascular and visceral injury occurs in association with closed laparoscopic technique. In a French study, approximately 75% of the vascular injuries were related to the insufflation needle and 25% to the T-CS.[56] It is unclear how many of these injuries could have been prevented with appropriate modifications in technique based on available clinical information such as previous lower abdominal or pelvic surgery. One group of investigators has suggested the use of a small-caliber endoscope that can be passed through an insufflation needle to confirm proper placement.[57] Nevertheless, such an approach would seem more likely to make an early visual diagnosis of injury, rather than to prevent it. Consequently, when proper placement of the insufflation needle cannot be achieved or the existence of a previous surgical incision precludes safe blind insertion of the insufflation needle, alternate approaches should be considered.

Once the insufflation needle is positioned, most clinicians infuse the distending gas until a target pressure of 12 to 15 mm Hg is reached. Some evidence suggests, however, that inflating to a higher level (25 to 30 mm Hg) may assist in separating the anterior abdominal wall from the intra-abdominal and retroperitoneal vessels and viscera, thereby reducing the risk of injury.[58] Of note, if maintained for prolonged periods of time, such pressures increase the risk of hypercapnia and acidemia[59]; therefore, if higher pressures are used, they should be returned to 12 mm Hg or less once the access ports have been established, to minimize the risks of hypercarbia.[60]

Alternate Insertion Sites

If previous surgery has been performed in the abdomen, and particularly if an incision was located anywhere near the umbilicus, an alternate site should be chosen for positioning the insufflation needle. In view of the risks of visceral and vascular injury in the patient with previous abdominal or pelvic surgery, use of one of the following approaches should be considered:

• Left upper quadrant[61-63]
• Cul-de-sac of Douglas
• Uterine fundus

Any of these approaches also may be of particular value in the obese patient.[64]

An extremely useful alternative site is in the left upper quadrant, usually in the midclavicular line just below the costal margin (see Fig. 4–18).[61] Drainage of the stomach with an orogastric or nasogastric tube should precede left upper quadrant insertion of an insufflation needle. In the upper abdominal wall, the existence of separate anterior and posterior rectus fascia, in addition to the peritoneum, creates three distinct layers to traverse in insertion of the needle. An appropriately sized incision generally is made in the midclavicular

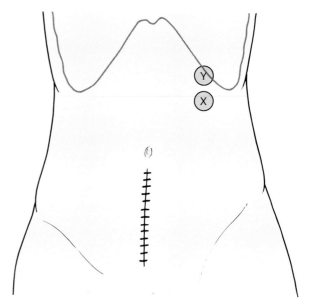

Figure 4–19 ■ **Left upper quadrant access.** The spot marked X is *Palmer's point*, described by the French laparoscopist of the same name. It generally is preferable to position the insufflation needle higher, just below the costal margin (Y), and to use a 2.7-mm trocar-cannula system that allows insertion of a 2-mm laparoscope (see Fig. 4–10). In such circumstances, correct placement can be confirmed before insufflation. This technique must not be used in patients who have undergone previous left upper quadrant surgery. The stomach should be decompressed with a nasogastric or oralgastric tube before placement of the laparoscope.

line just below the costal margin. The needle is inserted at a relatively steep angle (60 to 80 degrees) and slightly (approximately 10 degrees) toward the midline. Insertion in this location may not be appropriate if the patient has undergone previous left upper quadrant surgery.

Other sites for insufflation needle placement include the cul-de-sac of Douglas[65,66] and the uterine fundus.[67] Before using the cul-de-sac of Douglas for insufflation, the surgeon should be as certain as possible that this area is free of masses or adhesions such as those encountered with previous surgery or in severe endometriosis, in which the sigmoid colon can be fused to the posterior uterus. The patient is placed in Trendelenburg's position, and a vaginal speculum is inserted and a tenaculum attached to the posterior lip of the cervix, which is then placed in traction and lifted anteriorly, putting the posterior fornix on the stretch (Fig. 4–19). A long insufflation needle (150 mm) is aligned with the axis of the cervical canal (thereby avoiding the sigmoid colon) and purposefully passed into the peritoneal cavity. Tests for appropriate positioning are similar to those employed for insertion elsewhere.

If adhesions involve or potentially involve the umbilicus, the left upper quadrant, and the cul-de-sac, transfundal insufflation can be considered (Fig. 4–20). After the patient has been placed in Trendelenburg's position and a vaginal speculum has been inserted, the anterior lip of the cervix is grasped with a tenaculum and the cervix placed in traction. As with insufflation through the cul-de-sac, a long insufflation needle is required and is placed through and colinear with the axis of the cervical canal. As the needle is pushed through the uterine

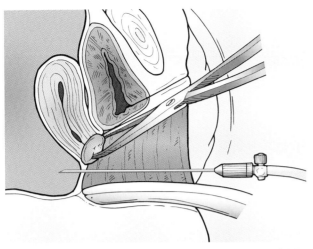

Figure 4–20 ▪ **Insufflation through the cul-de-sac of Douglas.** If abdominal access is prevented, cul-de-sac insufflation can be performed, provided that no obstructions such as adhesions are present, binding the rectosigmoid to the posterior cervix. The posterior lip of the cervix is held under anterior traction, and the needle is inserted while avoiding the sigmoid.

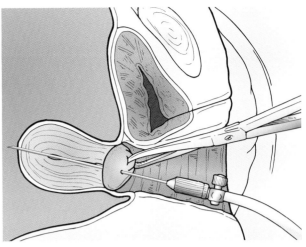

Figure 4–21 ▪ **Transfundal insufflation.** This approach is a last resort in the event that abdominal or cul-de-sac access is impossible or fraught with too much risk. The uterus should be relatively small and the cavity structurally normal, and the risk of adhesions to the corpus, as would occur from past surgery (e.g., myomectomy), must be essentially zero.

fundus, the corpus is anteverted. Tests of proper positioning are similar to those for other insertion sites. This approach should be avoided when the endometrial cavity is distorted with myomas, when the corpus is significantly enlarged, or when the presence of adhesions to the uterus is likely, such as after abdominal or laparoscopic myomectomy. For both cul-de-sac and transfundal insufflation, the needle should be removed under direct vision.

Placement of the Primary Cannula

When an appropriate intraperitoneal pressure is reached, the initial or primary cannula is positioned. As discussed in the section on instrumentation, devices of varied design are available with different mechanisms for penetrating the abdominal wall. The traditional approach is to use a T-CS that possesses a pyramidal or conical trocar for penetration of the abdominal wall after creation of a small skin incision with a scalpel. In the absence of previous pelvic or abdominal surgery, the device is passed through the intraumbilical incision, held in a sagittal plane, and directed purposefully toward the hollow of the sacrum, as described for insufflation needles. In obese patients, it may be necessary to direct the T-CS closer to a vertical plane, but extreme care should be exerted to ensure that adequate space exists between the abdominal wall and the great vessels and that the length of trocar that passes into the peritoneal cavity is controlled (Fig. 4–21). The T-CS is held with the thenar eminence of the dominant hand over the trocar hub and with the remaining fingers and thumb positioned around the hub and on the proximal shaft of the cannula.

It is important to limit the amount of the system that enters the peritoneal cavity, to reduce the risk of injury, particularly to the retroperitoneally located great vessels. The amount of allowable length will vary somewhat based on abdominal wall thickness, but if the incision is placed in the umbilicus, this length generally will range from 3 to 5 cm. For surgeons with large hands who are using relatively short cannulas, a functional "stop" can be created by extending the index finger of the dominant hand (Fig. 4–22). For those with smaller hands, however, or for anyone using relatively long instruments, such a technique will be insufficient. Consequently, adding the second hand is necessary to limit the length of trocar and cannula that is inserted into the peritoneal cavity (see Fig. 4–22). For many surgeons, including female surgeons, this hand also may be used to add to the insertion force while preserving safety of insertion.

Twisting motions generally are not necessary with pyramidal or other sharp-tipped devices. A number of devices, however, require specific insertion techniques. The ADAPT system (Taut Inc., Geneva, Illinois) has a blunt-tipped obturator that requires a pronounced rotational action to allow penetration of the abdominal wall (see Fig. 4–5). The surgeon's dominant hand is rotated clockwise and then counterclockwise in 180-degree arcs, with relatively moderate axial pressure. It may take 10 to 15 seconds to achieve penetration with this technique. The EndoTIP device (Karl Storz Endoscopy America) has no trocar (see Fig. 4–9). Instead, the subcutaneous tissue is dissected away, and the device is used to engage the fascia by means of the blunt-tipped screw tip on the side of the cannula. The device is twisted in, with an endoscope in its lumen that guides the insertion until the peritoneum is breached and the peritoneal cavity visualized. Originally the manufacturer suggested that an incision be made in the fascia, but such a step now seems unnecessary. The Step trocar (Autosuture Division of United States Surgical Corp.) (see Fig. 4–5) requires that a proprietary sheath be positioned with an insufflation needle. After positioning of the needle, the sheath is pushed as far as possible into the abdominal wall. Then the needle is removed and the obturator-cannula system is introduced into the flute-shaped proximal aspect of the sheath. Now, using two hands, and usually with a twisting motion, the operator passes the obturator into the peritoneal cavity by dilating the initially small incision

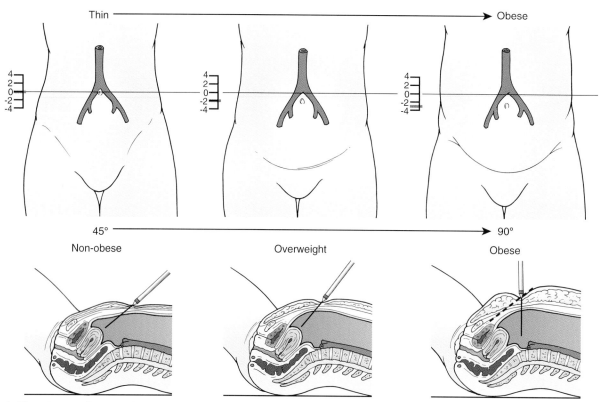

Figure 4–22 ▪ **Impact of patient obesity on insertion angle.** The *bottom series* of figures depicts the fate of an insufflation needle placed at the same 45-degree angle in non-obese, overweight, and obese persons—it is preperitoneal in the obese patient. The *top series* of figures (after Hurd et al[83]) shows the changing relationship between the umbilicus and the bifurcation in similar patients. Note that with obese patients, the umbilicus typically (but not always—note the error bars) is 2-3 cm caudal to the bifurcation, permitting the safe insertion of the needle in a vertical orientation.

made by the insufflation needle. A relatively large amount of force is required to achieve this step, especially when large-caliber (10- to 12-mm) devices are used.

The risk of injury to intraperitoneal structures may be associated with loss of control of a sharp trocar during attempts to penetrate the abdominal wall. When the abdominal wall is finally breached, the trocar may suddenly "pop" into the peritoneal cavity in an uncontrolled fashion, and with considerable force. In a survey of Canadian gynecologists done before the introduction of disposable T-CSs, up to a third admitted to experiencing "difficulty" in applying sufficient force during insertion of either the primary or ancillary T-CS. Injuries occurred twice as often in procedures in which the operator had experienced such difficulty.[68] Determining the cause of the difficulty is not possible at this point, of course, but likely contributing factors include suboptimal technique, unfamiliarity with or less advantageous instrument design, and, in the case of reusable instrumentation, poorly maintained and dull trocar tips. One interpretation of this information is that unless the surgeon can control the T-CS carefully, the risk of injury may increase—a perception that led to the dissemination of the unproven concept that sharper trocars would be associated with reduced risk of injury.[69] This may be true if the trocar is sharp enough to enter the bowel but not sharp enough to traverse the abdominal wall efficiently. The advent of so-called blunt trocars (see Fig. 4–5) challenges that concept, however. It is clear that these devices

generally require more force by which to gain entry,[6] but the devices may be too blunt to damage the great vessels. Consequently, and especially if these devices can be inserted with control, they may reduce significantly the incidence of vascular injury associated with closed techniques.

A number of factors may influence control of the T-CS as it is inserted. One such factor is height of the operating room table as a work surface for the surgeon. If the table is set to a height that requires the surgeon to elevate the arms markedly, the result is reduced control, with perhaps a greater risk for injury. Consequently, it seems important for the surgeon to drop the table to the level of the waist or, if this maneuver does not establish the appropriate relationship, to achieve the same goal by standing on a platform of adequate height. In view of the high intraperitoneal pressure necessary for insertion of the cannula, use of a relatively short cannula is recommended, and the fingers of the second hand should be applied to the shaft to limit the length of the device entering the peritoneal cavity (Fig. 4–23). Adherence to these precautions likely minimizes the risk of vascular injury.

It seems intuitively obvious that blunt-tipped trocars should carry less risk of vascular injury than that reported for pyramidal trocars or even those with a sharp conical design. Some evidence suggests, however, that even the type of sharp trocar tip may influence the risk of major vascular injury. For example, Hurd, in an animal model, demonstrated that a conical trocar would have to score a "direct hit" on a mesen-

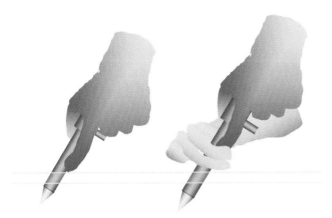

Figure 4–23 ▪ **Limiting insertion distance.** Limitation of insertion distance is one key component of safe positioning of laparoscopic ports. If the surgeon's hand is large enough, or if the cannula is short enough, the index finger may serve as a stopper *(left)*. In other circumstances, however, the index finger may not suffice, and the index and middle fingers must be combined with the thumb of the other hand to accomplish this task *(right)*.

teric vessel to cause vascular injury, whereas the 10 mm pyramidal device of the same diameter caused significant vessel trauma if it struck virtually anywhere in a radius of four millimeters.[70]

Consequently, in view of the apparent superiority of the threaded cannula and conical or blunt-tipped trocars with respect to wound parameters, and a potential if not probable reduced risk of vascular injury, they should be strongly considered for routine use with closed techniques.

CLOSED INSERTION WITHOUT PREINSUFFLATION

It is evident that when vascular injury occurs in association with closed laparoscopic technique, at least a large proportion and perhaps a majority of such injuries can be ascribed to the insufflation needle. In a French study, approximately 75% of the vascular injuries were related to the insufflation needle and 25% to the T-CS.[56] At least in selected patients, therefore, this step probably could be omitted. Reasonably good evidence suggests that insertion of the initial or primary cannula can be safely accomplished without preinsufflation, provided that the patient has no history of previous peritonitis or abdominal or pelvic intraperitoneal surgery.[71-74] The technique requires that the abdominal wall be lifted to provide counterpressure against the vector of force created by the trocar, if a trocar is used. Although surgeons with relatively large hands may safely insert a T-CS with one hand while holding the abdomen with another, a safer option may involve the use of two hands on the T-CS as described previously, with the fingers of the nondominant hand on the cannula serving to prevent entry of too much of the device into the peritoneal cavity. In such instances, a capable assistant provides the needed lift of the anterior abdominal wall.

An effective closed insertion technique is the use of a modified Veress needle, with a removable sprung obturator, which allows a small-caliber endoscope to be inserted into the peritoneal cavity. This technique is especially useful in the presence of lower abdominal incisions, if the patient has not previously undergone surgery in the left upper quadrant. The device is inserted subcostally in the left midclavicular line, after decompression of the stomach with a nasogastric or orogastric tube.[61,75,76]

OPEN LAPAROSCOPY

Cannulas can be inserted after the creation of a minilaparotomy incision, an approach introduced by Hasson's "open laparoscopy." Although this approach appears to entail less risk of injury to blood vessels, it is clear that such injuries can occur, particularly in thin patients.[21,77,78] In these circumstances, it is assumed that while working in the confines of such a small incision, the surgeon may inadvertently grasp the posterior peritoneum and enter great vessels with scissors or a knife. It is not clear that open laparoscopy confers better protection against intestinal injury in comparison with other techniques such as left upper quadrant access, described elsewhere in this chapter—if adherent to the anterior abdominal wall, intestine can be entered inadvertently, no matter how small or big the laparotomy incision.

Inserting Ancillary Cannulas

Ancillary cannulas are necessary for the performance of most diagnostic and operative laparoscopic procedures. Most of the currently available disposable ancillary access ports are identical to those designed for use as primary cannulas, but are of smaller caliber, reflecting the generally smaller diameter of hand instruments. Proper and safe positioning of these ancillary ports depends on insight regarding surgical strategy and a sound knowledge of the vascular anatomy of the anterior abdominal wall and that of the underlying great vessels and viscera.

Access-related bladder injury can largely be prevented by preprocedural drainage with a transurethral catheter. With previous lower abdominal surgery performed through transverse incisions, however, the bladder may be pulled up to an abnormally high level. In the presence of such incisions, it may be most appropriate to keep the incision at or above the level of the previoius incision.[79]

Lower-quadrant cannulas usually are necessary for operative laparoscopy in the female pelvis, but the deep inferior epigastric vessels present an obstacle that must be avoided (Fig. 4–24). Although intraperitoneal transillumination may reveal the location of the superficial inferior epigastric vessels in a majority of instances, it is less accurate in dark-skinned persons and persons with increasing body mass.[80] Furthermore, it is not useful for identifying the deep inferior epigastric vessels that lie below the rectus muscle, presenting a much greater risk for significant hemorrhage.[81] The deep inferior epigastric artery is the last branch of the external iliac artery before it courses under the inguinal ligament. For the laparoscopist, the most consistent landmarks are the median umbilical ligament (obliterated umbilical artery) and the entry point of the round ligament into the inguinal canal through the internal inguinal ring. At the pubic crest, the deep inferior epigastric vessels begin their course cephalad between the medially located umbilical ligament and the laterally positioned exit point of the round ligament. In most instances the

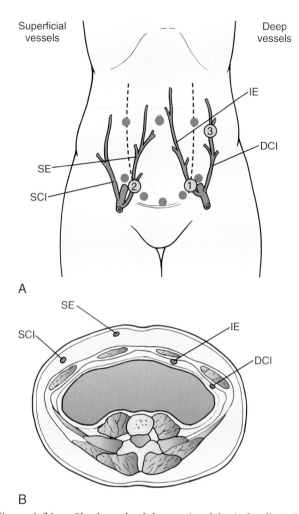

A

B

Figure 4–24 ▪ **Blood vessels of the anterior abdominal wall. A,** Four pairs of vessels require specific consideration in gynecologic laparoscopic procedures: the deep inferior epigastrics (1, IE), the superficial epigastrics (2, SE), the deep circumflex iliacs (3, DCI), and the superficial circumflex iliacs (SCI). The *dashed lines* depict the lateral edge of the rectus abdominis muscles. The *blue circles* represent the ideal cunnula placement sites. **B,** The vessels are shown in cross section at approximately 1 cm below the umbilicus. (**A** and **B** redrawn after Hurd et al.[14])

vessels can be seen, and frequently, arterial pulsation can be traced cephalad. Particularly in obese patients, however, the location often is obscured with fat, so that the deep vessels are seen in less than three fourths of the cases.[80]

The T-CS should be inserted well medial or lateral to the vessels if they are visualized. If the deep vessels can be seen, but obesity precludes accurate localization of an appropriate incision site and angle of insertion, a spinal needle can be placed to facilitate orientation. If the vessels cannot be seen and the cannula must be positioned in the lower quadrant, it should be placed approximately 8 cm lateral to the midline, 5 cm above the symphysis.[14] Care should be taken to avoid an insertion site that is too laterally located, which may endanger the deep circumflex epigastric artery (see Fig. 4–24). Lower abdominal ancillary ports can be inserted approximately 4 cm from the midline if they are 3 cm above the symphysis.[14] In inserting the port, care must be taken not to direct the lower-

quadrant T-CS medially, where it may strike the deep inferior epigastric vessels despite attempts to avoid such an injury. Instead, the entry is perpendicular or nearly perpendicular to the skin surface, preferably with an intraperitoneal pressure at 25 mm Hg and placing the fingers of the nondominant hand on the shaft of the cannula. Then, after creation of the skin incision, the T-CS is carefully inserted in controlled fashion.

Wound Management

The tip design of the T-CS may be important in evaluating the risk of a number of complications, including bleeding at the insertion site, hernia and dehiscence, and injury to abdominal and pelvic vessels and viscera. Some data support an increased frequency of incisional hernia and dehiscence associated with use of pyramidal tips. A group of investigators from Germany, in a nonrandomized comparative study, showed that the risk of incisional hernia was more than 10 times greater when a disposable pyramidal device was used than when access was gained with reusable conical T-CS (1.83% versus 0.17%).[41] Our group has described a mechanism that may explain these differences by evaluating the effect of tip design on laparoscopic wound parameters in a swine model.[3] A randomized and observer-blinded study demonstrated that the pyramidal and bladed devices evaluated created significantly larger fascial defects than those observed with use of the two disposable conical devices; these findings apparently were confirmed by other investigators.[82] Subsequent work has shown that substantial movement of the device in surgery does not seem to change the parameters of wounds created with conical devices.[7]

One obvious question is whether the fascial defects should be closed in an attempt to reduce the risk of dehiscence or hernia when T-CSs with an ID of 10 mm or more are used. The answer is not clear, but in view of the relative frequency of incisional hernia associated with devices with an ID of more than 10 mm, it seems prudent to close and then suture both the fascia and the underlying peritoneum, the latter to prevent Richter's hernia. The influence of screw-like anchoring systems on wound size has not been reported, but it would be reasonable to surmise that they may add to the trauma, so that if they are used in association with 10-mm-ID devices and perhaps even 8-mm-ID cannulas, routine closure should be considered. The apparent reduced impact of conical devices on wound parameters, and thus on the risk of hernia and dehiscence, invites contemplation about the need to close such wounds, even if devices up to 12 mm in diameter are used. One group of investigators performed an RCT comparing a pyramidal design with a radially expanding system that appears to create wounds that are similar in size and other characteristics to those produced by a conical device of similar diameter.[8] The incisions of greater than 10 mm diameter made with the pyramidal systems were routinely closed, whereas those associated with the radially dilating system were not. Although the numbers were relatively small, no incisional defects developed in the conical group. In a recent series, a 12-mm blunt conical system created fascial defects similar to those observed with use of an 8-mm-ID pyramidal system, and the extent of the muscle injury was even less.[7] Thus, routine closure of these 12-mm-device–related incisions may be unnecessary.

The type of trocar tip also may have an impact on postoperative outcomes short of hernia and dehiscence. One well-designed trial using a radially expanding system and a pyramidal device demonstrated that incisions were smaller and patient perception of pain was significantly less when the radially expanding system was used. In view of the similarities in wound parameters between blunt conical devices and the radially dilating device,[3] it seems likely that any of these tissue-dilating systems would achieve similar results.

CONCLUSIONS

Access to the peritoneal cavity is critical to the performance of any laparoscopic procedure. Often overlooked are the potential complications associated with peritoneal access, largely because they are relatively uncommon, and the fact that most surgeons will encounter relatively few, if any, of the serious, life-threatening variety in their professional careers. Clearly, vascular and visceral injury together constitute the most sinister of the complications, and the diagnosis of each may not be made until some time later—a situation that often compounds the severity of the situation. A review of the currently available literature suggests that overall, major vascular injury, although rare, is more common with closed techniques for positioning the primary cannula than with open laparoscopy. Nevertheless, major vascular injury may occur with open laparoscopy, and it is possible that closed techniques may be at least equally safe if they are modified by use of alternate insertion sites and access devices associated with lower risk, such as threaded cannulas or conical or blunt trocars. These approaches may be particularly important in reducing the risk of access-based visceral injury in the face of previous surgery—a complication for which the risk may not be affected by open laparoscopy.

Other complications, such as wound dehiscence and hernia, also are more prevalent than was previously thought and may be reduced in incidence by proper closure of selected fascial and peritoneal defects or by use of access systems that minimize the size and configuration of myofascial wounds. Wound size may be limited by using smaller-caliber instrumentation with smaller-diameter access cannulas, or by selecting access systems that minimize trauma to the anterior abdominal wall. Admittedly, the evidence supporting the notion that such approaches will reduce these risks is preliminary at best, but absent the existence of RCTs, it would seem prudent to use the results of available animal and clinical studies to guide clinical practice. Furthermore, some clinical advantages may accrue to use of these devices, such as reduced pain and incisional bleeding and bruising, and smaller-caliber access systems should be associated with a reduced cosmetic impact.

The issue of metastatic seeding of access port incisions is not yet resolved. First of all, an association with increased risk of such seeding has not been convincingly demonstrated, and if such a risk exists, its impact on prognosis has not been determined. Some evidence indicates that careful handling of the surgical specimen, using bags for removal and, if possible, ensuring that the instruments do not come in contact with the malignant tissue, may reduce the incidence of port-related metastatic disease. Clearly, however, more careful and comparative basic and clinical research will be necessary to further elucidate the relevance of this recently perceived potential problem.

References

1. Uen YH, Liang AI, Lee HH. Randomized comparison of conventional carbon dioxide insufflation and abdominal wall lifting for laparoscopic cholecystectomy. J Laparoendosc Adv Surg Tech A 2002;12:7.
2. Horvath KD, Whelan RL, Lier B, et al. The effects of elevated intra-abdominal pressure, hypercarbia, and positioning on the hemodynamic responses to laparoscopic colectomy in pigs. Surg Endosc 1998;12:107.
3. Tarnay CM, Glass KB, Munro MG. Incision characteristics associated with six laparoscopic trocar-cannula systems: A randomized, observer-blinded comparison. Obstet Gynecol 1999;94:89.
4. Bhoyrul S, Vierra MA, Nezhat CR, et al. Trocar injuries in laparoscopic surgery. J Am Coll Surg 2001;192:677.
5. Sharp HT, Dodson MK, Draper ML, et al. Complications associated with optical-access laparoscopic trocars. Obstet Gynecol 2002;99:553.
6. Tarnay CM, Glass KB, Munro MG. Entry force and intra-abdominal pressure associated with six laparoscopic trocar-cannula systems: A randomized comparison. Obstet Gynecol 1999;94:83.
7. Munro MG, Tarnay CM. The impact of trocar-cannula design and simulated operative manipulation on incisional characteristics: A randomized trial. Obstet Gynecol 2004;103:681.
8. Bhoyrul S, Payne J, Steffes B, et al. A randomized prospective study of radially expanding trocars in laparoscopic surgery. J Gastrointest Surg 2000;4:392.
9. Ternamian AM. Laparoscopy without trocars. Surg Endosc 1997;11:815.
10. Ternamian AM, Deitel M. Endoscopic threaded imaging port (EndoTIP) for laparoscopy: Experience with different body weights. Obes Surg 1999;9:44.
11. Glass KB, Tarnay CM, Munro MG. Randomized comparison of the effect of manipulation on incisional parameters associated with a pyramidal laparoscopic trocar-cannula system and the EndoTIP cannula. J Am Assoc Gynecol Laparosc 2003;10:412.
12. Glass KB, Tarnay CM, Munro MG. Intraabdominal pressure and incision parameters associated with a pyramidal laparoscopic trocar-cannula system and the EndoTIP cannula. J Am Assoc Gynecol Laparosc 2002;9:508.
13. Matthews BD, Heniford BT, Sing RF. Preperitoneal Richter hernia after a laparoscopic gastric bypass. Surg Laparosc Endosc Percutan Tech 2001;11:47.
14. Hurd WW, Bude RO, DeLancey JO, Newman JS. The location of abdominal wall blood vessels in relationship to abdominal landmarks apparent at laparoscopy. Am J Obstet Gynecol 1994;171:642.
15. Baadsgaard SE, Bille S, Egeblad K. Major vascular injury during gynecologic laparoscopy. Report of a case and review of published cases. Acta Obstet Gynecol Scand 1989;68:283.
16. Nordestgaard AG, Bodily KC, Osborne RW Jr, Buttorff JD. Major vascular injuries during laparoscopic procedures. Am J Surg 1995;169:543.
17. Riedel HH, Lehmann-Willenbrock E, Conrad P, Semm K. German pelviscopic statistics for the years 1978-1982. Endoscopy 1986;18:219.
18. Catarci M, Carlini M, Gentileschi P, Santoro E. Major and minor injuries during the creation of pneumoperitoneum. A multicenter study on 12,919 cases. Surg Endosc 2001;15:566.
19. Champault G, Cazacu F, Taffinder N. Serious trocar accidents in laparoscopic surgery: A French survey of 103,852 operations. Surg Laparosc Endosc 1996;6:367.
20. Bonjer HJ, Hazebroek EJ, Kazemier G, et al. Open versus closed establishment of pneumoperitoneum in laparoscopic surgery. Br J Surg 1997;84:599.
21. Soderstrom RM. Injuries to major blood vessels during endoscopy. J Am Assoc Gynecol Laparosc 1997;4:395.
22. Vilos GA. Litigation of laparoscopic major vessel injuries in Canada. J Am Assoc Gynecol Laparosc 2000;7:503.
23. Corson SL, Chandler JG, Way LW. Survey of laparoscopic entry injuries provoking litigation. J Am Assoc Gynecol Laparosc 2001;8:341.
24. Hurd WW, Pearl ML, DeLancey JO, et al. Laparoscopic injury of abdominal wall blood vessels: a report of three cases. Obstet Gynecol 1993;82 (4 Pt 2 Suppl):673.

25. Audebert AJ, Gomel V. Role of microlaparoscopy in the diagnosis of peritoneal and visceral adhesions and in the prevention of bowel injury associated with blind trocar insertion. Fertil Steril 2000;73:631.
26. Vilos GA. Laparoscopic bowel injuries: Forty litigated gynaecological cases in Canada. J Obstet Gynaecol Can 2002;24:224.
27. Deziel DJ, Millikan KW, Economou SG, et al. Complications of laparoscopic cholecystectomy: A national survey of 4,292 hospitals and an analysis of 77,604 cases. Am J Surg 1993;165:9.
28. Wolfe BM, Gardiner BN, Leary BF, Frey CF. Endoscopic cholecystectomy. An analysis of complications. Arch Surg 1991;126:1192.
29. Thompson BH, Wheeless CR Jr. Gastrointestinal complications of laparoscopy sterilization. Obstet Gynecol 1973;41:669.
30. Bishoff JT, Allaf ME, Kirkels W, et al. Laparoscopic bowel injury: Incidence and clinical presentation. J Urol 1999;161:887.
31. Gayer G, Apter S, Garniek A, et al. Complications after laparoscopic gynecologic procedures: CT findings. Abdom Imaging 2000;25:435.
32. Ho AC, Horton KM, Fishman EK. Perforation of the small bowel as a complication of laparoscopic cholecystectomy: CT findings. Clin Imaging 2000;24:204.
33. Berry MA, Rangraj M. Conservative treatment of recognized laparoscopic colonic injury. JSLS 1998;2:195.
34. Angle HS, Young SB. Conservative management of incidental cystotomy at laparoscopy. A report of two cases. J Reprod Med 1995;40:809.
35. Lamaro VP, Broome JD, Vancaillie TG. Unrecognized bladder perforation during operative laparoscopy. J Am Assoc Gynecol Laparosc 2000;7:417.
36. Godfrey C, Wahle GR, Schilder JM, et al. Occult bladder injury during laparoscopy: Report of two cases. J Laparoendosc Adv Surg Tech A 1999;9:341.
37. Nezhat CH, Seidman DS, Nezhat F, et al. Laparoscopic management of intentional and unintentional cystotomy. J Urol 1996;156:1400.
38. Karram M, Partoll L, Miklos J, Goldwasser S. Suprapubic bladder drainage after extraperitoneal cystotomy. Obstet Gynecol 2000;96:234.
39. Montz FJ, Holschneider CH, Munro MG. Incisional hernia following laparoscopy: A survey of the American Association of Gynecologic Laparoscopists. Obstet Gynecol 1994;84:881.
40. Plaus WJ. Laparoscopic trocar site hernias. J Laparoendosc Surg 1993;3:567.
41. Leibl BJ, Schmedt CG, Schwarz J, et al. Laparoscopic surgery complications associated with trocar tip design: Review of literature and own results. J Laparoendosc Adv Surg Tech A 1999;9:135.
42. Maio A, Ruchman RB. CT diagnosis of postlaparoscopic hernia. J Comput Assist Tomogr 1991;15:1054.
43. Sotrel G, Hirsch E, Edelin KC. Necrotizing fasciitis following diagnostic laparoscopy. Obstet Gynecol 1983;62(3 Suppl):67s.
44. Lane G, Tay J. Port-site metastasis following laparoscopic lymphadenectomy for adenosquamous carcinoma of the cervix. Gynecol Oncol 1999;74:130.
45. Lavie O, Cross PA, Beller U, et al. Laparoscopic port-site metastasis of an early stage adenocarcinoma of the cervix with negative lymph nodes. Gynecol Oncol 1999;75:155.
46. Tjalma WA, Winter-Roach BA, Rowlands P, et al. Port-site recurrence following laparoscopic surgery in cervical cancer. Int J Gynecol Cancer 2001;11:409.
47. Wang PH, Yen MS, Yuan CC, et al. Port site metastasis after laparoscopic-assisted vaginal hysterectomy for endometrial cancer: Possible mechanisms and prevention. Gynecol Oncol 1997;66:151.
48. Leminen A, Lehtovirta P. Spread of ovarian cancer after laparoscopic surgery: Report of eight cases. Gynecol Oncol 1999;75:387.
49. Bacha EA, Barber W, Ratchford W. Port-site metastases of adenocarcinoma of the fallopian tube after laparoscopically assisted vaginal hysterectomy and salpingo-oophorectomy. Surg Endosc 1996;10:1102.
50. Bouvy ND, Marquet RL, Jeekel H, Bonjer HJ. Impact of gas(less) laparoscopy and laparotomy on peritoneal tumor growth and abdominal wall metastases. Ann Surg 1996;224:694.
51. Cavina E, Goletti O, Molea N, et al. Trocar site tumor recurrences. May pneumoperitoneum be responsible? Surg Endosc 1998;12:1294.
52. Hopkins MP, Dulai RM, Occhino A, Holda S. The effects of carbon dioxide pneumoperitoneum on seeding of tumor in port sites in a rat model. Am J Obstet Gynecol 1999;181:1329.
53. Agostini A, Robin F, Jais JP, et al. Impact of different gases and pneumoperitoneum pressures on tumor growth during laparoscopy in a rat model. Surg Endosc 2002;16:529.
54. Allardyce RA. Is the port site really at risk? Biology, mechanisms and prevention: A critical view. Aust N Z J Surg 1999;69:479.
55. Lacy AM, Delgado S, Garcia-Valdecasas JC, et al. Port site metastases and recurrence after laparoscopic colectomy. A randomized trial. Surg Endosc 1998;12:1039.
56. Mintz M. Risks and prophylaxis in laparoscopy: A survey of 100,000 cases. J Reprod Med 1977;18:269.
57. Schaller G, Kuenkel M, Manegold BC. The optical "Veress-needle"—initial puncture with a minioptic. Endosc Surg Allied Technol 1995;3:55.
58. Reich H, Ribeiro SC, Vidali A. Hysterectomy as treatment for dysfunctional uterine bleeding. Baillieres Best Pract Res Clin Obstet Gynaecol 1999;13:251.
59. Sharma KC, Kabinoff G, Ducheine Y, et al. Laparoscopic surgery and its potential for medical complications. Heart Lung 1997;26:52.
60. Gutt CN, Oniu T, Mehrabi A, et al. Circulatory and respiratory complications of carbon dioxide insufflation. Dig Surg 2004;21:95.
61. Childers JM, Brzechffa PR, Surwit EA. Laparoscopy using the left upper quadrant as the primary trocar site. Gynecol Oncol 1993;50:221.
62. Parker J, Reid G, Wong F. Microlaparoscopic left upper quadrant entry in patients at high risk of periumbilical adhesions. Aust N Z J Obstet Gynaecol 1999;39:88.
63. Parker J, Rahimpanah F. The advantages of microlaparoscopic left upper quadrant entry in selected patients. Aust N Z J Obstet Gynaecol 2001;41:314.
64. Pasic R, Levine RL, Wolf WM Jr. Laparoscopy in morbidly obese patients. J Am Assoc Gynecol Laparosc 1999;6:307.
65. Neely MR, McWilliams R, Makhlouf HA. Laparoscopy: Routine pneumoperitoneum via the posterior fornix. Obstet Gynecol 1975;45:459.
66. van Lith DA, van Schie KJ, Beekhuizen W, du Plessis M. Cul-de-sac insufflation: An easy alternative route for safely inducing pneumoperitoneum. Int J Gynaecol Obstet 1980;17:375.
67. Wolfe WM, Pasic R. Transuterine insertion of Veress needle in laparoscopy. Obstet Gynecol 1990;75(3 Pt 1):456.
68. Yuzpe AA. Pneumoperitoneum needle and trocar injuries in laparoscopy. A survey on possible contributing factors and prevention. J Reprod Med 1990;35:485.
69. Corson SL, Batzer FR, Gocial B, Maislin G. Measurement of the force necessary for laparoscopic trocar entry. J Reprod Med 1989;34:282.
70. Hurd WW, Wang L, Schemmel MT. A comparison of the relative risk of vessel injury with conical versus pyramidal laparoscopic trocars in a rabbit model. Am J Obstet Gynecol 1995;173:1731.
71. Byron JW, Markenson G, Miyazawa K. A randomized comparison of Verres needle and direct trocar insertion for laparoscopy. Surg Gynecol Obstet 1993;177:259.
72. Woolcott R. The safety of laparoscopy performed by direct trocar insertion and carbon dioxide insufflation under vision. Aust N Z J Obstet Gynaecol 1997;37:216.
73. Borgatta L, Gruss L, Barad D, Kaali SG. Direct trocar insertion vs. Verres needle use for laparoscopic sterilization. J Reprod Med 1990;35:891.
74. Yim SF, Yuen PM. Randomized double-masked comparison of radially expanding access device and conventional cutting tip trocar in laparoscopy. Obstet Gynecol 2001;97:435.
75. Penfield AJ. How to prevent complications of open laparoscopy. J Reprod Med 1985;30:660.
76. Reich H. Laparoscopic bowel injury. Surg Laparosc Endosc 1992;2:74.
77. Hanney RM, Carmalt HL, Merrett N, Tait N. Use of the Hasson cannula producing major vascular injury at laparoscopy. Surg Endosc 1999;13:1238.
78. Voitk A, Rizoli S. Blunt Hasson trocar injury: Long intra-abdominal trocar and lean patient—a dangerous combination. J Laparoendosc Adv Surg Tech A 2001;11:259.
79. Godfrey C, Wahle GR, Schilder JM, et al. Occult bladder injury during laparoscopy: Report of two cases. J Laparoendosc Adv Surg Tech A 1999;9:341.
80. Hurd WW, Amesse LS, Gruber JS, et al. Visualization of the epigastric vessels and bladder before laparoscopic trocar placement. Fertil Steril 2003;80:209.
81. Quint EH, Wang FL, Hurd WW. Laparoscopic transillumination for the location of anterior abdominal wall blood vessels. J Laparoendosc Surg 1996;6:167.
82. Kolata RJ, Ransick M, Briggs L, Baum D. Comparison of wounds created by non-bladed trocars and pyramidal tip trocars in the pig. J Laparoendosc Adv Surg Tech A 1999;9:455.
83. Hurd WH, Bude RO, DeLancey JO, et al. Abdominal wall characterization with magnetic resonance imaging and computed tomography. The effect of obesity on the laparoscopic approach. J Reprod Med 1991;36:473.

Vascular Injuries

Barbara Levy

5

Laparoscopic surgery has, in many ways, revolutionized gynecology over the past several decades. Surgical procedures that previously required large abdominal incisions and prolonged recovery times may now be performed through minimally invasive incisions, resulting, for the most part, in equivalent outcomes and markedly reduced recovery times. Access to the peritoneal cavity for laparoscopy carries with it, however, a unique set of complications. This chapter addresses the vascular injuries most commonly encountered at laparoscopic surgery.

The incidence of major vessel injury at laparoscopy varies, ranging in the recent literature from a low of 0.1 per 1000[1] to a high of 6.4 per 1000 procedures.[2] When devastating and life-threatening retroperitoneal vessel injuries are considered, the rate is approximately 0.1 per 1000 to 1 per 10,000 cases. This means that most gynecologists will, thankfully, never see this complication during their surgical careers. From a national standpoint, however, several hundred of these dangerous injuries can be expected each year.

In the remainder of this chapter, injuries occurring during abdominal access are differentiated from those that occur during the surgical dissection. Laparoscopy has been asociated with both of these problems.

ABDOMINAL ACCESS–RELATED INJURIES

Insertion of the Veress needle and of the primary trocar is a unique step in laparoscopic surgery. Injury to the large retroperitoneal vascular structures has been reported with both open and closed laparoscopic entry techniques, as well as with the use of either reusable or disposable trocars. Bhoyrul and colleagues[3] reviewed the U.S. Food and Drug Administration (FDA) database of endoscopic complications and found manufacturer-reported or hospital-reported major vessel injuries related to all types and brands of laparoscopic trocars. "Safety shields" do not consistently deploy to protect intraperitoneal or retroperitoneal structures, and even the optical viewing disposable trocars have been implicated in devastating injuries to major vessels. Sharp and associates[4] reported 37 major vessel injuries related to newer optical trocars. These included injuries to the aorta, vena cava, and

iliac vessels. The lesson here is well stated by Hulka and Reich in their textbook of laparoscopic surgery: "The magic is in the magician and not in the wand."[5] In the FDA search conducted by Bhoyrul and colleagues,[3] an examination of the device associated with vessel injury was performed in 41 cases. Malfunction of the trocar was demonstrated in only 1 case.

Technical errors account for a majority of the cases of catastrophic retroperitoneal injury. Such errors include the following:

- Inadequate skin incision
- Failure to note anatomic landmarks
- Abnormal or inappropriate patient positioning
- Failure to adequately stabilize the abdominal wall
- Forceful thrusting motion for insertion
- Perpendicular or lateral insertion of the needle or trocar
- Failure to control the depth of penetration

Experience of the surgeon clearly is a factor as well. Most laparoscopic injuries have been reported to occur in a surgeon's first 100 procedures.

Related Anatomy

Baggish[6] reported on 31 cases of major vessel injury at laparoscopy and found that the vast majority of injuries (71%) occurred in overweight or obese women (those with a body mass index [BMI] greater than 25). An additional 19% of the cases occurred in underweight women (BMI less than 20), with only 10% of cases in women of normal body habitus. Clearly, gynecologic surgeons must have a heightened awareness of the more difficult anatomy in obese women and take great care during abdominal access in thin patients. Either situation may predispose to retroperitoneal injury.

Excellent familiarity with and careful identification of anatomic landmarks and their association with the aortic bifurcation also are essential. In 75% of people, the aortic bifurcation occurs at the level of L4. Although the sacral promontory and aortic pulse may not be palpable in obese women, the summits of the iliac crests usually are identifiable. The bifurcation will be within 1.25 cm above or below an imaginary line connecting the iliac crests in 80% of people.[7] The position of the umbilicus is quite variable and should not be used to predict the location of the retroperitoneal vessels. Nezhat and colleagues[8] have studied the relationship among patient position, obesity, and the position of the umbilicus with respect to the aortic bifurcation during laparoscopic surgery. They found that the position of the bifurcation varied, ranging between 5 cm cephalic and 3 cm caudal to the umbilicus in the supine position and between 3 cm cephalic and 3 cm caudal to the umbilicus in the Trendelenburg position. Of interest, obesity was not correlated with a statistically significant alteration in position of the aorta relative to the umbilicus; however, in non-overweight women and in the Trendelenburg position, the aortic bifurcation was significantly more likely to be located caudal to the umbilicus. In the supine position, the aortic bifurcation was caudal to the umbilicus in only 11% of patients. This increased to 33% of patients once they were placed in the Trendelenburg position. This has obvious implications for the appropriate angle and direction of the Veress needle or trocar inserted in blind fashion.

Narendran and Baggish[9] looked at the depth of the retroperitoneal vessels relative to the umbilical trocar entry site. They found a significant difference in both the depth of the abdominal wall (not a big surprise!) and the depth of the great vessels in obese women. As the BMI increased, the dis-

tance to the aorta increased as well. The patient's height also was correlated with distance to the great vessels—the taller the patient, the greater the distance to the retroperitoneal structures. In their analysis, no difference was noted in the depth of the structures related to patient positioning. Data would therefore suggest that placement of the patient into the Trendelenburg position before needle and trocar insertion should modify the angle but not the depth of insertion. With the aortic bifurcation located caudal to the umbilicus in 33% of patients in the Trendelenburg position, however, it would seem prudent to maintain the patient flat on the table to minimize the risk of injury when placing sharp instruments blindly and aiming toward the pelvis (Fig. 5–1A-C).

Finally, it is important for the operating surgeon to position the patient on the operating table personally. Not only will this permit a clear assessment of anatomic landmarks before the sterile drapes are applied and the points of reference obscured, but it also will afford an opportunity to ensure protection of the patient's arms, hands, and legs. Anesthesiologists, in an effort to be helpful, will often place the patient into the Trendelenburg position while the surgeon is scrubbing. It is critical for the surgeon to document for himself or herself the proper position of the patient and the anatomic

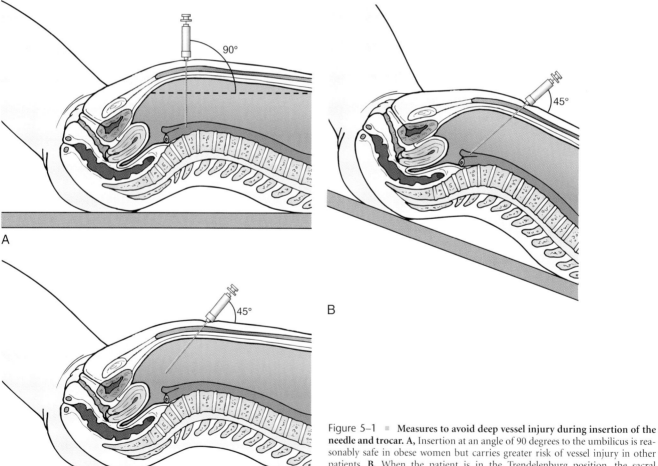

Figure 5–1 ▪ **Measures to avoid deep vessel injury during insertion of the needle and trocar. A,** Insertion at an angle of 90 degrees to the umbilicus is reasonably safe in obese women but carries greater risk of vessel injury in other patients. **B,** When the patient is in the Trendelenburg position, the sacral promontory is rotated closer to the umbilicus, and a needle inserted at 45 degrees can skewer the vessels. **C,** With the patient lying flat, the needle will avoid the deep vessels.

landmarks once again before inserting a scalpel, needle, or trocar.

Abdominal Entry Techniques

Once adequate anesthesia has been established and the surgeon is prepared to gain entry into the peritoneal cavity, the superior aspect of the iliac crest should be palpated and an effort made to assess the position of the aorta and its bifurcation. Infiltration of the proposed insertion site with a local anesthetic agent permits fine needle exploration of the structures that lie beneath. Not only will this give the surgeon a sense of the depth of the peritoneal cavity at the chosen location, but it also may allow identification of bowel adhesions beneath the proposed area of entry. Aspiration of either blood or succus entericus will warn the surgeon before significant harm to the patient has occurred. An alternate access site may then be considered. A skin incision should be made that is adequate to permit easy movement of the trocar sleeve. An inadequate skin incision may create a situation in which excessive force will be required to place the trocar. Before using either disposable or reusable laparoscopic devices, the surgeon should inspect and test them for proper function.

If carbon dioxide insufflation is to be accomplished, the Veress needle should be inserted with the valve in the open position. This allows room air to enter immediately on entry into the peritoneal cavity, thereby allowing the bowel and its mesentery to fall away. This also will permit egress of blood in the event that intravascular placement has occurred.

Many techniques may be used to elevate and stabilize the abdominal wall to facilitate needle or direct trocar insertion. Manual elevation of the lower abdominal wall, placement of towel clips into the umbilical incision, and severe anteflexion of the uterus with a manipulator, using the fundus to provide countertraction from inside the peritoneal cavity, all are useful techniques (Fig. 5–2). Vigorous bites with towel clips, however, have been associated with bowel perforation; therefore, as always, the anatomy of the patient and the

potential for subumbilical adhesions must be considered. Surgeons must find the method that affords them the most control and best stabilization of the abdominal wall. This probably will vary depending on the surgeon's height, strength, and hand size.

With the abdominal wall stabilized, the Veress needle or trocar should be firmly, but gently, guided into the peritoneal cavity while aiming for the hollow of the sacrum, or toward the fundus of the uterus if the landmarks have been difficult to identify. The depth of penetration must be controlled and sharp thrusting motions avoided. Correct placement may be verified by several techniques. No test, however, is 100% reliable. If difficulty or excessive opening pressure with insufflation is encountered, the surgeon must entertain the possibility that placement is inappropriate. This possibility should prompt consideration of an alternate access site such as the left upper quadrant, or of an alternate access method such as open laparoscopy.

Although one would think that Hasson's open laparoscopy technique would avoid injury to the aorta, vena cava, and iliac vessels, penetration of these vessels has occurred even with this technique. Thin patients are obviously at highest risk for this complication of open laparoscopy, and care must be taken to avoid penetration into the abdominal cavity with the scalpel in thin, frail, and multiparous patients, who may have significant rectus muscle diastasis. Jansen and associates evaluated the incidence of complications related to open versus closed laparoscopic entry techniques.[10] In approximately 52,000 cases, no differences in vascular complications were found between open and closed laparoscopy. These investigators concluded that surgeons who become skilled with blind insertion techniques are able to avoid major vessel injuries under most circumstances. These findings underscore that proper technique, accurate identification of anatomic landmarks, and recognition of high risk situations, with appropriate modifications in technique, will permit safe peritoneal access independent of the surgical approach chosen.

Greater than half of the reported major vessel injuries are incurred during insertion of either the primary or the ancillary trocars. Once peritoneal access has been gained, insertion of any additional instruments should occur *only* under direct vision. If a surgical assistant is controlling the camera, the surgeon must verify that the point of trocar insertion is within the field of view. Once again, infiltration of local anesthetic into the incision area permits penetration of the peritoneal space by a small needle and maps the pathway of the trocar to follow. The angle of insertion should be toward the midline, avoiding the pelvic sidewall. Placement of secondary trocars lateral to the rectus muscles will avoid injury to the epigastric vessels; however, this placement does put the external iliac vessels at risk if the direction of insertion is not carefully monitored (Fig. 5–3).

Careful control of the instruments to limit the depth of insertion also is critical to avoiding injuries. Baggish and co-workers[11] studied the force required to insert various laparoscopic access devices. They determined that it took on average 17.5 lb of pressure to insert a sharpened reusable 11-mm trocar, compared with 10 lb for a pyramidal-tipped disposable trocar of the same diameter. These findings have several implications. Although it may be easier to insert a trocar when less

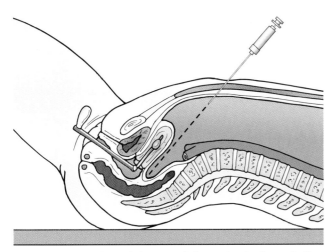

Figure 5–2 ■ **Mechanical elevation of the uterine fundus to facilitate abdominal wall penetration.** Pushing down on the handle of a uterine manipulator elevates the fundus of the uterus and pushes the peritoneum up against the abdominal wall, making it easier to penetrate.

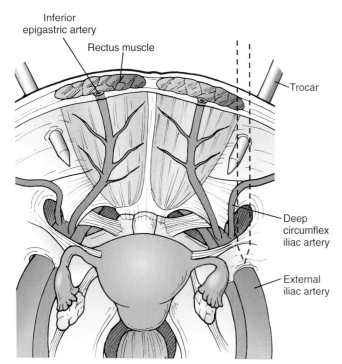

Figure 5–3 ▪ Caudal view of the pelvis and anterior abdominal wall, depicting the relative positions of the lower accessory trocar sites in relation to the deep circumflex iliac artery, external iliac artery, and rectus muscles.

force is required, surgeons who are accustomed to reusable equipment may inadvertently apply excess pressure when using unfamiliar disposable devices. Similarly, those who are used to disposable trocars may find themselves unable to insert a reusable trocar, especially one that has not been recently sharpened, without applying what seems to be excessive force. Trocar insertion in women who have undergone previous abdominal procedures presents a greater challenge in that the fascia is likely to be scarred and thickened in the midline. Nicking the fascia with the tip of the scalpel blade is a convenient trick for reducing the pressure required to insert any trocar through tough fascia. This also gives the surgeon a secure anchor into the fascia in order to direct the force in the proper direction and for the appropriate depth.

A review of cases of retroperitoneal vessel injury suggests that difficult anatomy (e.g., in the obese patient with obscured landmarks) predisposes to challenges in stabilizing the abdominal wall, as well as determining the appropriate depth of penetration. In addition, the so-called safety shields— plastic sheaths that spring over the sharp blade once pressure against the blade is released—may be too large to penetrate the fascia and peritoneum easily. They will "hang up" in the abdominal wall, causing the surgeon to apply additional force for them to pass through the smaller opening created by the blade. When they do pop through, the blade remains uncovered for the split second required to traverse the abdominal cavity and lodge in the retroperitoneum. Once again, women with abdominal incisions and dense scarring may be at highest risk for this technical problem to occur. It may be prudent to consider open laparoscopy, or an alternate site for trocar insertion, if difficulty is encountered at the umbilicus.

MAJOR VESSEL INJURIES

Recognizing Vessel Injury

Retroperitoneal bleeding may be difficult to visualize initially in a patient with major vessel injury. Large hematomas may track superiorly outside the pelvis and outside the visual field of the surgeon. A small amount of unexplained intraperitoneal bleeding, visualized at first inspection with the laparoscope, should prompt the surgeon to inspect the retroperitoneum carefully. This may require repositioning the patient in order to visualize the origin of the mesenteric vessels and great vessels without interference by the small bowel.

Any sudden deterioration in vital signs (decrease in end-tidal carbon dioxide, decreased blood pressure and increased heart rate) after needle or trocar insertion should be treated as a catastrophic major vessel accident until proved otherwise. Anesthesiologists may be tempted to attribute the patient's deterioration to anaphylaxis or gas embolism. The surgeon's role, however, is to assume that this represents a vascular injury and prepare for immediate laparotomy. Delay in controlling the rapid blood loss may lead to serious sequelae. Both Bhoyrul and colleagues[3] and Baggish,[6] in cataloguing the consequences of major vessel injuries, report substantial mortality associated with these injuries. Baggish noted a 23% fatality rate. Of interest, all of the deaths were related to venous injuries. In addition, major morbidity, including postoperative vascular insufficiency, stroke, and infection, was reported in a substantial number of survivors. In Bhoyrul and colleagues' series, 26 deaths occurred among 408 patients; 87% of the injuries resulting in death occurred with the use of disposable trocars and safety shields. Of the different trocars used, 9% were disposable with a direct viewing feature. It is clear that manufacturers' attempts to provide safer instrumentation to access the peritoneal cavity have thus far been unsuccessful.

Management of Vessel Injury

Thankfully, most gynecologists will never encounter the complication of vessel injury during their surgical careers. The consequences of a major vessel injury are so serious for the patient, however, that each gynecologic surgeon should have a "game plan" rehearsed in case such a complication occurs. Such preparation is particularly important for surgeons who perform laparoscopic procedures in free-standing surgicenters without the availability of hospital services such as the laboratory and blood bank. It may be prudent to store several units of type O–negative blood on site in such facilities.

Management of vessel injury by the gynecologic surgeon must proceed without hesitation. Rapid recognition and response to this emergency may make a significant difference in patient outcome. Specialized equipment, retractors, and instruments are not required for appropriate intervention, which entails the following:

• Perform laparotomy through a midline incision.
• Call for help, preferably from a vascular surgeon, as soon as possible. An experienced general surgeon can substitute for a vascular surgeon if the latter is not available.

- Apply pressure using laparotomy sponges to the retroperitoneal space while the anesthesiologist and nursing team resuscitate the patient.
- Do not attempt to open the retroperitoneal space or clamp the bleeding vessel(s).
- Send blood for emergency type and crossmatch, hemoglobin, hematocrit, and clotting studies.
- Infuse O-negative blood if available.
- Consider the use of heparin to prevent thrombosis and occlusion of distal vessels if the vascular surgeon is not immediately available to repair the injury.

Abdominal Wall Vessel Injuries

Most significant injuries to the major vessels (deep or superficial epigastrics) occur with the use of large pyramidal trocars. Hurd and colleagues[12] looked at the risk of abdominal wall vessel injury in an animal model related to the size and shape of trocar used. When the vessel was directly punctured (0 cm between the tip of the trocar and the midportion of the vessel wall), the rates of injury were identical. As the distance increased from the central portion of the vessel, however, large-diameter pyramidal trocars were significantly more likely to lacerate a vessel wall, even at a distance of 4 to 5 mm.

Strategies to reduce the risk of vessel injury in the abdominal wall include placement of the smallest possible trocars laterally, with 10- to 12-mm trocars remaining in the midline as much as possible. In thin patients, the inferior epigastric vessels may be visualized and transilluminated in the anterior abdominal wall. In larger patients, attempts at transillumination will be fruitless; however, placing the ancillary trocars outside the rectus muscles should avoid injury to these vessels, which traverse the underside of the muscle bellies. Engaging the trocar tip into the fascia before the application of force will help to avoid slippage of the instrument and inadvertent puncture of the vessels. Again, the direction of insertion is toward the midline to avoid damaging the pelvic sidewall structures. Slow, steady pressure should be applied, while the path of the trocar is visualized continuously. If slow pressure causes the trocar shield to deploy, the spike may be removed and the peritoneum punctured with a blunt instrument inserted through the trocar sleeve.

It is not always possible to completely avoid the abdominal wall vasculature. Inspection of all trocar sites for persistent bleeding with the abdomen deflated at the end of the procedure will permit the surgeon to identify and treat injuries to these vessels. Bipolar coagulation or suture may be used for control. Tamponade alone may be inadequate and predispose to delayed hemorrhage.

NON–MAJOR VESSEL INJURIES: PREVENTION AND MANAGEMENT OF BLEEDING

Damage to large and small blood vessels also may occur during the operative portion of the laparoscopic procedure after the trocars have been safely placed. Anatomic landmarks may be distorted by the patient's disease process, and the magnification that is often the surgeon's friend in identifying pathologic conditions may become an enemy if working within a small, magnified, visual field causes the surgeon to lose track of anatomic geography. Dissection of the retroperitoneum for treatment and excision of deep infiltrating endometriosis, lymph node dissection, and extensive "adhesiolysis" place the pelvic sidewall vessels and great vessels at risk. Unintended injuries have occurred with sharp dissection, as well as with a multitude of energy sources. The pneumoperitoneum, by potentially collapsing the veins, makes identification and protection of the large venous structures more difficult at laparoscopic surgery.

Strict attention to detail and careful observation of anatomic landmarks will help to avoid bleeding complications in most cases. When severe adhesive disease or endometriosis obscures normal anatomic planes, it is useful to pull the scope back and find an area in the abdomen or pelvis where the anatomy is clear. From that perspective, then, the retroperitoneum may be entered and the distorted anatomy clarified. This approach demands a solid understanding of pelvic anatomy, as well as the use of slow, deliberate, sharp dissection. The principles of surgical technique apply to laparoscopic surgery and to open surgery as well. Traction with atraumatic instruments will demonstrate the appropriate plane for sharp dissection. Having an instrument ready to apply discreet energy for hemostasis also is important. All energy sources, cords, and instruments must be hooked up and tested before dissection is initiated. It is disconcerting for a surgeon to find out that the bipolar cautery is not functional while watching a pumping vessel!

Many standard as well as new instruments are available to provide hemostasis when bleeding is encountered during laparoscopic surgery. Monopolar graspers, needle or hook electrodes, bipolar forceps of various sizes with or without cutting capabilities, newer pulsed bipolar systems, ultrasonic instrumentation, and vessel-sealing devices all are available and may be used effectively under most circumstances. It is essential that the surgeon become knowledgeable about the instrumentation available in his or her operative environment. Each modality has some advantages and disadvantages; however, the key to safe application of any of them is the careful dissection and identification of the bleeding source, followed by discreet application of energy. Mechanical occlusion of the vessel before the application of energy will permit control of the bleeding using the least amount of energy. This approach will limit collateral damage as much as possible.

Most of the bleeding encountered during gynecologic surgery may be controlled with any one of these systems. At times, however, the infundibulopelvic ligament or the uterine artery may be too large for consistent hemostasis with ultrasonic or bipolar technology. These systems have been shown to reliably control bleeding from vessels 1 to 3 mm in diameter. The pulsed bipolar system (Gyrus) uses standard cutting current but pulses the energy to allow heat to dissipate from the surrounding tissue. Use of this device may decrease the thermal damage to tissues adjacent to bleeding vessels, but it still cannot seal vessels larger than approximately 1 to 3 mm. Vessel-sealing technology (Ligasure), which utilizes the combination of mechanical pressure and high-amperage, low-voltage radiofrequency energy, will seal vessels up to 7 mm. Whichever systems are deployed, the surgeon must be confidently knowledgeable about their use before the procedure begins. Having a "fall-back" choice also is recommended in the event that the surgeon's standard instruments malfunction. The surgeon should have the instruments hooked up, tested, and accessible before initiating the procedure, with the standard instrument of choice immediately available for use in the abdomen. Both bipolar and monopolar standard graspers may conveniently be used to obtain rapid hemostasis. In addition, mechanical devices such as staples, sutures, preformed suture loops, and clips should not be overlooked. At times, these may be necessary to secure hemostasis.

The principal surgical steps for safe management of bleeding remain the same whichever technique is used to establish control of the vessel:

1. Recognition of anatomic landmarks
2. Visualization of the bleeding vessel
3. Discreet mechanical control of the vessel
4. Coaptation of the vessel

Use of a consistent approach to control bleeding and avoidance of indiscriminate use of energy will prevent most collateral tissue damage.

DELAYED HEMORRHAGE

Significant damage to retroperitoneal or pelvic vessels may not be immediately apparent to the surgical team as a result of any of several factors:

- Increased intra-abdominal pressure (pneumoperitoneum)
- Decreased venous pressure associated with the Trendelenburg position
- Retroperitoneal dissection and tamponade

As with any surgical procedure, careful observation of the patient in the recovery room and post-recovery area is essential. Tachycardia, decreasing blood pressure, increasing abdominal distention, and oozing from the abdominal wounds should prompt suspicion of an ongoing uncontrolled bleeding source. Laboratory specimens should be drawn and the anesthesiologist notified. Recommended laboratory studies include complete blood count, platelet count, determination of prothrombin time and partial thromboplastin time, and type and crossmatch studies. If ultrasonography is readily available, a pelvic and abdominal ultrasound examination will be useful in identifying large amounts of intraperitoneal fluid. This approach is less helpful, of course, if fluid was intentionally left in the pelvis.

Once the decision to reoperate has been made, the surgeon must determine whether laparoscopic exploration is an appropriate option. If the patient is relatively hemodynamically stable and the surgeon feels confident that appropriate equipment is available, laparoscopic re-exploration is quite reasonable. If, however, the patient is "crashing" and the operating room is short-staffed, it may be prudent to proceed with immediate laparotomy to achieve rapid control of the situation. Under these circumstances, a midline incision often is the most appropriate to permit quick access to the major retroperitoneal vessels.

Whichever route is chosen, the surgeon must have a plan to identify and control the source(s) of bleeding. At laparoscopy it is useful to place a 10-mm ancillary trocar through which standard suction tubing may be inserted to rapidly remove clots and pooled blood. The end of the suction tubing is cut off, and a hole is created in the tubing approximately 15 inches from the end so that the amount of suction can be controlled. This modification will enable rapid removal of large clots, which can be challenging with standard suction irrigation devices. Once visualization is achieved either laparoscopically or by laparotomy, a systematic exploration of the abdomen must be performed, with specific attention to the abdominal wall, the pelvis, the retroperitoneum, the omentum, and the mesentery of the bowel. The exploration should begin with the access sites and proceed logically through the area of surgery to the retroperitoneum. It is important to look carefully for subtle but expanding retroperitoneal hematomas.

If an area of bleeding is identified, it may be somewhat more difficult to isolate a discrete source of bleeding because edema and small clots may obscure visualization. Once again, deliberate dissection of the anatomy and isolation of the bleeding pedicle will help to avoid collateral damage. For control of areas of oozing without a clear-cut vascular pedicle, topical agents may be useful. The hospital pharmacist should be consulted preoperatively to determine which agents are available. Topical thrombin frequently is helpful for controlling oozing deep in the pelvis. Avitene, Surgicel, Floseal, Tisseal, and other hemostatic aids, in addition to mechanical pressure, also are useful for achieving hemostasis. The surgeon should make certain these products are available before surgery.

If an area of bleeding cannot be identified, the pelvis is filled with fluid and the area is observed "underwater." This maneuver often will reveal an area of continued bleeding. If glycine or sorbitol is used in lieu of saline for this purpose, coagulation may be performed through the liquid medium, facilitating rapid control. At laparotomy, it is important to check for bleeding in areas that may be "packed away," such as the omentum.

Once hemostasis appears adequate, the patient is observed for several more minutes to rule out any additional bleeding. At laparoscopy, the pneumoperitoneum should be released for several minutes and then the abdomen reinsufflated to search for venous bleeding that may have been obscured. Surgical closure is performed only when the operator is satisfied that hemostasis has been achieved.

At times, massive hemorrhage may lead to disseminated intravascular coagulation (DIC), a condition that will lead to diffuse bleeding. The coagulopathy may be recognized first by the anesthesia team, who will note bleeding from the intravenous access sites. The fastest way to diagnose DIC is to draw a tube of blood and watch for it to coagulate. Failure to form a clot is clear-cut evidence for disruption in the clotting cascade. Infusion of fresh frozen plasma will replenish most of the depleted clotting factors. Consultation with a hematologist to optimize use of blood and factors usually is indicated for these patients. If postoperative hemorrhage is suspected and treated rapidly, massive blood loss resulting in DIC usually is avoidable.

CONCLUSIONS

Major vessel injuries are uncommon in gynecologic laparoscopic procedures and are avoidable in most circumstances.

Patients in whom difficult access at the umbilicus may be encountered typically are obese women, especially those who have healed abdominal incisions from previous surgery. Anatomic landmarks must be identified in each patient before any attempt at peritoneal entry, and the patient's position on the table verified. If an initial attempt at peritoneal entry is unsuccessful, consideration should be given to use of an alternate technique or entry site.

Insertion of the Veress needle and trocars requires a slow, deliberate motion, with positive control to prevent deep penetration. The angle of insertion may vary by patient anatomy, but the direction of insertion should be toward the hollow of the sacrum or the fundus of the uterus. Secondary trocars should be inserted laterally, aimed medially, and placed only under continuous direct vision to avoid pelvic sidewall and abdominal wall vessels. The principles of surgery should be meticulously followed during laparoscopic surgery to avoid uncontrolled bleeding during operative dissection. Recognition of anatomic planes of dissection, traction, sharp dissection, and isolation of vessels all are important in rapidly achieving hemostasis.

Finally, prompt recognition of major vessel injuries can be lifesaving. Laparoscopic surgeons must have an awareness of this rare complication and respond with a rapid diagnosis, fluid resuscitation, and immediate midline laparotomy in order to minimize the consequences for the patient.

References

1. Harkki-Siren P, Kruki T. A nationwide analysis of laparoscopic complications. Obstet Gynecol 1997;89:108.
2. Chapron CM, Lacroix PF, Querleu D, et al. Major vascular injuries during gynecologic laparoscopy. J Am Coll Surg 1997;185:461.
3. Bhoyrul S, Vierra MA, Nezhat DR, et al. Trocar injuries in laparoscopic surgery. J Am Coll Surg 2001;192:677.
4. Sharp HT, Dodson MK, Draper ML, et al. Complications associated with optical-access laparoscopic trocars. Obstet Gynecol 2003;19:63.
5. Hulka JF, Reich H. Textbook of laparoscopy, 2nd ed. Philadelphia: WB Saunders, 1994;85.
6. Baggish MS. Analysis of 31 cases of major-vessel injury associated with gynecologic laparoscopy operations. J Gynecol Surg 2003;19:63.
7. Gray H. The blood-vascular system. In Goss GM, ed. Anatomy of the human body, 28th ed. Philadelphia: Lea & Febiger, 1966;646.
8. Nezhat F, Brill AI, Nezhat CH, et al. Laparoscopic appraisal of the anatomic relationship of the umbilicus to the aortic bifurcation. J Am Assoc Gynecol Laparosc 1998;5:135.
9. Narendran M, Baggish MS. Mean distance between primary trocar insertion site and major retroperitoneal vessels during routine laparoscopy. J Gynecol Surg 2002;18:121.
10. Jansen FD, Kolkman W, Bakkum EA, et al. Complications of laparoscopy: An inquiry about closed- versus open-entry technique. Am J Obstet Gynecol 2004;190:634.
11. Baggish MS, Gandhi S, Kasper G: Force required by laparoscopic trocar devices to penetrate the human female's anterior abdominal wall. J Gynecol Surg 2003;19:1.
12. Hurd WW, Pearl ML, DeLancey JOL, et al. Laparoscopic injury of abdominal wall blood vessels: A report of three cases. Obstet Gynecol 1993;82:673.

Laparoscopic Bowel Injuries

6

Stephanie N. Morris and Charles H. Koh

BACKGROUND

Although gastrointestinal injuries associated with laparoscopy are rare, they represent a significant cause of morbidity and mortality. Bowel injuries account for between 13% and 51% of all major laparoscopic complications[1-4] and constitute the third leading cause of death from laparosopy, after major vascular injuries and anesthesia.[5] Many of the bowel injuries are not recognized at the time of the primary surgical procedure, leading to increased morbidity and mortality. To decrease the morbidity of laparoscopic bowel injury, the surgeon must routinely use techniques to minimize complications, maintain a high index of suspicion, and have a good understanding of different types of gastrointestinal injury, their clinical presentations, and appropriate treatment options.

Tremendous advances in laparoscopy have occurred since the 1970s, when laparoscopy was used primarily as a diagnostic tool. As new techniques are developed and technologic advancements are made, minimally invasive surgery is becoming more complex and is establishing itself as an alternative method for performing many gynecologic procedures. With increasingly complex laparoscopic procedures, higher overall rates of complications, including bowel injuries, have been reported.[2-4,6,7] When laparoscopic procedures are performed by more experienced surgeons, however, the rate of bowel complications is lower. A study by Chapron and colleagues[2] demonstrates the interplay of operative complexity and surgeon experience. Complication rates were calculated for two periods, 1987 to 1991 and 1992 to 1995; a significant drop in the number of bowel injuries occurred during the latter period despite the larger proportion of advanced laparoscopic surgical procedures performed.[2] This decrease was attributed to improved surgical skill and techniques. However, even with advanced laparoscopic skills and appropriate precautions, bowel injuries can still occur.

INCIDENCE OF BOWEL INJURY

The risk of gastrointestinal injuries occurring during gynecologic laparoscopy has been reported to be between 0.06% and 0.65%.[1-3,6,8-13] Two large studies, one a survey of almost 37,000 operative gynecologic laparoscopies in the United States (the 1988 American Association of Gynecologic Laparoscopists [AAGL] Membership Survey)[1] and the other a retrospective review from France of data for 29,966 gynecologic laparoscopy patients,[2] both reported a 0.16% incidence of bowel injury. Other studies report much lower complication rates.[3] The discrepant complication rates between studies may be related to the proportion of complex operative procedures included in the study and to underreporting of complications.

The general complication rate, as well as the rate of bowel injury, has been significantly correlated with the complexity of the laparoscopic surgery.[2-4,6,7] Difficulty of the procedure is a major predictor of complications.[14] Only 20% of bowel injuries occur during diagnostic or "minor" cases, whereas 80% occur during "major" or "advanced" operative laparoscopy, defined as surgery for ectopic pregnancy, pelvic inflammatory disease, benign or malignant ovarian masses, moderate or severe endometriosis, extended adhesiolysis, hysterectomy, myomectomy, and genital prolapse.[7] Diagnostic and minor procedures carry a risk of bowel injury between 0.06% and 0.19%, whereas operative procedures carry a higher risk of 0.15% to 0.80%.[2,6,9,15] A retrospective study from Finland reviewing 32,205 gynecologic laparoscopies from the period 1995 to 1996 revealed intestinal injury rates of 0.03%, 0.04%, and 0.16% for diagnostic, sterilization, and operative laparoscopy, respectively.[4] A survey of 1165 laparoscopic hysterectomies performed in Finland between 1993 and 1994 found a 0.4% rate of bowel injury.[10] Similarly, the AAGL Membership Survey reported a bowel complication rate of 0.26% for laparoscopy-assisted hysterectomies.[11] The higher complication rates noted in these two studies are likely a reflection of the increased complexity of the surgical procedures being examined (laparoscopic hysterectomies), rather than the inherent risk of the procedure itself. Bowel injury rate is higher not with laparoscopic hysterectomies per se but with more complex procedures, of which laparoscopic hysterectomy is an example that is commonly cited.

In addition to the complexity of the procedure, surgeon experience affects laparoscopic complication rates: Complication rates are lower for experienced laparoscopic surgeons than for inexperienced ones.[2,12] Specifically, with increasing surgeon experience, a significant decrease is observed in the number of bowel injuries.[2,9,15] Despite the overall lower intestinal complication rate, the rate of injury during the entry phase of laparoscopy was not affected by surgeon experience,[15] highlighting the inherent risk of injury during this portion of the procedure.

TYPES OF BOWEL INJURY

Laparoscopic bowel complications can be classified as those occurring during the *entry* phase and those occurring during the *operative* portion of the procedure. Anywhere from 29% to 83% of gastrointestinal injuries occur during the access phase of the procedure, depending on the study cited.[2-4,9,15] Chapron and associates[7] found that approximately one third of bowel injuries occurred during creation of the pneumoperitoneum and trocar placement. The remaining two thirds of the bowel injuries occurred during the operative part of the surgery—during dissection, electrocauterization, or grasping.[7] In the same study, 18% of the bowel injuries that occurred during the operative portion of the procedure were due to electrosurgery, and 82% were related to sharp dissection.[7] These findings are in contrast with those in several other studies that report much higher rates of bowel injury due to electrocautery. In one retrospective study of complications occurring with laparoscopic hysterectomy, all of the bowel injuries were attributed to electrocoagulation.[10] A large nationwide review of 32,205 gynecologic laparoscopic procedures reported that 54% of bowel injuries were caused by electrocautery.[4] The literature seems to indicate that in expert centers, the contribution of electrosurgery to bowel injuries is low. It is important that practitioners using electrosurgery be thoroughly aware of the properties of electrothermal energy and the potential for injury when using this modality.

Several possible mechanisms of thermal injury from the use of electrocautery or laser are recognized. Direct thermal injury can result from unintentionally touching the bowel with an active electrode or if a defect in the insulation of the instrument allows current to escape and damage the surrounding tissue.[16] Direct thermal injuries also can occur when the zone of coagulation extends beyond the intended area. Some authors have reported that when monopolar electrosurgery is used, tissue damage can occur up to 3 to 5 cm beyond the point of contact. Although using bipolar cautery decreases the amount of thermal spread to approximately 5 mm, a risk of direct extension injury is still present.[17] Direct coupling is another possible mechanism of thermal injury. Direct coupling occurs when the electric current is diverted away from its intended route by a metal instrument that is in contact with an active monopolar instrument.[16] For example, if the monopolar instrument is touching a metal blunt probe, the current can be redirected down the probe, causing thermal injury to adjacent tissues. Regardless of the specific mechanism, thermal injury to bowel can result in tissue necrosis potentially leading to intestinal perforation 72 to 96 hours after the initial injury.[18]

Gastrointestinal injuries also can occur with grasping or manipulating the bowel, during dissection or lysis of adhesions, and with movement of instruments into and out of the operative field. Finally, intentional bowel injury can occur during excision of areas of rectal endometriosis. For such procedures, the patient should always undergo preoperative mechanical bowel preparation.

The most common location for bowel injury varies according to different studies. Chapron and associates reported that almost half of bowel injuries involve the large intestine (48.4%), one third (33.9%) involve the small bowel, and 16% involve the omentum.[7] A prospective multicenter survey of 1165 laparoscopic hysterectomies reported rates of injury to small bowel, large bowel, and stomach at 59%, 36%, and 5%, respectively.[3]

RECOGNITION AND DIAGNOSIS OF BOWEL INJURY

One of the keys to recognition of bowel injuries during laparoscopy is heightened awareness and diligence during every step of the surgery. Patients with previous abdominal surgery or known adhesions are at an elevated risk, and a high index of suspicion for bowel injury should be maintained.

The creation of the pneumoperitoneum with the Veress needle and placement of the trocars can lead to bowel injury. Although Veress needle injuries often go undiagnosed because the area of perforation is small and can heal spontaneously, indications of damage may be present at the time of the procedure. The following findings may indicate the occurrence of a bowel injury during placement of the Veress needle:

- Leakage of bowel contents through the Veress needle.
- Aspiration of gastric or feculent material through the Veress needle.
- An initial opening pressure greater than 8 mm Hg. Normal intra-abdominal pressure is 8 mm or lower, with a mean of 4 mm Hg. Colonic pressures have been reported to be between 10 and 12 mm Hg.[19]
- Unusual tactile sensation during the placement of the Veress needle. Normally the surgeon feels two "pops" with passage of the needle through the fascia and the peritoneum and some mobility of the Veress needle after the second pop. If the second pop is not encountered or limited mobility is felt, the tip of the Veress needle may be in bowel, a blood vessel, or adhesions.

If the trocar is placed in bowel, the bowel lumen may be directly visualized when the laparoscope is inserted. With laparoscopically guided trocar placement, an injury to bowel may be recognized at the time of initial placement (Fig. 6–1A). Occasionally the umbilical trocar can go completely through and through a loop of bowel and is recognized only when the laparoscope is removed under direct visualization, or if the primary port site is visualized from a secondary port. If the umbilical trocar is withdrawn with the laparoscope inside it, the surgeon can see parietal peritoneum before the trocar is withdrawn completely, confirming that the trocar was not inadvertently placed through a loop of bowel. By placing the laparoscope in an auxiliary port, the surgeon can visualize the umbilical trocar and confirm the absence of evidence for bowel injury (Fig. 6–2A-D). These maneuvers should be performed if a survey of the abdomen after insertion of the

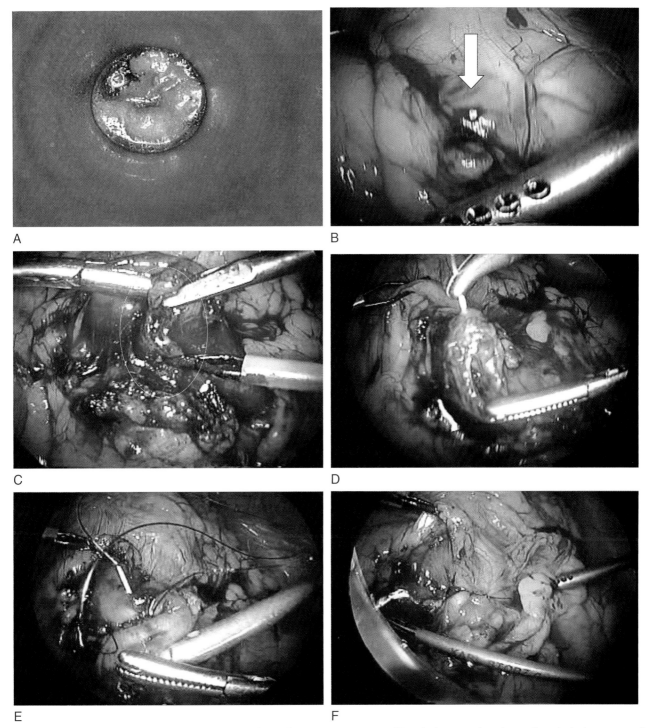

Figure 6–1 ▪ **Umbilical trocar injury of the transverse colon and repair. A,** Appearance of intestinal rugae and stool, seen through the laparoscope after the umbilical trocar was placed into the lumen of the transverse colon during direct trocar insertion without previous pneumoperitoneum. **B,** View of the transverse colon after pneumoperitoneum was created. The only sign of bowel injury is evidence of a hematoma *(arrow)* covered by mesenteric fat. **C,** After dissection of the mesenteric fat, the muscularis is exposed, revealing a 1-cm defect. **D,** The first suture is placed through the mucosa and muscularis using 3-0 polydioxanone suture (PDS). Four continuous throws are made to close the defect, running from left to right. **E,** Using the same suture, a second layer through the muscularis and serosa was used to imbricate the first layer of suture. This layer ran from right to left and was tied to the original tail of the suture on the left. **F,** Completed two-layer continuous closure of the transverse colon using a single 3-0 PDS. The defect is repaired in a transverse fashion to prevent luminal constriction.

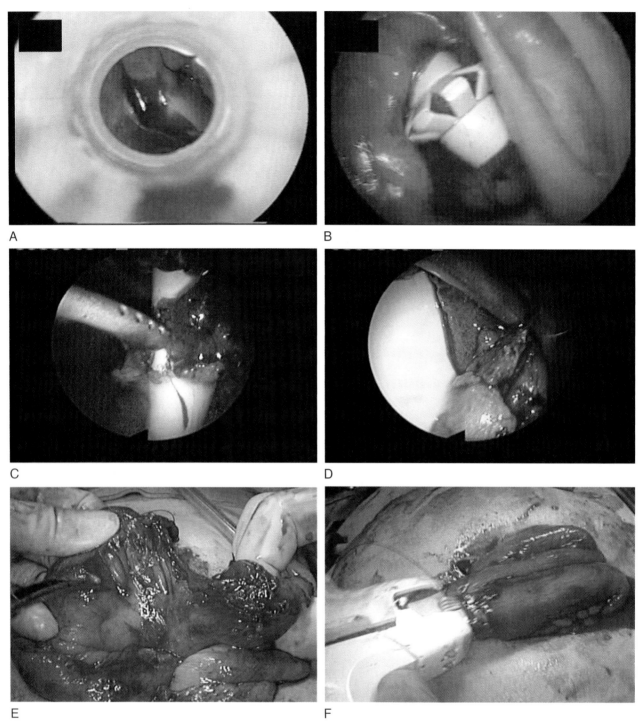

Figure 6–2 ▪ **Umbilical trocar injury to the ileum repaired through mini-laparotomy. A,** Laparoscopic view following blind direct trocar placement at the umbilicus. No obvious evidence of bowel injury is apparent, although a small amount of blood is present. **B,** View of the umbilical port from the right lateral port. Although no clear evidence of bowel perforation is present, bowel appears adherent to the anterior abdominal wall, raising concern for the possibility of a through-and-through bowel injury. **C,** View of the umbilical port from the right lateral port. Lysis of adhesions around the umbilical trocar. **D,** View of the umbilical port from the right lateral port. Intestinal mucosa is evident after lysis of adhesions, confirming that the umbilical trocar caused a through-and-through injury to the ileum. **E,** The injured ileum is exteriorized after the umbilical port site incision is enlarged. **F,** Side-to-side anastomosis of the ileum.

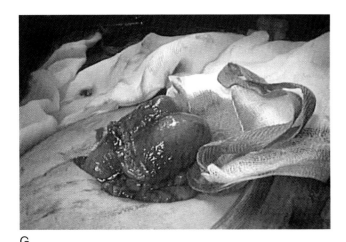

G

Figure 6–2 cont'd ▪ **G,** Completed side-to-side anastomosis. The bowel is returned to the abdominal cavity, and the planned procedure is completed laparoscopically.

laparoscope reveals evidence of adhesions of bowel or omentum to the anterior abdominal wall. Additionally, feculent material seen in the abdominal cavity or a hematoma in the bowel serosa indicates bowel injury[17] (see Fig. 6–1B).

Injuries resulting from the operative portion of the procedure also are frequently missed. An obvious sign of bowel injury is evidence of bowel contents in the abdominal cavity. Most bowel injuries are not so readily identified, however. A finding strongly suggestive of bowel injury is visualization of areas of deserosalized bowel after lysis of adhesions or removal of endometriotic lesions. Atraumatic bowel graspers can be used to "milk" bowel contents to the suspected area of injury to identify any leakage, which would indicate a full-thickness injury. If injury of the sigmoid or rectum is suspected, the pelvis can be filled with fluid and the rectum distended with air; bubbles in the pelvis indicate a full-thickness defect in the bowel.

It often is easier to recognize gastrointestinal injuries caused by dissection than those caused by thermal damage, because the extent of thermal injuries may not be immediately apparent and perforation may not occur until several days later. Thermal injury may be evident by blanching of the tissue. Even if thermal injury is recognized, it may be challenging to identify the extent of the damage, because a large area may be involved, with areas of delayed necrosis.

Prompt recognition of bowel injuries is imperative for appropriate treatment and to reduce morbidity. Unfortunately, a significant number of bowel injuries go undiagnosed at the time of the primary procedure, with one report of delayed diagnosis in 100% of cases![10] Depending on the study cited, between 24% and 100% of complications are missed at the time of the initial procedure.[2-4,7,9,10] Chapron and associates reported that only one third (35.7%) of laparoscopic bowel injuries were recognized at the time of surgery, with a mean time to diagnosis of 4 days (range 0 to 23 days).[7] Patients may be asymptomatic for several days before the development of signs or symptoms of bowel perforation. As a general rule, 24 to 48 hours after laparoscopy, patients should progressively feel better; with persistent or worsening clinical manifesta-

tions such as pain, nausea, vomiting, or fever, the index of suspicion for injury should be high.

Harkki-Siren and Kurki[3] looked specifically at time to diagnosis of small bowel and large bowel injury depending on the mechanism of the injury. Only 1 of the 26 small bowel injuries (3.9%) was diagnosed at the time of primary laparoscopy, with an average time to diagnosis of 3.3 days for all injuries. The time to diagnosis was longer for injuries caused by electrocautery (4.8 days, range 1 to 10 days) than for injuries caused by a trocar or Veress needle (1.7 days, range 0 to 5). Diagnosis was delayed in 56% of large bowel injuries; complications were recognized earlier if the cause of injury was traumatic, as from a Veress needle or trocar (1.3 days, range 0 to 4), than if the injury was caused by electrocautery (10.4 days, range 0 to 38).[3] In summary, traumatic mechanical injuries usually manifest earlier than thermal injuries to bowel,[3] because it can take 72 to 96 hours after thermal insult for tissue necrosis to cause intestinal perforation.[18]

Patients with gastrointestinal injuries will often present several days after surgery with signs and symptoms of peritonitis, such as abdominal pain, nausea, vomiting, fever, and leukocytosis. Imaging studies are of variable usefulness in the diagnosis of bowel perforation. An abdominal radiograph to evaluate for free air under the diaphragm is of limited use, because patients commonly demonstrate residual pneumoperitoneum after laparoscopy.[20-23] Presence of free air under the diaphragm has been demonstrated a few hours to several weeks postoperatively.[22] A computed tomography (CT) scan with water-soluble oral contrast can be helpful to aid diagnosis, especially if extravasation of dye into the peritoneal cavity is seen. Additionally, water-soluble rectal contrast can be used if rectal or sigmoid injury is suspected, although if with enough time, oral contrast can be sufficient to evaluate the lower gastrointestinal tract. Finally, intravenous contrast can be added to evaluate for ureteral injuries as a source of the patient's symptoms.

Gastrointestinal complications can lead to significant morbidity and even death, with a mortality rate as high as 21% in cases of delayed diagnosis.[15] Not only can these delays lead to significant morbidity and mortality, but they also represent a major cause for litigation after laparoscopy.[24]

MANAGEMENT OF BOWEL INJURIES

Intraoperative management of bowel injuries depends on the type of injury and the experience and comfort level of the surgeon. Most patients with gastrointestinal injury undergo a laparotomy for repair. In a Finnish nationwide review of 32,205 gynecologic laparoscopic procedures, no bowel injuries were treated laparoscopically; 23 out of 24 cases were treated with laparotomy, and one rectovaginal fistula healed without further surgical management.[4] Chapron and associates[7] also reported that the vast majority (83.9%) of patients underwent laparotomy for repair of the gastrointestinal injury, with the remainder undergoing laparoscopic repair.[7]

The management of bowel injuries depends on the location, extent, and mechanism of the injury and on whether preoperative mechanical bowel preparation was performed. Most bowel injuries that are recognized at the time of the initial procedure can be repaired in primary fashion; diversion usually is not required. This decision is best made in conjunction with a consulting general surgeon, unless the gynecologist has had ample experience dealing with bowel injuries. The decision whether to perform the repair through laparoscopy or laparotomy also relies on the judgment of the gynecologist and the general surgeon according to their respective experience. If intraperitoneal spillage occurs in a patient who has not undergone preoperative mechanical bowel preparation, vigorous lavage should be performed after laparoscopic repair. If the contamination is extensive, a laparotomy may be needed to adequately perform peritoneal toilet. In the case of delayed diagnosis, especially with peritonitis or abscess formation, bowel diversion usually is performed at the time of repair through a laparotomy. In general, an attempt at laparoscopic bowel repair should be performed only by practitioners who have ample suturing and surgical experience. Consultation with a general surgeon is indicated if the gynecologist is not comfortable with evaluation or repair of bowel injuries or if any question remains regarding the optimal manage-ment plan.

Small Bowel Injury

Mechanical Injury

The management of bowel injuries caused by mechanical trauma—such as from the Veress needle or trocar or from dissection or lysis of adhesions—varies depending on the extent of the damage. Defects limited to the serosa or seromuscular layer of bowel with an intact mucosa can be oversewn using a small-caliber (3-0 to 6-0) polydioxanone suture (PDS) with an SH or BV-1 needle. Most of these superficial injuries occur during dissection or lysis of adhesions

Although small punctures may be expectantly managed, larger injuries should always be surgically repaired. Expectant management in these situations can lead to peritonitis, reoperation, and significant morbidity.[17] Injuries requiring surgical repair may result from a Veress needle laceration or a trocar puncture or may be secondary to dissection and lysis of adhesions.

Some authors advocate that if an injury is less than 5 mm in diameter, such as a Veress needle injury, the perforation may heal spontaneously, and medical management including broad-spectrum antibiotics and close surveillance may be sufficient.[3,9,17,18,25] Nevertheless, Veress needle injuries frequently have been implicated as the cause of bowel injury and subsequent morbidity. Such injuries should be repaired with a simple figure-of-eight suture. Larger lacerations may be repaired using a two-layer closure, to help avoid subsequent morbidity.

If a trocar or laparoscope enters the lumen of a loop of bowel, it should be left in place to limit contamination of the abdominal cavity and to help identify the site of the defect.[18] Once the site of injury is identified and controlled to prevent spillage of bowel contents, the instrument can be removed and the repair completed.

The extent of the injury and the skill and comfort level of the surgeon will help dictate whether repairs can be done laparoscopically or if a laparotomy should be performed. An experienced surgeon can treat isolated small bowel injuries laparoscopically. With an extensive injury or multiple areas

of damage, bowel resection with anastomosis may be performed by laparoscopy or laparotomy. Alternatively, a mini-laparotomy can be performed to exteriorize the damaged segment of bowel, followed by resection of the compromised areas with side-to-side reanastomosis. For example, by extending the umbilical trocar site, a small incision can be made through which an adequate repair can be performed (see Fig. 6–2E-G). The morbidity associated with such a procedure is low, with a short postoperative recovery period.

Thermal Injury

The treatment of thermal injury depends on the extent of the damage, which often is difficult to assess at the time of injury. Thermal injury may be identified intraoperatively as an area of blanching; however, the area of injury is not always clear, and the full extent often is not immediately apparent.

Superficial serosal burns can be observed expectantly for signs and symptoms of peritonitis or oversewn with a size 3-0 PDS suture. More extensive injury warrants immediate treatment, and bowel resection may be required. The extent of injury is proportional to the surgical dosage applied. *Surgical dosage* is defined as watts × duration (time of contact) and is influenced by the size of the electrode. The most dangerous injury is caused by monopolar current, which may contact bowel for a prolonged period of time without the surgeon's being aware of it. It is prudent in these cases to resect the compromised area with margins well beyond the area of blanching, because the thermal damage can extend beyond its apparent border. When thermal injury is witnessed directly, the surgical dosage is evident and the damage not as extensive. We prefer oversewing, rather than expectant management, for witnessed injuries.

Case Study 6–1 ▪ SMALL BOWEL INJURY CASE PRESENTATION

A 43-year-old healthy woman with multiple uterine fibroids and uterine enlargement (to a size consistent with 18 weeks of gestation) causing bladder pressure and dyspareunia desired surgical managment. A total laparoscopic hysterectomy was scheduled, and the patient performed a mechanical bowel preparation before her scheduled surgery.

During blind direct puncture with a 5-mm nonoptical trocar, trauma was noted on the uterus, raising suspicion of an impalement injury (Fig. 6–3A). Once all the trocars were inserted, the bowel was examined along its length laparoscopically from the ileocecal junction to the duodenum (see Fig. 6–4B). Atraumatic bowel graspers can be used to "milk" ileal contents to help identify the area of injury. The small bowel was found to have a through-and-through puncture, with an additional hole approximately 4 inches away where the ileum had been bunched together. The larger lacerations were repaired with a two-layer closure using 4-0 PDS in a continuous fashion. It is imperative that the defect be closed in a transverse fashion to avoid narrowing of the intestinal lumen (Fig. 6–4; see also Fig. 6–3C and D). The smaller puncture sites were closed with a single figure of eight suture using 4-0 Prolene (see Fig. 6–3E and F). The defects were closed transversely, to avoid narrowing and constriction of the intestinal lumen. After repair of the ileum, laparoscopic hysterectomy with ovarian conservation was carried out, and the patient had an uncomplicated postoperative course.

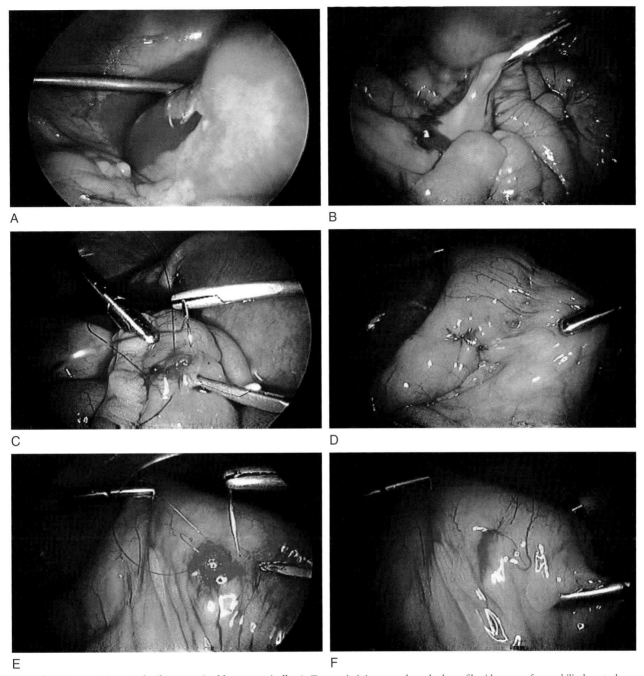

Figure 6–3 ▪ **Trocar injury to the ileum repaired laparoscopically. A,** Traumatic injury noted on the large fibroid uterus after umbilical port placement raises suspicion for potential bowel injury. **B,** The full length of the bowel was examined, revealing three puncture sites, including a through-and-through injury. **C,** The injury is repaired using a continuous 4-0 Prolene suture in two layers. **D,** Completed repair. Note that the repair of the defect is completed in a transverse fashion, perpendicular to the longitudinal axis of the bowel, to avoid narrowing of the intestinal lumen. **E,** The other side of the same through-and-through injury is repaired in figure-of-eight fashion using 6-0 Prolene. **F,** The completed repair.

Large Bowel Injury

Mechanical Injury

As with small bowel injuries, the management of injuries to the large bowel varies depending on the extent of the damage. Serosal or seromuscular defects of the colon and sigmoid can be repaired by oversewing the damaged area, as described earlier for management of small bowel injuries.

Full-thickness injury to the large intestines can be managed with either laparoscopic or open techniques, depending on the extent of the injury, surgeon experience, whether a preoperative mechanical bowel preparation was performed, and how much spillage of bowel contents has occurred. Management preferences vary, and an intraoperative general surgery consultation should be considered if any questions remain about optimal management or if the repair

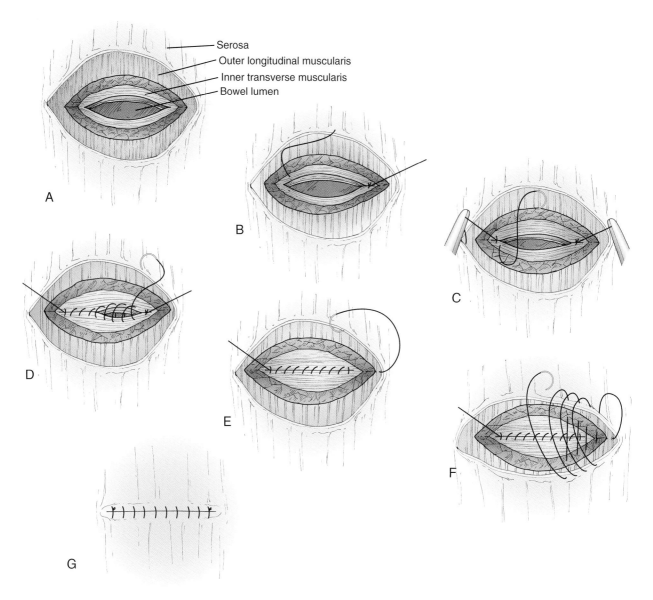

Serosa
Outer longitudinal muscularis
Inner transverse muscularis
Bowel lumen

Figure 6–4 ▪ **Repair of full-thickness defect of the bowel.** The defect may result from an intentional resection of endometriosis or inadvertent injury to the bowel. Regardless of the mechanism, the repair can be performed as described. **A,** The bowel is composed of an outer serosal layer, the muscularis, and the mucosa. The muscularis consists of an outer longitudinal and an inner transverse, or circular, muscle layer. **B,** A single interrupted stitch is placed on the right side of the defect for reference. Using 3-0 to 6-0 (depending on the location of the injury) polydiaxinone suture (PDS) starting on the *left*, a running suture includes the mucosa and transverse muscularis layers. A long tail is left on the running suture for traction and is used to tie the second layer of suture (see **F**). **C,** Occasional traction on the reference stitch on the *right* allows clear definition of the extent of the defect and an even closure. It is important to perform the closure in a transverse fashion, perpendicular to the longitudinal axis of the bowel. **D,** Completion of the first layer of the running suture for the length of the defect. **E,** Once the first suture layer is complete, the needle and suture should emerge approximately 1 cm lateral to the right wound edge. **F,** Using the same suture, a second continuous layer is performed, placing the suture 1 cm lateral to the previous suture in order to imbricate the first layer. This layer may include the outer longitudinal muscularis alone, or the outer longitudinal muscularis and the serosa. **G,** The suture from the second layer is tied to the tail that was left long from the initial knot from the first layer. Thus, the defect is closed with a single suture.

of the large bowel injury is beyond the scope of the gynecologist's experience.

In a patient in whom a preoperative bowel preparation has been performed, damage to large bowel can be closed primarily, if appropriate. Patients with an "unprepped" bowel or significant spillage, however, may require a diverting colostomy. The need for a bowel resection depends on the extent of the bowel injury.

If a trocar or laparoscope enters the lumen of a loop of bowel, it should be left in place as a "seal" to limit contamination of the abdominal cavity until the defect can be repaired.[18] If the repair will be attempted laparoscopically, alternate sites should be used for insufflation, visualization, and manipulation. If the repair will be performed by laparotomy, the trocar or laparoscope should not be removed until the incision is made, the injured bowel has been located, and

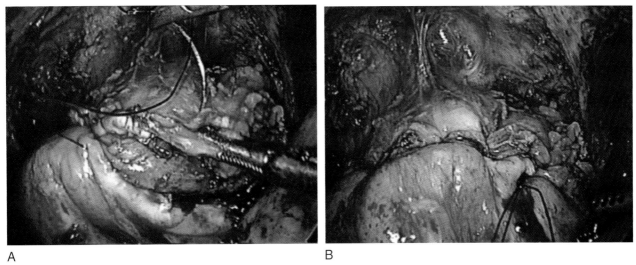

A   B

Figure 6–5 ▪ **Partial-thickness large bowel injury and repair. A,** Partial-thickness excision of area of endometriosis on the sigmoid is repaired by using 3-0 polydiaxinone suture (PDS) in a single continuous layer to oversew the defect. **B,** Completed repair. Note the transverse orientation of the suture line in the oversewn repair.

the defect isolated to prevent spillage of bowel contents into the abdominal cavity.

Intentional bowel injury can occur during the excision of areas of rectal endometriosis or for cul-de-sac obliteration with rectovaginal adherence. Such procedures require preoperative bowel preparation. (See "Prevention" section for a bowel preparation regimen.) Superficial endometriotic lesions on the bowel manifest as external bulges on the bowel surface without associated narrowing of the bowel lumen. During the excision of these lesions using either the laser or scissors, a defect is made in the bowel wall to the level of the inner longitudinal muscularis. The defect created by the partial-thickness resection is oversewn using a single or double layer of continuous 3-0 PDS (Fig. 6–5A and B). Intramural endometriosis penetrates the inner transverse, or circular, muscle layer (Fig. 6–6A). If these lesions are less than 3 cm across, they can be excised with a full-thickness disk excision (see Fig. 6–6B), followed by closure using 3-0 Prolene in two or three layers. The first layer is continuous and incorporates the bowel mucosa and muscularis (see Fig. 6–6C and D); the second layer also is continuous and incorporates the sero-muscularis (see Figs. 6–6E and F and 6–4). A third layer, either continuous or interrupted, can be used to imbricate the sero-muscularis over the previous suture line (see Fig. 6–4). The same technique just described for repair of intentional injuries to bowel can be used to repair inadvertent injuries to bowel as well.

After the repair of partial- or full-thickness excision, a test for leakage should be performed. An atraumatic bowel grasper is used to compress the bowel proximal to the repair and the operating table is flattened to horizontal. The pelvis is filled with fluid and a proctoscope is inserted into the rectum; air is insufflated through the proctoscope to distend the rectum. The absence of bubbles indicates a secure repair. An alternative method to air distention is to instill povidone-iodine (Betadine) through a large Foley catheter inserted into the rectum. The pelvic fluid must be very clear to allow detection of leakage of Betadine from the wound. Because this method

is not always practicable, the use of air to test for leakage is preferable.

Thermal Injury

The treatment of thermal injuries to large bowel is similar to that for small bowel. Superficial serosal burns can be observed

---

Case Study 6–2 ▪ LARGE BOWEL INJURY CASE PRESENTATION

A 34-year-old gravida 1 para 0 with pelvic pain and a history of known endometriosis presented with recurrent, worsening pain. Seven years ago she underwent laparoscopic fulguration of endometriosis, which resulted in significant pain relief for almost 6 years. She has a history of pelvic inflammatory disease, and her past surgical history includes exploratory laparotomy for a ruptured ectopic pregnancy. She performed a bowel preparation before her scheduled surgery for treatment of her pelvic pain and endometriosis.

During the peritoneal access procedure using a 5-mm Optiview (Ethicon Endosurgery, Cincinnati, Ohio) trocar, injury to the transverse colon was recognized instantly by a view of the classic rugae of intestinal mucosa and fecal material (see Fig. 6–1A). In this case, another Optiview trocar was inserted laterally and a pneumoperitoneum created. During this process, the injured bowel fell away from the umbilical trocar. The puncture location could be readily visualized. The umbilical trocar was replaced and the laparoscope moved to this port. Two 5-mm trocars placed on the patient's right side allowed laparoscopic suture of the injury. The only clue to the area of damage was a mild hematoma in the omentum (see Fig. 6–1B); if the injury had not been identified as it occurred, it could easily have been missed.

The omentum was dissected using bipolar forceps and scissors until the muscle of the intestine was seen, at which time the 1-cm hole was evident (see Fig. 6–1C). The puncture was repaired laparoscopically using two layers of 3-0 PDS in a continuous fashion (see Figs. 6–1D–F and 6–4). Vigorous peritoneal lavage was performed at the end of the repair. The planned procedure, ablation of endometriotic lesions, then was carried out, without further complications. The patient made an uneventful recovery.

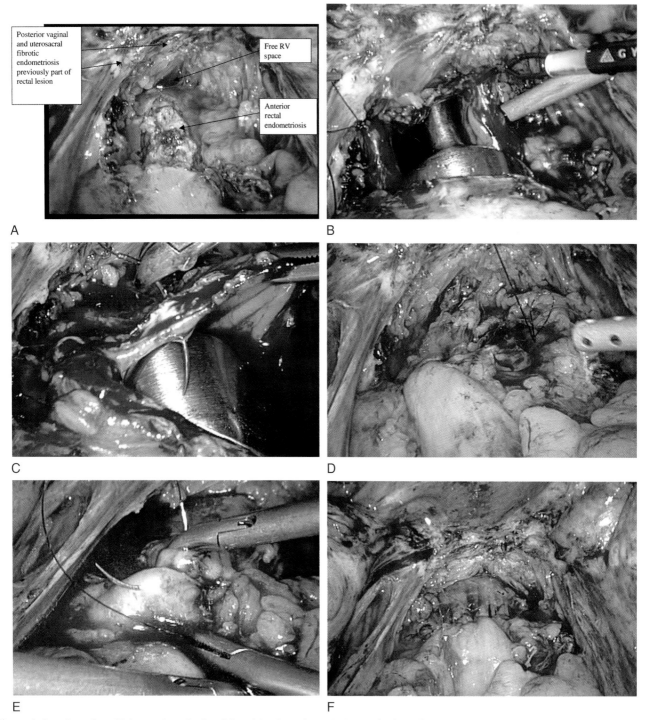

Figure 6–6 ▪ **Large bowel injury and repair after disk excision for endometriosis. A,** After lysis of adhesions and separation of the rectum from the posterior vagina, an area of rectal endometriosis is evident as a *white* lesion. RV, rectovaginal. **B,** A rectal defect is created after a full-thickness disk excision of the area of endometriosis. An end-to-end anastomosis sizer is left in the rectum to provide better visibility. The "tail" of the suture is left long to help identify the most lateral edge of the defect. **C,** The first layer includes the rectal mucosa and the muscularis. The repair is performed using 3-0 Prolene on an SH needle and a Storz macro-needle holder starting at the left aspect of the defect. **D,** The first layer of continuous suture is completed and tied on the right margin of the defect. **E,** Using the same suture, the second layer of the closure is performed. This layer includes the muscularis and imbricates the first layer. This suture is tied to the original "tail" of the first knot. **F,** Completed two-layer closure of the rectal defect. Note the transverse direction of the repair, which helps avoid luminal narrowing and constriction.

expectantly for signs and symptoms of peritonitis[16,17] or over-sewn with 3-0 PDS. More extensive injury warrants immediate treatment, and bowel resection may be required, possibly with a diverting colostomy in a patient in whom preoperative bowel preparation was not performed.[16]

PREVENTION OF BOWEL INJURY

Prevention of gastrointestinal injury is one of the keys to decreasing the morbidity and mortality of laparoscopic surgery. The surgeon should employ both preoperative and intraoperative strategies to help prevent bowel injuries. Unfortunately, even if all appropriate precautions are taken, complications will still arise. In such cases, a high index of suspicion and prompt recognition are of utmost importance.

Several studies have demonstrated a significant decrease in the number of laparoscopic complications,[24,25] and of bowel injuries specifically,[2] with increasing surgeon experience. This finding highlights the importance of training and good surgical technique.

Thorough preoperative planning and selective bowel preparation for patients who are at high risk for bowel injury are recommended. Risk factors include a history of surgery, endometriosis, and known or suspected adhesions. Mechanical injury to the large or small bowel is 10 times more likely in patients with previous intraperitoneal inflammation or abdominal surgery.[26] Although a preoperative bowel preparation may not prevent an injury, it can allow primary repair if an injury does occur. If no bowel preparation is done, a diverting colostomy may be required, depending on the location and type of injury. One suggested bowel preparation regimen is as follows:

1. Clear liquid diet the day before surgery
2. Sodium phosphate (Fleet Phospho-Soda) 45 mL orally twice, the day and the evening before surgery
3. Sodium phosphate enema (Fleet Enema) once on the morning of surgery

To diminish the risk of bowel injury during the entry phase, several precautions can be taken. Gastric emptying before the abdominal cavity is entered can prevent injury to an overinflated stomach. Some experts advocate routine use of a nasogastric or orogastric tube for every case, whereas others empty the stomach only if left upper quadrant entry is planned, after a difficult intubation, or if signs of gastric distention are present.[7,26]

Additionally, in patients with known or suspected adhesions, alternative sites for insufflation should be considered. The possibility of bowel adhesions is increased in patients who have had previous surgery, leading to concern for potential bowel injury during insertion of the umbilical trocar. Rates for incidence of umbilical bowel adhesions in patients with a previous vertical midline incision, after a low transverse incision, and after laparoscopy have been reported to be 52%, 20%, and 1.6%, respectively.[27]

Left upper quadrant entry, initially described by Palmer in 1974,[28] can be used as an alternative for patients in whom presence of umbilical bowel adhesions is likely (Fig. 6–7). Once placement of the left upper quadrant port has been accomplished, it can hold the laparoscope for the remainder

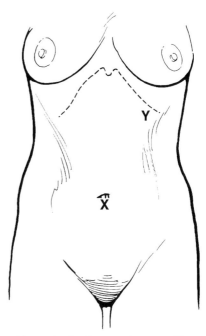

Figure 6–7 ■ **Alternative sites for port placement.** The umbilicus (X) is the usual site for Veress needle and initial port placement. The left upper quadrant (Y) can be used as an alternative site for Veress needle and initial port placement when presence of subumbilical or umbilical adhesions is known or suspected.

of the procedure. Alternatively, successful entry at the left upper quadrant allows the insertion of a second 5-mm port through which adhesiolysis and enterolysis can be performed, freeing new areas for more secondary ports to be inserted and ultimately for the laparoscope to be inserted in the cleared umbilical area. This technique of sequential and serial placement of ports may be necessary in women whose entire anterior abdominal wall has dense bowel adhesions (Fig. 6–8). Other options include creating the pneumoperitoneum through the posterior fornix of the vagina or the fundus of the uterus.[26,29]

The fact that approximately a third of gastrointestinal injuries occur during the initiation phase of laparoscopy[7] draws attention to the method of entry used. Many different access techniques have been described. The techniques most commonly used are (1) the closed (or Veress) technique, with blind insertion of the Veress needle to create the pneumoperitoneum, followed by blind insertion of the trocar, (2) blind direct trocar placement without previous pneumoperitoneum, and (3) the open (Hasson) method. In the limited studies comparing techniques, no one technique has been clearly demonstrated to be superior.[29-31] Of note, although proponents of each technique will advocate its benefits, major vascular and visceral injuries have been reported with all of these techniques.[5,31]

Although the open or Hasson technique may reduce the risk of major vascular injuries, it does not prevent bowel injuries.[30-34] In fact, several studies report an increased risk of bowel injury with the open access technique.[31,32] This finding may be due to patient selection bias—surgeons may be more likely to use the open technique in patients at higher risk for bowel adhesions. In addition, the risk of bowel injury may

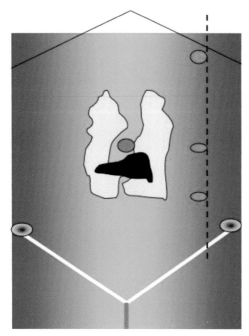

Figure 6–8 ▪ **Alternative port site placement.** Once placement of the left upper quadrant port has been accomplished, it can hold the laparoscope for the remainder of the procedure. Alternatively, successful entry at the left upper quadrant allows the insertion of a second 5-mm port through which adhesiolysis and enterolysis can be performed, freeing new areas for more secondary ports to be inserted and ultimately for the laparoscope to be inserted in the cleared umbilical area. This technique of sequential and serial placement of ports may be necessary in women whose entire anterior abdominal wall has dense bowel adhesions.

be higher in general surgery procedures than in gynecologic procedures. One proposed advantage to the open technique is rapid identification of bowel injury if it does occur. A third of small intestine injuries caused by this technique, however, are not diagnosed at the time of the primary procedure.[29,33]

Another commonly used method of entry is direct insertion of the trocar without creation of a pneumoperitoneum, to avoid the additional blind step required with the Veress needle. Comparisons of the blind and the Veress techniques fail to show an advantage of either method.[5,31,32] In addition, new technologies and instrumentation such as optical trocars, retractable shields, and radially expanding access systems have been developed in attempts to minimize complications. Bowel injuries have been reported with all of these modalities, however, and no large-scale studies have established any significant advantage of one over any other method.[17,31,35,36]

Most laparoscopists use the technique that they were initially taught. A majority of gynecologists use the Veress technique.[31] In view of the lack of conclusive data supporting one particular entry method over another, familiarity with several entry techniques is recommended, so that the surgeon can use the method most appropriate for the individual patient.

Regardless of the entry method used, it is important to systematically inspect the bowel after the primary trocar is placed. If adhesions to the anterior abdominal wall are present, the laparoscope should be placed in another port to visualize the site of the primary trocar. Although the most common access injuries are caused by the Veress needle or the primary trocar, 16% of bowel perforations that occur during the access phase of laparoscopy are caused by auxiliary trocars.[7] Directly visualizing the entry of the secondary trocars, to ensure they are inserted in a place that is free from adhesions and away from bowel, can help reduce inadvertent bowel injury and allow instant recognition should it occur. The skin incision should be large enough to avoid excessive tissue resistance, which can lead to uncontrolled entry when the skin suddenly gives way. Occasionally, the bowel needs to be pushed away from the path of the trocar if the sharp tip comes dangerously close to the bowel.

Care also should be taken during dissection and adhesiolysis; furthermore, the surgeon should carefully inspect all areas after performing lysis of adhesions. Viewing adhesions from different ports may help delineate the extent of bowel adhesions and help operative planning. For example, a 5-mm laparopscope initially placed in the umbilical port can be moved to an ancillary lateral 5-mm port in order to get a better view of midline anterior abdominal wall adhesions and allow for safer dissection. Increasing the magnification during dissection by bringing the laparopscope closer to the operative field also can help with identifying correct planes and safe areas for dissection (Fig. 6–9A and B). If electrocautery is used during the focus on the operative field, care must be taken to ensure that no inadvertent thermal injuries have been created outside of the visualized area. Blunt dissection also can be used to help lyse adhesions and define surgical planes; however, caution is in order, because aggressive blunt dissection also can lead to inadvertent bowel injury. Placing the scissors or other instrument behind adhesions to determine if they are transparent (and thus do not contain bowel) can help identify areas that can be safely dissected. If dense bowel adhesions to the anterior abdominal wall are seen, part of the adhesion and the parietal peritoneum can be taken down with the bowel to avoid compromising the bowel serosa and muscularis. Care must be taken not to completely de-peritonealize the anterior abdominal wall, because this can lead to re-formation of the adhesions. Similar operative techniques can be employed in lysis of large bowel adhesions. Although the transverse colon can be adherent to the anterior abdominal wall and the ascending and descending colon can be adherent to the lateral abdominal wall, rectosigmoid adhesions are most commonly encountered and treated in gynecologic surgery. The rectosigmoid often is adherent to the ovaries and posterior uterus as a result of pelvic inflammatory disease, endometriosis, or previous surgery by laparoscopy or laparotomy for fibroids or endometriosis.

If the possibility of rectal perforation after lysis of adhesions is a concern, the pelvis can be filled with saline, and air injected into the rectum. Any air bubbles will help identify a defect in the bowel. Of note, bowel injuries caused by electrocautery may not be identified with this method, because necrosis does not lead to immediate perforation.

Lysis of dense bowel adhesions should be attempted only by an experienced laparoscopist. If the surgery cannot be performed safely laparoscopically, the surgeon has the option of performing a laparotomy.

Thermal injury from electrocautery has been implicated in a significant proportion of bowel injuries. Instruments should be inspected before use to rule out any defects in the insulation and should be removed from the abdominal cavity

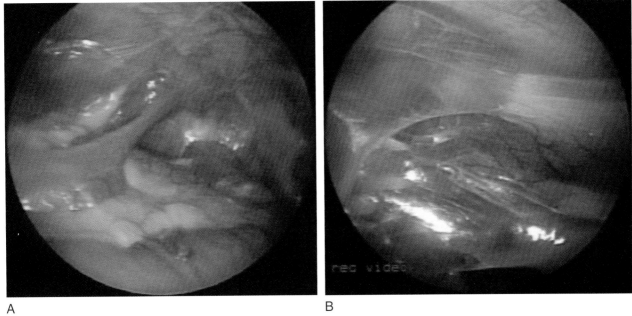

A   B

Figure 6–9 ■ Increasing magnification can help identify safe surgical planes for dissection. **A,** Overall view of anterior abdominal wall adhesions. **B,** Increasing magnification by bringing the laparoscope closer to the adhesions and the operative field can help identify operative planes and safe areas for dissection.

when not being used, to prevent direct thermal injuries caused by inadvertently touching tissue with an active electrode. The entire active portion of the instrument should be visualized in the operative field, and care should be taken to make sure that the active electrode is not in contact with any conducting instruments. Both bipolar and monopolar electrocautery can cause bowel injury and thermal extension. Of note, however, the thermal extension with monopolar electrosurgery is up to 5 cm (compared with 5 mm with bipolar), and this modality should be used with caution.[17] To reduce the risk of thermal spread to unintended tissues, areas that are going to be coagulated must be isolated and elevated, with care taken to ensure an adequate margin of tissue.

INCISIONAL HERNIAS

Herniation of bowel through a laparoscopic incision site is a rare occurrence but should be considered in the differential diagnosis if a patient presents postoperatively with obstructive gastrointestinal symptoms, nausea, vomiting, abdominal distension, pain, and fever or chills. On average, the time to diagnosis and surgical treatment of incisional hernias is 8.5 days (range 2 to 42 days).[37]

Overall, hernias appear more common in extraumbilical port sites[11,37,38] and with larger port sizes.[38-40] The incidence of incisional hernias varies depending on the study cited. A large nationwide review of 32,205 gynecologic laparoscopies revealed an incisional hernia rate of 0.03%, occurring in 5- to 12-mm port sites.[4] In a large retrospective study done by the AAGL in 1994, 933 hernias were reported from an estimated 4,385,000 laparoscopic procedures (0.02%).[41] Eighty-six percent of these incisional hernias occurred in port sites 10 mm in diameter or greater.[41] Approximately one fifth of the

reported hernias occurred despite fascial closure.[41] A survey of laparoscopy-assisted vaginal hysterectomies in 2000 reported a 0.23% hernia rate; the vast majority of these (85%) occurred with trocars larger than 10 mm.[11] Risk of herniation was higher with extraumbilical ports than with umbilical port sites.[11] A retrospective review by Kadar and colleagues of 3560 laparoscopies examined the frequency of incisional hernias at extraumbilical 10- and 12-mm trocar insertion sites and reported a 0.17% rate of incisional hernia per insertion site; these hernias were reported most frequently with 12-mm ports and if the fascia was left open.[39]

To correctly and promptly diagnose an incisional hernia after laparoscopy, the possibility of postoperative bowel or omental herniation must always be kept in mind. The index of suspicion should be higher in patients who have undergone laparoscopic procedures requiring extensive manipulation through trocar sites, multiple entries of the trocar into the incision, or removal of a specimen from an incision resulting in stretching of the fascia. Diagnosis of bowel or omental herniation can be made by clinical examination, CT scan, or upper gastrointestinal series.[37]

Some methods are useful to help reduce the incidence of incisional hernias. Because of the increased risk of herniation with larger port sizes,[38-40] the fascia should always be closed when 10-mm or larger trocars are used. Accurate identification of fascial edges is important but often can be challenging because of limited visibility. Laparoscopic guidance may be helpful to ensure adequate closure of the fascia. Additionally, the surgeon should consider using trocars with smaller diameters when possible. Although closing the fascia of these larger ports is thought to decrease the incidence of hernias, incisional hernias have been described despite fascial closure in multiple cases.[37,40-42] Although quite unusual, herniation of bowel through 5-mm port sites also has been reported. Nevertheless, most surgeons do not close the fascia on 5-mm incisions as it is technically challenging and a rare occurrence.

Removing ports under direct visualization, slow decompression of the pneumoperitoneum when the sheath is removed, and inserting a blunt probe into the trocar as it is withdrawn all have been proposed as methods to decrease the occurrence of bowel herniation through the trocar incisions.[40]

CONCLUSIONS

Bowel complications resulting from laparoscopic surgery are rare; however, they are associated with significant morbidity. Methods should be employed both preoperatively and intraoperatively to reduce the occurrence of bowel injuries. Even when all possible precautions are observed, complications still can occur. Prompt diagnosis and appropriate, timely management will limit the subsequent morbidity associated with these complications.

References

1. Peterson HB, Hulka JF, Phillips JM. American Association of Gynecologic Laparoscopists 1988 membership survey on operative laparoscopy. J Reprod Med 1990;35:587.
2. Chapron C, Querleu D, Bruhat MA, et al. Surgical complications of diagnostic and operative gynaecological laparoscopy: A series of 29,966 cases. Hum Reprod 1998;13:867.
3. Harkki-Siren P, Kurki T. A nationwide analysis of laparoscopic complications. Obstet Gynecol 1997;89:108.
4. Harkki-Siren P, Sjoberg J, Kurki T. Major complications of laparoscopy: A follow-up Finnish study. Obstet Gynecol 1999;94:94.
5. Philips PA, Amaral JF. Abdominal access complications in laparoscopic surgery. J Am Coll Surg 2001;192:525.
6. Wang PH, Lee WL, Yuan CC, et al. Major complications of operative and diagnostic laparoscopy for gynecologic disease. J Am Assoc Gynecol Laparosc 2001;8:68.
7. Chapron C, Pierre F, Harchaoui Y, et al. Gastrointestinal injuries during gynaecological laparoscopy. Hum Reprod 1999;14:333.
8. Lehmann-Willenbrock E, Riedel HH, Mecke H, Semm K. Pelviscopy/laparoscopy and its complications in Germany, 1949-1988. J Reprod Med 1992;37:671.
9. Jansen FW, Kapiteyn K, Trimbos-Kemper T, et al. Complications of laparoscopy: A prospective multicentre observational study. Br J Obstet Gynaecol 1997;104:595.
10. Harkki-Siren P, Sjoberg J, Makinen J, et al. Finnish National Register of Laparoscopic Hysterectomies: A review and complications of 1165 operations. Am J Obstet Gynecol 1997;176(1 Pt 1):118.
11. Kives SL, Levy BS, Levine RL, American Association of Gynecologic Laparoscopists. Laparoscopic-assisted vaginal hysterectomy: American Association of Gynecologic Laparoscopists' 2000 membership survey. J Am Assoc Gynecol Laparosc 2003;10:135.
12. Shen CC, Wu MP, Kung FT, et al. Major complications associated with laparoscopic-assisted vaginal hysterectomy: Ten-year experience. J Am Assoc Gynecol Laparosc 2003;10:147.
13. Garry R, Fountain J, Mason S, et al. The eVALuate Study: Two parallel randomised trials, one comparing laparoscopic with abdominal hysterectomy, the other comparing laparoscopic with vaginal hysterectomy. [Erratum appears in BMJ 2004;328:494.] BMJ 2004;328:129.
14. Mirhashemi R, Harlow BL, Ginsburg ES, et al. Predicting risk of complications with gynecologic laparoscopic surgery. Obstet Gynecol 1998;92:327.
15. Brosens I, Gordon A, Campo R, et al. Bowel injury in gynecologic laparoscopy. J Am Assoc Gynecol Laparosc 2003;10:9.
16. Voyles CR, Tucker RD. Unrecognized hazards of surgical electrodes passed through metal suction-irrigation devices. Surg Endosc 1994;8:185.
17. Donnez J. Complications of laparoscopic surgery in gynecology. In: Donnez J, Nisolle M, eds. An atlas of operative laparoscopy and hysteroscopy, 2nd ed. New York: Parthenon Publishing Group, 2001;373.
18. Nawnoum AB, Murphy AA. Diagnostic and operative laparoscopy. In: Rock JA, Jones HW, eds. TeLinde's operative gynecology, 9th ed. Philadelphia: Lippincott Williams & Wilkins, 2003;353.
19. Vilos GA, Vilos AG. Safe laparoscopic entry guided by Veress needle CO_2 insufflation pressure. J Am Assoc Gynecol Laparosc 2003;10:415.
20. Grainger DAA, Gershenson DM, DeCherney AH, et al. Postoperative care: Endoscopic surgery. In: Zorab R, ed. Operative gynecology, 2nd ed. Philadelphia: WB Saunders, 2001;81.
21. Farooqui MO, Bazzoli JM. Significance of radiologic evidence of free air following laparoscopy. J Reprod Med 1976;16:119.
22. Adcock J, Martin DC. Resolution of subdiaphragmatic gas. J Am Assoc Gynecol Laparosc 1999;6:501.
23. Thomson AJ, Abbott JA, Lenart M, et al. Assessment of a method to expel intraperitoneal gas after gynecologic laparoscopy. J Minim Invasive Gynecol 2005;12:125.
24. Soderstrom RM. Bowel injury litigation after laparoscopy. J Am Assoc Gynecol Laparosc 1993;1:74.
25. Townsend CM, Beauchamp RD, Evers BM, Mattox KL, eds. Sabiston textbook of surgery, 17th ed. Philadelphia: Elsevier Saunders, 2004;452.
26. Munro MG, Brill AI. Gynecologic endoscopy. In: Berek J S, Hillard PJA, Adashi EY, eds. Novak's gynecology, 13th ed. Philadelphia: Lippincott Williams & Wilkins, 2002;711.
27. Audebert AJ, Gomel V. Role of microlaparoscopy in the diagnosis of peritoneal and visceral adhesions and in the prevention of bowel injury associated with blind trocar insertion. Fertil Steril 2000;73:631.
28. Palmer R. Safety in laparoscopy. J Reprod Med 1974;13:1.
29. Rosen DM, Lam AM, Chapman M, et al. Methods of creating pneumoperitoneum: A review of techniques and complications. Obstet Gynecol Surv 1998;53:167.
30. Chapron C, Cravello L, Chopin N, et al. Complications during set-up procedures for laparoscopy in gynecology: Open laparoscopy does not reduce the risk of major complications. Acta Obstet Gynecol Scand 2003;82: 1125.
31. Molloy D, Kaloo PD, Cooper M, Nguyen TV. Laparoscopic entry: A literature review and analysis of techniques and complications of primary port entry. Aust N Z J Obstet Gynaecol 2002;42:246.
32. Merlin TL, Hiller JE, Maddern GJ, et al. Systematic review of the safety and effectiveness of methods used to establish pneumoperitoneum in laparoscopic surgery. Br J Surg 2003;90:668.
33. Penfield AJ. How to prevent complications of open laparoscopy. J Reprod Med 1985;30:660.
34. Bonjer HJ, Hazebroek EJ, Kazemier G, et al. Open versus closed establishment of pneumoperitoneum in laparoscopic surgery. Br J Surg 1997;84:599.
35. Sharp HT, Dodson MK, Draper ML, et al. Complications associated with optical-access laparoscopic trocars. Obstet Gynecol 2002;99:553.
36. Oshinsky GS, Smith AD. Laparoscopic needles and trocars: An overview of designs and complications. J Laparoendosc Surg 1992;2:117.
37. Boike GM, Miller CE, Spirtos NM, et al. Incisional bowel herniations after operative laparoscopy: A series of nineteen cases and review of the literature. Am J Obstet Gynecol 1995;172:1726.
38. Lajer H, Widecrantz S, Heisterberg L. Hernias in trocar ports following abdominal laparoscopy. A review. Acta Obstet Gynecol Scand 1997;76:389.
39. Kadar N, Reich H, Liu CY, et al. Incisional hernias after major laparoscopic gynecologic procedures. Am J Obstet Gynecol 1993;168:1493.
40. Rabinerson D, Avrech O, Neri A, Schoenfeld A. Incisional hernias after laparoscopy. Obstet Gynecol Surv 1997;52:701.
41. Montz FJ, Holschneider CH, Munro MG. Incisional hernia following laparoscopy: A survey of the American Association of Gynecologic Laparoscopists. Obstet Gynecol 1994;84:881.
42. Azurin DJ, Go LS, Arroyo LR, Kirkland ML. Trocar site herniation following laparoscopic cholecystectomy and the significance of an incidental preexisting umbilical hernia. Am Surg 1995;61:718.

Urologic Injuries in Laparoscopic Surgery

Peter L. Rosenblatt and Edward Stanford

7

The venial sin is injury to the ureter; the mortal sin is failure of recognition.

DR. THOMAS GREEN

INCIDENCE OF UROLOGIC INJURIES

The incidence of urinary tract injuries during gynecologic laparoscopy is estimated at approximately 1 to 2 injuries per 1000 procedures.[1] This rate appears to be similar to the published rates of urinary tract injury reported after laparotomy.[2] As with laparotomy, the risk of injury during laparoscopy appears to increase with the increasing complexity of the procedure. Ureteral injury has been described in association with a variety of gynecologic procedures, including laparoscopic-assisted vaginal hysterectomy (LAVH), oophorectomy, tubal sterilization, pelvic lymphadenectomy, excision and cautery of endometriotic lesions, and adhesiolysis. In the 1995 American Association of Gynecologic Laparoscopists (AAGL) survey of LAVH procedures, cystotomy occurred at a rate of 10 per 1000 procedures and ureteral injury at a rate of 3 per 1000.[3] Shen and colleagues reported a rate of bladder injury at 4 per 1000 procedures and ureteral injury at 1 per 1000.[4] Although the rates for incidence of ureteral injury seem to be similar whether laparoscopic or open hysterectomy is performed, the incidence of cystotomy may be higher with the laparoscopic approach.[3]

The incidence of bladder injury with vaginal hysterectomy is similar to that for LAVH and total abdominal hysterectomy, but the incidence of ureteral injury is lower for the vaginal approach. Immediate recognition of urinary tract injuries clearly reduces morbidity from these complications; however, most of these injuries are not recognized intraoperatively. Therefore, a high index of suspicion must be maintained during all laparoscopic procedures, and diagnostic tests to determine if an injury has occurred should be performed whenever such a complication is suspected.

ANATOMIC CONSIDERATIONS

A thorough understanding of pelvic anatomy is essential not only for performance of advanced laparoscopic procedures but also to reduce the likelihood of intraoperative complications. The ureter, which measures about 25 to 30 cm long, is divided into an abdominal and a pelvic component, which are approximately equal in length (Fig. 7–1). The abdominal ureters course retroperitoneally along the anteromedial surface of the psoas muscle and enter the pelvis bilaterally, as they cross over the bifurcation of the common iliac vessels at the pelvic brim. Each ureter then courses superficially along the medial leaf of the broad ligament (lateral to the uterosacral ligaments) and usually can be identified in this location by its peristalsis. The ureter then passes under the uterine artery in its connective tissue tunnel within the cardinal ligament, about 1.5 cm lateral to the cervix. Once under the uterine artery, the ureter passes anteromedially over the lateral vaginal fornix and enters the bladder at the trigone. Blood supply to the ureter is quite variable—coming from several sources throughout the course of the ureter in the abdomen and pelvis. Branches directly from the aorta, as well as from the renal and ovarian arteries, provide a blood supply to the abdominal segment of the ureter through the adventitial layer within its sheath. The pelvic segment of the ureter is supplied by branches from the hypogastric artery, as well as from the superior and inferior vesical arteries.

The bladder is a hollow organ that acts as a reservoir for urine. The bladder wall is made up of muscular fibers that travel in many directions, although at the bladder neck, three discrete layers—the inner longitudinal, middle circular, and outer longitudinal layers—can be identified. The superior and upper posterior surface of the bladder is covered with visceral peritoneum. The anterior bladder is extraperitoneal and is found in the retropubic space. The bladder is collapsed and flat in its empty state, becoming more globular and discrete when distended with urine. The superior margin of the full bladder can easily be seen laparoscopically, which is a useful landmark when the retropubic space is entered for reconstructive surgery (Fig. 7–2). The urethra can be seen laparoscopically only after dissection into the retropubic space. The urethra is approximately 4 cm in length, traveling from the trigone distally toward the external meatus as it perforates the perineal membrane. The urethra is firmly attached to the adventitia of the anterior vaginal wall and can easily be palpated with the help of an indwelling catheter.

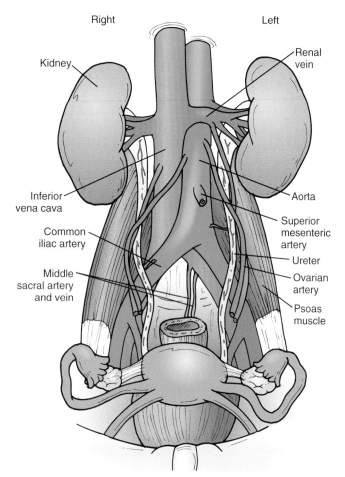

Figure 7–1 ▪ **Anatomy of the ureter.** The abdominal ureters originate from the renal pelvis and descend along the anterior surface of the psoas muscles, posterior to the ovarian vessels. After they cross the pelvic brim at the bifurcation of the common iliac arteries, they are referred to as the pelvic ureters, and they descend along the posteriolateral pelvic sidewall, lateral to the sacrum. Each ureter then passes under the uterine artery 1 to 2 cm lateral to the internal cervical os and then travels medially and anteriorly to enter the bladder at the trigone.

The laparoscopic surgeon also must be aware of potential alterations in the anatomy of the urinary tract, whether the anatomic variants are the result of congenital anomalies, such as pelvic kidneys, duplicated ureters, and urachal remnants, or are changes secondary to pathologic conditions of the pelvis such as endometriosis, fibroids, or pelvic adhesions from previous surgery or infection. Preoperative imaging with intravenous pyelography (IVP) or computed tomography (CT) may be useful in documenting congenital or other structural abnormalities involving the urinary tract, although their use has never been shown to reduce the incidence of urinary tract injuries.[5]

PREVENTION OF UROLOGIC INJURIES

Identification of the Ureter

Prevention of ureteral injury during laparoscopic surgery begins with careful identification of the course of the ureter, which is most easily performed at the start of the procedure, on initial inspection of the pelvis. The laparoscopic surgeon should make a point of identifying anatomic structures including the course of the ureter in even the most straightforward cases, so that this maneuver becomes routine in more difficult ones. The ureter usually can be found along the pelvic sidewall, anterior to the uterosacral ligaments and posterior to the adnexa (Fig. 7–3). Identification should be confirmed with visualization of peristalsis of the ureter, because the ureter may be confused with other structures such as the hypogastric vessels. Identification of the ureter usually is more difficult later on in a laparoscopic procedure, because the

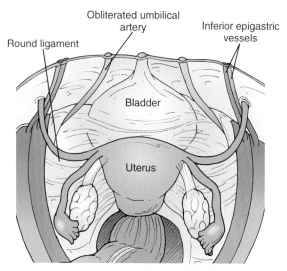

Figure 7–2 ▪ **Laparoscopic view of distended bladder.** Retrograde filling of the bladder during laparoscopic surgery clearly delineates the superior margin of the bladder.

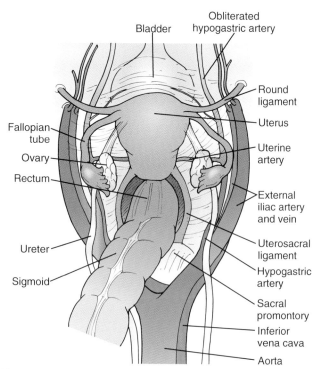

Figure 7–3 ▪ **Laparoscopic view of ureter.** The ureter is most easily identified at the pelvic brim as it descends into the pelvis along the pelvic sidewall, lateral to the uterosacral ligaments.

peritoneum becomes more opaque (i.e., less translucent). This phenomenon is thought to result from a reaction between the CO_2 introduced for the pneumoperitoneum and water within the peritoneum, which results in the formation of carbonic acid.

The course of the ureters is not identical bilaterally. The right ureter tends to be closer to the infundibulopelvic ligament and the uterosacral ligament than on the left. In addition, congenital bowel attachments to the pelvic sidewall, which are more common on the left side, may obsure the identification of anatomic landmarks.[6] When attempting to identify the course of the ureter, the surgeon should keep in mind that lesions of endometriosis may be more commonly found on the left side.[7]

When tracking of the course of the ureters is more difficult, such as with distorted anatomy or retroperitoneal scarring, dissection at or above the pelvic brim usually will allow for adequate identification.[8] Because laparoscopic surgery is simply a means of access for performing surgery, the surgical principles are the same as for an open, abdominal approach. In a stepwise fashion, lateral dissection of the peritoneum at the round ligament leads to easy access to the retroperitoneum (Fig. 7–4). Using blunt dissection or hydrodissection, the peritoneum is incised and the retroperitoneum is further exposed. Usually this maneuver allows identification of the ureter above the pelvic brim. Gentle dissection with medial traction can be employed to free the ureter within the retroperitoneum. In difficult cases, identification of the retroperitoneal structures may facilitate dissection, removal, or ablation of intraperitoneal pathology because vital structures are now within the surgeon's control. Unfortunately, even with proper identification, injury to the ureters, nerves, and vessels may be unavoidable.

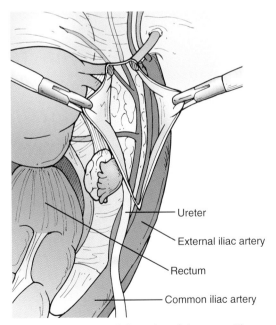

Figure 7–4 ▪ **Retroperitoneal dissection of the ureter.** The ureter can be identified by transection of the round ligament and blunt dissection of the paravesical space, where it is located on the medial leaf of the parietal peritoneum.

Minimizing Risk Factors Associated with Urinary Tract Injury

Although injury to the urinary tract can occur with any laparoscopic procedure, several risk factors are recognized as being associated with an increased likelihood of these complications. As with open surgery, bleeding may obscure anatomic landmarks, and in effort to achieve hemostasis, inadvertent clamping or suture ligation may obstruct or partially obstruct the ureter. Therefore, meticulous attention to hemostasis is essential to permit proper visualization throughout laparoscopic surgery.

Pelvic adhesions from previous surgery, infection, endometriosis, or pelvic tumors not only may distort anatomy but also may involve the ureter or bladder, increasing the likelihood of injury.[9] Lysis of adhesions between the bladder and the anterior abdominal wall should be performed sharply, to avoid tearing of the bladder if significant tension is applied.

Although some urinary tract injuries are unavoidable as a result of involvement of urinary tract structures in the disease process, adherence to sound surgical principles should reduce the incidence of many types of injuries. Frequent assessment of anatomic structures during the procedure may reorient the surgeon, thereby helping to prevent inadvertent injury, even though the structures were identified at the start of the procedure. If the ureter cannot be identified on the pelvic sidewall, it often is helpful to examine the pelvic brim, where the ureter crosses over the bifurcation of the common iliac artery, and then trace its path more distally.

Bladder Catheterization

Injury to the bladder during laparoscopic procedures is most likely to occur when the bladder has not been catheterized before the procedure, or if continuous bladder drainage with an indwelling catheter is not used during prolonged procedures. As little as 100 mL of urine in the bladder may increase the risk of injury during laparoscopic surgery.[10] Bladder catheterization should therefore be performed before all laparoscopic procedures, and consideration should be given to the use of an indwelling catheter for operative laparoscopic procedures.

Retrograde filling of the bladder with saline or sterile water stained with indigo carmine also can be performed to delineate the margins of the bladder during operative laparoscopic surgery (Fig. 7–5). This technique commonly is used to identify the superior margin of the bladder during dissection in the retropubic space for paravaginal repair and Burch colposuspension. It also can be used during procedures that require that the bladder be mobilized off the lower uterine segment, as with hysterectomy, or off the vaginal cuff, as with laparoscopic sacrocolpopexy.

Ureteral Stenting

Ureteral stents can be used during laparoscopic surgery to assist with the identification of the ureter, especially if the normal anatomy is distorted by fibroids, adhesions, endometriosis, or other pelvic masses. In general, it appears that the routine use of ureteral stents is not beneficial in gynecologic procedures. In one prospective study, 3071 patients

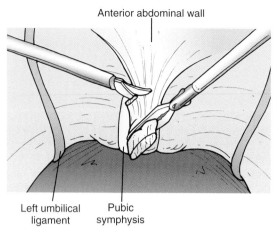

Anterior abdominal wall

Left umbilical   Pubic
  ligament   symphysis

Figure 7–5 ▪ **Entry into retropubic space.** The surgeon may enter the retropubic space by incising the peritoneum above the superior margin of the distended bladder with electrocautery or other energy source. By keeping the dissection between the obliterated umbilical arteries, the surgeon may prevent injury to the inferior epigastric vessels. This technique may be used for a laparoscopic Burch or paravaginal cystocele repair.

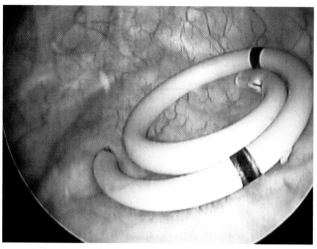

Figure 7–6 ▪ Ureteral stent in the right ureter. (Courtesy of Edward Stanford, MD, MS.)

undergoing either laparotomy or laparoscopy were randomly assigned to one of two groups, with one group receiving prophylactic ureteral stents. Four ureteral injuries occurred in the study, with an equal number occurring in both groups, suggesting no advantage from the stents.[11] Furthermore, complications from ureteral stent placement have been reported.[12] Lighted ureteral stents are available and can best be seen if the light source of the laparoscope is manually reduced. Although lighted ureteral stents can easily be seen as the ureter courses along the pelvic sidewall, the light usually is not visible as the ureter enters its tunnel in the cardinal ligament.

Surgeons performing advanced or difficult pelvic surgery should consider learning how to place ureteral stents. Use of a 7F double-J stent placed over a flexible guidewire usually is adequate for most patients. During cystoscopy, the bladder is distended until the ureteral orifices are easily identified. To avoid urethral injury, the cystoscopic sheath is introduced with a blunt obturator. A 70-degree cystoscope with a deflector then is inserted into the sheath. The flexible guidewire is gently placed into the ureteral orifice and pushed up into the ureter. The scope is removed while the flexible guidewire is controlled to avoid contamination and inadvertent removal. The double-J stent is straightened using the plastic sheath and placed over the guidewire, tapered end first. The stent then is introduced until the distal end is just proximal to the urethra. Cystoscopy is repeated to confirm placement so that the distal end of the stent is protruding through the ureter and coiled in the bladder (Fig. 7–6). Fluoroscopy is done to confirm that the stent is positioned correctly, with the upper part of the stent coiled in the renal pelvis.

Most laparoscopic procedures are done on tables not equipped for radiologic evaluations. Therefore, placement of the patient lower on the table before retraction of the femoral support allows for a C-arm fluoroscope to be used. If needed, a lateral view may suffice when the femoral support is placed after the patient is already in dorsal lithotomy position.

Peritoneal Relaxing Incisions

Endometriotic or other lesions requiring treatment may lie in proximity to the course of the ureter. In an effort to avoid ureteral injury, many surgeons choose to ignore these lesions, potentially resulting in inadequate surgical treatment. A better approach is to make a peritoneal relaxing incision between the lesion and the ureter, thereby allowing complete resection of lesions without fear of injuring the ureter. This maneuver is perhaps more familiar as used with uterosacral ligament suspension for uterine or vaginal vault prolapse: If the ureter lies too close to the ligament, a peritoneal relaxing incision can be made between the structures, and blunt dissection can further separate the ligament from the ureter.

Hydrodissection techniques can be used to prevent bladder or ureteral injuries if the surgeon needs to excise or coagulate endometriosis overlying the structures. A small cut is made in the peritoneum, and an irrigation instrument is inserted through this incision, which separates the peritoneum from the underlying structure and creates a fluid buffer that protects the underlying structures.

ETIOLOGY OF URINARY TRACT INJURIES

Trocar injuries to the bladder are frequent and sometimes result from failure to empty the bladder before the procedure (Fig. 7–7). Although injuries of this type typically are reported with primary trocar placement, bladder injuries occur just as commonly as the result of secondary suprapubic trocar placement.[13] Some authors recommend that suprapubic trocars be placed at a minimum of 4 cm above the pubic symphysis, in order to reduce the chances of this type of injury. An important point is that accessory trocar injuries may involve both an entrance and an exit defect, both of which need to be considered in planning the repair. If the space of Retzius has been previously dissected, as with a laparoscopic Burch procedure, the suprapubic trocar may be placed as close to the pubic symphysis as desired, because the bladder falls away from this area after the dissection. Injury can occur with

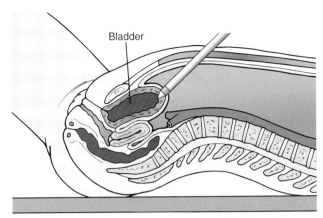

Figure 7–7 ▪ **Mechanism of trocar injury to the bladder.** Injury to the bladder may occur if a trocar is inserted before the bladder is drained, or if a secondary suprapubic trocar is placed too inferiorly.

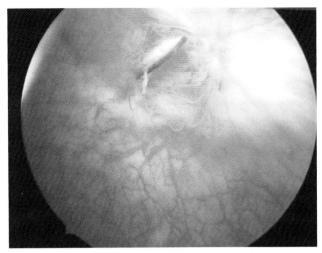

Figure 7–8 ▪ Foreign body in the bladder. (Courtesy of Peter L. Rosenblatt, MD.)

other instruments as well, including the Veress needle, endoscopic scissors, and instruments that transmit energy, such as monopolar and bipolar cautery devices, laser, or harmonic scalpel. Such injuries may result from coagulation of implants of endometriosis in the anterior cul-de-sac.

Bladder injuries also may be caused by foreign bodies, such as tacks, clips, rubber bolsters, or permanent sutures.[14,15] Staples from endoscopic gastrointestinal anastomosis (GIA) devices also have been found in the bladder on postoperative cystoscopy.[16] Complications involving the urinary tract have been described for every type of anti-incontinence procedure. For example, properly placed Stamey bolsters clearly placed outside of the bladder have been recognized to erode into the bladder over time.[17] Spiral tacks to secure permanent mesh have been used for laparoscopic retropubic urethropexy, paravaginal repair, or sacrocolpopexy. Several case reports have described postoperative discovery of intravesical metal tacks on cystoscopy.[18,19] Either these metal tacks were inadvertently placed intravesically during the procedure and were not recognized at that time, or they eroded over time. Theoretically, the fixed metal tack or other material may "rub" against the perivesical tissue during filling and emptying of the bladder, predisposing the tissue to potential erosion. Presenting symptoms include recurrent urinary tract infection, hematuria, and suprapubic pain. Permanent sutures also have been found on cystoscopy, usually misplaced at the time of retropubic urethropexy.[20] All foreign bodies need to be removed, whether by operative cystoscopy, laparoscopy, or laparotomy (Fig. 7–8).

Vesicovaginal fistulas are an uncommon complication of laparoscopic surgery but have been reported after laparoscopy-assisted vaginal hysterectomy.[21] This injury can occur if the bladder is inadvertently sutured or coagulated near the vaginal cuff. Patients may become symptomatic immediately or after several weeks as tissue breakdown occurs. Patients may experience continuous leakage of urine or report an odor of urine from the vagina.

Ureteral injury also can occur with use of instruments that transmit energy, as mentioned previously. Ureters also can be ligated or transected by sutures, clips, or staples during hysterectomy or adnexectomy. In one series of five patients with ureteral injuries, most of the injuries were due to

unipolar or bipolar electrocoagulation near the uterosacral ligaments for endometriosis.[22] Ureteral injury also may occur during laparoscopic uterosacral nerve ablation (LUNA) for chronic pelvic pain. If the injury is not detected intraoperatively, patients usually present within 2 to 3 days with lower back, flank, or abdominal pain. In addition, they may have a fever, ileus, or other signs of peritonitis. Laboratory testing may reveal leukocytosis, and the serum creatinine level may be slightly elevated.[23] Other sequelae of ureteral injury may include pseudocysts, urinary ascites, hydronephrosis, fistula or stricture formation, renal damage, and death.[24]

A majority of patients with ureteral injuries have no identifiable predisposing risk factors.[25] Most ureteral injuries (greater than 50%) occur in the lower third of the ureter, followed by the upper and middle thirds.[26] As with open gynecologic surgery, injury to the ureter most often occurs at one of four locations during laparoscopic surgery: (1) at the pelvic brim where the ureter passes over the hypogastric vessels and under the infundibulopelvic ligament, (2) along the pelvic sidewall under the ovarian fossa, (3) lateral to the cervix where the ureter passes under the uterine arteries, and (4) lateral to the vaginal fornices.[27] Injury near the infundibulopelvic ligament can occur during adnexectomy,[28] especially if any adhesions or scarring is present between the adnexa and the pelvic sidewall. Injuries to this portion of the ureter can occur with use of electrocautery devices, linear staplers, or the harmonic scalpel, or with laparoscopic suturing. It is not uncommon to find endometriotic lesions or fibrocollagenous scarring in the ovarian fossa leading to an altered operative field along the course of the ureter, where dissection may lead to injury. The ureter also may be injured during laparoscopic hysterectomy or myomectomy as it passes underneath the uterine artery, especially when bleeding obscures the field or distortion of anatomy occurs as a result of fibroids, endometriosis, or pelvic adhesions. This portion of the ureter also may be injured or obstructed by procedures that involve the uterosacral ligament, such as laparoscopic uterosacral nerve ablation or uterosacral ligament uterine or vaginal suspension. Resection of endometriosis or lysis of adhesions in the cul-de-sac also can injure the ureter in this location. The most distal portion of the ureter, near its insertion into the bladder, may be injured during reconstructive pelvic surgery, such as laparoscopic urethropexy or paravaginal repair.[29]

Most ureteral injuries are not identified intraoperatively, and the diagnosis is therefore made postoperatively.[30] Several methods are described to detect ureteral injury. Administration of intravenous indigo carmine can be used to rule out ureteral injury by looking for leakage laparoscopically or to document ureteral efflux during cystoscopy. Other intraoperative methods to detect ureteral injury may include surgical dissection of the ureter to visualize its course and peristalsis, retrograde dye injection, intraoperative stent placement, and IVP. Urethral injury occurs infrequently during laparoscopic surgery but can occur during laparoscopic Burch colposuspension, either with dissection in the retropubic space or from paraurethral sutures that inadvertently penetrate the urethral wall. Laparoscopic retropubic urethropexy should be performed only with use of an indwelling urethral catheter to confirm the location of the urethra during the procedure. Slight medial retraction of the urethra during suture placement for the Burch procedure should protect the urethra during this procedure.

DETECTION OF URINARY TRACT INJURIES

As mentioned previously, early recognition of urinary tract injuries reduces morbidity associated with these complications. The laparoscopic surgeon should be vigilant for a possible injury, so that intraoperative assessment can be undertaken as indicated; then, if necessary, the surgeon can either correct the injury or obtain intraoperative urologic consultation.

Leakage of urine from the cystotomy or from a trocar site or distention of the bladder with carbon dioxide may be noticed by the surgeon during the procedure. In women with an indwelling catheter, injury to the bladder may cause the urine to become bloody, which usually is noted by the circulating nurse or the anesthesiologist.

Suspected bladder perforation injuries can be confirmed during laparoscopy by instilling 300 to 500 mL of indigo carmine or sterile milk in retrograde fashion through an indwelling urethral catheter, with spillage subsequently observed through the cystotomy. In this manner, bladder injuries can be precisely located and immediately repaired, and the integrity of the repair can be checked by refilling the bladder. The cystotomy may be large enough to allow direct laparoscopic visualization of the bladder mucosa, Foley balloon, and trigone.

Bladder perforation also has been discovered during laparoscopic surgery when the urine collection bag became distended with carbon dioxide. In one report, two such cases were recognized by the anesthesiologist, who then alerted the surgeons to the presence of the injury.[31]

Cystoscopy is an invaluable tool whose mastery is well within the scope of the gynecologic surgeon's practice. Preoperative cystoscopy performed after intravenous dye injection (e.g., indigo carmine) may be used as an alternative to an imaging study to ensure bilateral ureteral function in patients in whom ureteral compromise is suspected as a result of previous pelvic surgery or presence of extensive endometriosis.

Intraoperative cystoscopy may be performed to check ureteral function in select patients in whom ureteral compromise is in question.[32] Some surgeons routinely perform intraoperative cystoscopy after laparoscopic reconstructive procedures that can potentially cause ureteral compromise. These procedures include Burch colposuspension, paravaginal repair, uterosacral ligament suspension, and sacrocolpopexy.

To facilitate identification of ureteral function during cystoscopy, 5 mL of indigo carmine can be administered intravenously by the anesthetist. The dye will be present in the urine within 5 to 20 minutes, depending on the patient's hydration status. Simply observing blue urine in the Foley bag is inadequate, because unilateral obstruction will not be evident with use of this technique. In most cases, a 30- or 70-degree cystoscope is necessary to visualize the ureteral orifices during cystoscopy. Visualization of blue jets of urine coming from each ureteral orifice confirms ureteral patency, although delayed injury or obstruction after cauterization near the ureter has been reported, even after a functioning ureter has been visualized during surgery. If unilateral or bilateral obstruction is suspected because of failure to visualize ureteral jets, the surgeon should take steps to relieve the obstruction. Suspect sutures should be removed, and cystoscopy should be repeated to confirm ureteral patency. Obstruction most often is seen after uterosacral ligament suspension for uterine or vaginal vault prolapse. If ureteral function is still not visualized, retrograde pyelogram or placement of ureteral stents may be performed, with urologic consultation as needed.

Cystoscopy also can be used to check for the presence of bladder injuries, as well as their anatomic proximity to the ureters and trigone. After completion of the repair, cystoscopy also can be performed to confirm that the repair has not compromised ureteral function.

DELAYED DIAGNOSIS OF URINARY TRACT INJURIES

Delayed diagnosis of laparoscopic bladder injury frequently has been reported in the literature. Patients may present with a constellation of symptoms, including malaise, lethargy, nausea, and vomiting. Oliguria or anuria may be reported by the patient. Abdominal distention may indicate leakage of urine from either the bladder or the ureters intraperitoneally, resulting in urinary ascites, or retroperitoneally, in which case it collects as a urinoma. In this situation, women may be found to have extreme elevations of serum renal function test values, which rapidly return to normal after bladder drainage.

Management of this complication depends on the size and location of the cystotomy. A retroperitoneal injury, as may occur with laparoscopic Burch or paravaginal repair, may be treated with simple bladder drainage for 7 to 10 days, followed by retrograde cystogram to confirm healing of the defect. Many authors recommend that a transperitoneal cystotomy be treated with primary surgical repair, performed either laparoscopically or by laparotomy.

Laparoscopic surgery, particularly hysterectomy, carries the risk of fistula development. These lesions may include vesicovaginal and ureterovaginal fistulas. Vesicovaginal fistulas may manifest in the immediate postoperative period, although more commonly they develop during the first few weeks after surgery. Diagnosis of a vesicovaginal fistula may be made by several means, including retrograde cystogram, cystoscopy, IVP, or a simple tampon test.

For the *tampon test*, a tampon is placed in the vagina, the bladder is filled with saline mixed with indigo carmine, and the patient is asked to ambulate for at least 30 minutes. The tampon then is removed by the physician and examined. Bluish fluid located on the proximal end of the tampon confirms the diagnosis of vesicovaginal fistula.

An evaluation of the upper urinary tracts is recommended before surgical repair to rule out concomitant ureterovaginal fistula. In the absence of ureteral obstruction, fistula repair can be safely delayed until resolution of edema and inflammation, at which time the appropriate surgery to restore ureteral or vesical patency can be performed.[33]

Recognition of ureteral injuries usually is delayed from 3 to beyond 30 days.[34] Because ureteral injuries may include complete or partial transection, ligation, and stricture, a high index of suspicion is essential. Ureteral obstruction may result in unilateral or bilateral flank pain, fever and chills, or signs and symptoms of peritonitis in the postoperative period. In addition, unilateral ureteral obstruction resulting in loss of renal function in one kidney has been reported in asymptomatic patients. Urinalysis may reveal hematuria or leukocytosis. Radiologic imaging including IVP or abdominal or pelvic CT should be ordered to determine whether ureteral obstruction is present and, if it is, to determine the exact location and degree (complete versus partial). These two tests also can be used to diagnose ureterovaginal fistulas.

In addition, an office test similar to the tampon test as described earlier can be used to differentiate vesicovaginal from ureterovaginal fistulas. Phenazopyridine tablets are given orally to turn the urine orange, and an indigo carmine solution is instilled through a catheter into the bladder. Orange discoloration of the tampon indicates a ureterovaginal fistula; a bluish stain indicates a vesicovaginal fistula.

Ureterovaginal fistulas also have been reported as a complication of laparoscopic hysterectomy. Nouira and associates reported the development of this complication postoperatively in two women, which was managed with double-J stenting and ureteral reimplantation.[35] The use of unipolar cautery for the uterine arteries was implicated by these investigators as a possible cause of this complication. It is thought that ischemia and delayed necrosis of the ureteral wall may lead to the development of a urinoma, which then may drain through the vaginal cuff or percutaneously.

MANAGEMENT OF URINARY TRACT INJURIES

Bladder Injuries

Management of intraoperative bladder injuries depends on the size and location of the cystotomy. Cystotomies up to 10 mm in diameter, resulting from needles and laparoscopic trocars, have been successfully managed with simple bladder drainage for 5 to 14 days postoperatively.[36] Some surgeons recommend confirmation of bladder integrity with a retrograde cystogram performed after continuous bladder drainage.

Larger bladder injuries can be treated with laparoscopic or open repair, using any of a number of techniques. Laparoscopic repair of bladder injuries, although somewhat controversial, has been shown in a number of case reports and series to be a viable alternative to more invasive repairs performed by laparotomy.[37-39]

Before laparoscopic or open repair of a bladder injury is undertaken, the surgeon must ensure that the injury does not involve the trigone, because ureteral obstruction may result from misplaced sutures. The surgeon should remove any necrotic tissue, adhesions, or areas of endometriosis before repairing the defect. Interrupted or continuous absorbable sutures may be placed full thickness through the bladder wall. Both polyglactin and polydioxanone sutures have been used successfully for laparoscopic repair procedures. Some authors recommend a two-layer closure (mucosa and muscularis),[40] although more recently, a one-layer mass closure has been reported with success.[41] The repair should include both mucosa and muscularis, as well as serosa, unless the defect occurs retropubically, where visceral peritoneum is absent. In a review of results in 19 women who underwent laparoscopic bladder repair, the only complication was a vesicovaginal fistula that required reoperation.[42] Alternatively, a pre-formed suture loop (e.g., Endoloop [Ethicon Endosurgery, Cincinnati, Ohio]) may be placed over a small defect less than 5 mm across, which is elevated with a laparoscopic grasper.[42]

Intraoperative check of bladder integrity may be performed with retrograde filling of the bladder through an indwelling catheter. After the repair, cystoscopy should be performed in most cases to confirm ureteral integrity. Postoperative drainage for 7 to 10 days after repair of bladder injuries is recommended in most cases and may be followed by retrograde cystogram to confirm healing.

If the bladder injury occurs in a location near the trigone, ureteral stenting may be required to allow confirmation of ureter location during the repair, to avoid ureteral kinking or obstruction. Cystoscopy may be performed to check for the proximity of the defect to the ureter before the repair is started. Consultation with a urologist is recommended for those gynecologic surgeons who lack experience with this technique.

Injury to the urethra during laparoscopic reconstructive surgery (Burch or paravaginal repair) should be managed with removal of any permanent sutures and postoperative indwelling catheterization for 7 to 10 days.

Vesicovaginal Fistula

The timing of repair of vesicovaginal fistulas is a subject of much controversy and is beyond the scope of this chapter. Nevertheless, repair may be accomplished vaginally, with a Latzko partial colpocleisis, or abdominally. Successful laparoscopic vesicovaginal fistula repair has been described.[43]

Ureteral Injuries

Excluding intentional ureteral injury such as during renal transplant surgery, iatrogenic ureteral injury most commonly occurs during gynecologic surgery, with an incidence of approximately 1 in 200 cases. In addition, the rates of ureteral injury are similar in private centers and in university training

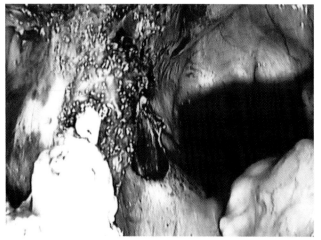

Figure 7–9 ▪ Ureteral injury with stent in place. (Courtesy of Edward Stanford, MD, MS.)

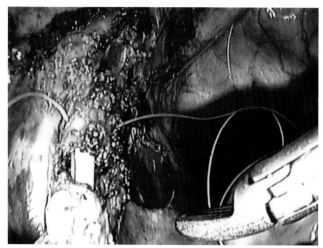

Figure 7–10 ▪ Full-thickness sutures placed laparoscopically. (Courtesy of Edward Stanford, MD, MS.)

centers.[44] Ureteral injuries identified during surgery can be treated with primary repair or end-to-end anastomosis, with good results.[45,46] The types of injuries include complete or partial transection, excision, ligation, and delayed injury such as after cautery or devascularization. Repair may require deligation of the ureter, ureteroureterostomy, or ureteroneocystostomy. Nephrectomy, ureterocutaneostomy, and ileal loop diversion are not commonly required to treat iatrogenic injuries. Failure of an initial ureteroureterostomy usually will lead to a ureteroneocystotomy.

Symptomatic ureteral obstruction should be repaired primarily after an attempt at ureteral stenting. If relief of the obstruction cannot be accomplished in a timely fashion, a percutaneous nephrostomy should be performed to preserve renal function. The usual setting for discovery of the injury is one in which the patient is undergoing radiologic evaluation for back pain or flank pain and is noted to have hydronephrosis secondary to ureteral obstruction. It may be beneficial to consider placing a nephrostomy drainage tube under radiologic guidance. Complications may include failure to place the nephrostomy tube due to technical difficulties and a lack of significant hydronephrosis.

Traditionally, ureteral injury most commonly is treated with laparotomy. Successful end-to-end ureteral reanastomosis has been reported laparoscopically in the gynecologic literature.[47-49] Tulikangas and associates reported four ureteral injuries, all of which were identified intraoperatively. Three of the four ureteral injuries were confirmed intraoperatively with the injection of intravenous indigo carmine.

After the ends of the transected ureter are spatulated to increase the circumference of the repair, to avoid the potential for stricture formation, interrupted full-thickness absorbable sutures are used to reanastomose the ureter over a double-J ureteral stent that was placed in a retrograde manner. The repaired ureter is covered with pelvic peritoneum, if possible (Figs. 7–9 to 7–11). The stents are removed in an outpatient procedure after 4 to 6 weeks, and ureteral patency is confirmed by fluoroscopy (Fig. 7–12). More recently, use of laparoscopic ureteroneocystotomy has been reported and may

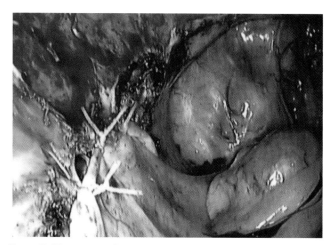

Figure 7–11 ▪ Ureteral repair is retroperitonealized. (Courtesy of Edward Stanford, MD, MS.)

be preferable if concern for ureteral stricture is a consideration because of poor blood supply to the area.[50] Reimplantation of the ureter into the bladder should not be performed if the ureter is under tension. A psoas hitch or Borari flap can be used in this situation to bring the bladder closer to the distal end of the healthy ureter.

CONCLUSIONS

As a result of the intimate anatomic relationship between the female urinary tract and reproductive system, injury to the urinary tract does occur during gynecologic surgery, whether the surgery is performed laparoscopically, through a vaginal approach, or by means of laparotomy. Every effort should be made to prevent injury, including routine preoperative bladder drainage, careful identification of anatomic structures, meticulous hemostasis, and preoperative imaging in selected cases. Liberal use of cystoscopy and other intraoper-

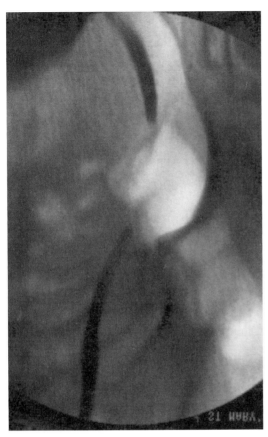

Figure 7–12 ▪ Retrograde pyelogram demonstrates post-repair ureteral patency. (Courtesy of Edward Stanford, MD, MS.)

ative diagnostic testing modalities should reduce the number of unrecognized injuries, which should reduce long-term morbidity. Finally, consideration should be given to repairing urinary tract injuries laparoscopically, if possible. Uncomplicated injuries to the bladder can be repaired by most operative laparoscopists who are familiar with laparoscopic suturing techniques. At present, only a few centers are repairing ureteral injuries laparoscopically, although certainly the potential exists for more widespread acceptance of these techniques.

References

1. Harkki-Sirne P, Sjoberg J, Makinen J, et al. Finnish National Register of Laparosopic Hysterectomies: A review and complications of 1165 operations. Am J Obstet Gynecol 1997;176:118.
2. Dicker RC, Greenspan JR, Strauss LT, et al. Complications of abdominal and vaginal hysterectomy among women of reproductive age in the United States. Am J Obstet Gynecol 1982;144:841.
3. Hulka JF, Levy BS, Parker WH, et al. Laparoscopic-assisted vaginal hysterectomy: American Association of Gynecologic Laparoscopists 1995 membership survey. J Am Assoc Gynecol Laparosc 1997;4:2.
4. Shen C, Wu M, Kung F, et al. Major complications associated with laparoscopic-assisted vaginal hysterectomy: Ten-year experience. J Am Assoc Gynecol Laparosc 2003;10:147.
5. Hurt G. Lower urinary tract injury: Prevention, recognition and management. In: Walters M, Karram M, eds. Urogynecology and reconstructive pelvic surgery. St Louis: Mosby, 1999.
6. Nezhat CH, Nezhat F, Brill AI, Nezhat C. Normal variations of abdominal and pelvic anatomy evaluated at laparoscopy. Obstet Gynecol 1999;94:238.
7. Ghezzi F, Beretta P, Franchi M, et al. Recurrence of ovarian endometriosis and anatomical location of the primary lesion. Fertil Steril 2001;75:136.
8. Berkmen F, Peker AD, Alagol H, et al. Treatment of iatrogenic ureteral injuries during various operations for malignant conditions. J Exp Clin Cancer Res 2000;19:441.
9. Taskin O, Wheeler JM. Laparoscopic repair of bladder injury and laceration. J Am Assoc Gynecol Laparosc 1995;2:227.
10. Smith S. Complications of laparoscopic and hysteroscopic surgery. In: Azziz R, ed. Practical manual of operative laparoscopy and hysteroscopy, 2nd ed. New York: Springer-Verlag, 1997.
11. Kuno K, Menzin A, Kauder JJ, et al. Prophylactic ureteral catheterization in gynecologic surgery. Urology 1998;52:1004.
12. Wood EC, Maher P, Pelosi MA. Routine use of ureteric catheters at laparoscopic hysterectomy may cause unnecessary complications. J Am Assoc Gynecol Laparosc 1995;3:393.
13. Smith S. Complications of laparoscopic and hysteroscopic surgery. In: Azziz R, ed. Practical manual of operative laparoscopy and hysteroscopy, 2nd ed. New York: Springer-Verlag, 1997.
14. Dwyer PL, Carey MP, Rosamilia A. Suture injury to the urinary tract in urethral suspension procedures for stress incontinence. Int Urogynecol J Pelvic Floor Dysfunct 1999;10:15.
15. Biyami CS, Upsdell SM. An unusual foreign body in the bladder 7 years after a Stamey endoscopic bladder neck suspension. Int Urogynecol J Pelvic Floor Dysfunct 1998;9:303.
16. Baughman SM, Sexton W, Bishoff JT. Multiple intravesical linear staples identified during surveillance cystoscopy after laparoscopic nephroureterectomy. Urology 2003;62:351.
17. Athanasopoulos A, Liatsikos EN, Perimenis P, Barbalias GA. Delayed suture intravesical migration as a complication of a Stamey endoscopic bladder neck suspension. Int Urol Nephrol 2002;34:5.
18. Kenton K, Fitzgerald MP, Brubaker L. Multiple foreign body erosions after laparoscopic colposuspension with mesh. Am J Obstet Gynecol 2002;187:252.
19. Hahnfeld L, Nakada S, Moon T. Identification of microtacks in the bladder after laparoscopic pelvic surgery. Urology 1999;54:162.
20. Stevenson KR, Cholhan HJ, Hartmann DM, et al. Lower urinary tract injury during the Burch procedure: Is there a role for routine cystoscopy? Am J Obstet Gynecol 1999;181:35.
21. Kadar N, Lemmerling L. Urinary tract injuries during laparoscopically assisted hysterectomy: Causes and prevention. Obstet Gynecol 1994; 170:47.
22. Grainger DA, Soderstrom RM, Schiff SF, et al. Ureteral injuries at laparoscopy: Insights into diagnosis, management, and prevention. Obstet Gynecol 1990;75:839.
23. Chan JK, Morrow J, Manetta A. Prevention of ureteral injuries in gynecologic surgery. Am J Obstet Gynecol 2003;188:1273.
24. Williams TJ. Urologic injuries. Obstet Gynecol Annu 1975;4:347.
25. Chan JK, Morrow J, Manetta A. Prevention of ureteral injuries in gynecologic surgery. Am J Obstet Gynecol 2003;188:1273.
26. Berkmen R, Peker AE, Alagol H, et al. Treatment of iatrogenic ureteral injuries during various operations for malignant conditions. J Exp Clin Cancer Res 2000;19:441.
27. Hurt WG, Jones CM III. Intraoperative ureteral injuries and urinary diversion. In: Nichols DH, ed. Gynecologic and obstetric surgery. St. Louis: Mosby, 1993;900.
28. Saidi M, Sadler R, Vancaille T, et al. Diagnosis and management of serious urinary complications after major operative laparoscopy. Obstet Gynecol 1996;87:272.
29. Ferland RD, Rosenblatt PL. Ureteral compromise after laparoscopic Burch colpopexy. J Am Assoc Gynecol Laparosc 1999;6:2;217.
30. Ostrzenski A, Radolinski B, Ostrzenska KM. A review of laparoscopic ureteral injury in pelvic surgery. Obstet Gynecol Surv 2003;58:794.
31. Schanbacher PD, Rossi LJ, Salem MR, Joseph NJ. Detection of urinary bladder perforation during laparoscopy by distention of the collection bag with carbon dioxide. Anesthesiology 1994;80:680.
32. Pettit PD, Petrou SP. The value of cystoscopy in major surgery. Obstet Gynecol 1994;84:318.
33. Nouira Y, Oueslati H, Reziga H, Horchani A. Ureterovaginal fistulas complicating laparoscopic hysterectomy: A report of two cases. Eur J Obstet Gynecol Reprod Biol 2001;96:132.
34. Oh B, Kwon D, Park K, et al. Late presentation of ureteral injury after laparoscopic surgery. Obstet Gynecol 2000;95:337.

35. Nouira Y, Oueslati H, Reziga H, Horchani A. Ureterovaginal fistulas complicating laparoscopic hysterectomy: A report of two cases. Eur J Obstet Gynecol Reprod Biol 2001;96:132.

36. Angle HS, Young SB. Conservative management of incidental cystotomy at laparoscopy: A report of two cases. J Reprod Med 1995;40:809.

37. Taskin O, Wheeler JM. Laparoscopic repair of bladder injury and laceration. J Am Assoc Gynecol Laparosc 1995;2:227.

38. Reich H, McGlynn F. Laparoscopic repair of bladder injury. Obstet Gynecol 1990;76:909.

39. Font GE, Brill AI, Stahldreher PV, et al. Endoscopic management of incidental cystotomy during operative laparoscopy. J Urol 1993;149:1130.

40. Taskin O, Wheeler JM. Laparoscopic repair of bladder injury and laceration. J Am Assoc Gynecol Laparosc 1995;2:227.

41. Nezhat CH, Seidman DS, Nezhat F, et al. Laparoscopic management of intentional and unintentional cystotomy. J Urol 1996;156:1400.

42. Nezhat CR, Nezhat FR, Luciano A, et al. Operative gynecologic laparoscopy: Principles and techniques. New York: McGraw-Hill, 1995.

43. Nezhat CH, Nezhat F, Nezhat C, Rottenberg H. Laparoscopic repair of a vesicovaginal fistula: A case report. Obstet Gynecol 1994;83:899.

44. Mann WJ, Arato M, Patsner B, Stone ML. Ureteral injuries in an obstetrics and gynecology training program: Etiology and management. Obstet Gynecol 1988;72:82.

45. Neuman M, Eidelman A, Langer R, et al. Iatrogenic injuries to the ureter during gynecologic and obstetric operations. Surg Gynecol Obstet 1991;173:268.

46. Oboro VO, Dare FO, Fadiora SO, et al. Ureteric injuries following pelvic operations. East Afr Med J 2002;79:611.

47. Tulikangas PK, Gill IS, Falcone T. Laparoscopic repair of ureteral injuries. J Am Assoc Gynecol Laparosc 2001;8:259.

48. Nezhat C, Nezhat F. Laparoscopic repair of ureter resected during operative laparoscopy. Obstet Gynecol 1992;80:542.

49. Liu CY, Kim JH, Bryant JF. Laparoscopic ureteroureteral anastomosis of the distal ureter. J Am Assoc Gynecol Laparosc 2001;8:412.

50. Andou M, Yoshioka T, Ikuma K. Laparoscopic ureteroneocystotomy. Obstet Gynecol 2003;102:1183.

Physiologic and Metabolic Complications

8

Simon Chau, Paul Cramp, and Peter J. O'Donovan

Laparoscopy and hysteroscopy are well-established techniques and are frequently performed procedures in gynecologic practice. Their increase in popularity with both surgeons and patients has been driven by the multiple clinical and economic benefits associated with these procedures. These benefits may include decreased postoperative pain as a result of smaller incisions, less postoperative pulmonary impairment, reduction in postoperative ileus, earlier ambulation, and shorter hospital stays. The advantages of a smaller surgical insult are obvious, but the physiologic and anesthetic-related changes induced during the procedure may be detrimental to the patient. Laparoscopy and hysteroscopy have significant effects on both cardiovascular and pulmonary physiology. Although these changes may be well tolerated in healthy persons, patients who are acutely unwell or have cardiovascular or pulmonary disease may find it difficult to cope with the subsequent respiratory and hemodynamic disturbances. It is not unusual for procedures to be terminated early as a result of patient compromise. These effects should be taken into account in assessing and selecting patients for endoscopic surgery.

PREOPERATIVE CONSIDERATIONS

Good preoperative care and planning are crucial for optimizing successful outcomes after surgery. A team approach that coordinates patient care provided by the surgeon, other physicians, the anesthetist, a physiotherapist, and nursing staff is recommended.

The internal medicine or primary care physician's role is particularly important in assessing the level of risk and recommending measures to reduce that risk, in consultation with the patient and other health care professionals, who also may be involved in planning postoperative care. It is not the role of these other health care professionals to clear the patient for surgery—this would imply no risk at all. Most requests for a medical consultation are specifically to help the anesthetist in the assessment of perioperative risk, with particular attention being paid to cardiac and respiratory status.

Physiologic reserve is an important concept in patients facing any kind of surgery. The cardiovascular system in particular has to mount a compensatory response to the physiologic stress. Patients who lack such compensatory capability because of impaired organ function have increased mortality risk, as demonstrated by the American Society of Anesthesiologists (ASA) classification of disease severity (Table 8–1).

Although many endoscopic procedures are carried out in office or outpatient environments in "healthy" persons in ASA class 1, it is still very important to provide appropriate preoperative assessment to reduce postoperative risk. Such assessment is particularly important in elderly or very sick patients, who often present with significant co-morbidity. Cardiovascular and respiratory diseases frequently are encountered in these patient populations.

Assessment of Patients with Cardiac Disease

The largest single cause of perioperative death is cardiac related. Cardiovascular disease affects 25% of the U.S. population. Much work has been done to try to assess cardiovascular risk before surgery, because perioperative myocardial infarction carries a 30% to 50% mortality rate. Seven main types of cardiac disease that may be present before surgery have been recognized:

- Ischemic heart disease
- Heart failure
- Valvular disease
- Cardiac arrhythmias, especially atrial fibrillation
- Hypertension
- Presence of a pacemaker
- Previous cardiac transplantation

The greater the cardiovascular stress during surgery, the greater the risk of cardiac complications (Table 8–2).

ISCHEMIC HEART DISEASE

Major clinical predictors of perioperative cardiac complications are recent (within 6 months) myocardial infarction, severe or unstable angina, and significant arrythmias. Many patients have controlled ischemic heart disease, however, and although a number of tests are available to assess this population, they are not necessarily helpful.

The American College of Cardiology and the American Heart Association have stratified predictors of perioperative cardiovascular risk into minor, intermediate, and major[1] (Table 8–3). These guidelines also discuss the appropriate use of echocardiography, exercise stress testing, radionuclide investigations, and coronary angiography and the subsequent need for medical and surgical intervention (percutaneous transluminal coronary angioplasty and coronary artery bypass grafting) before noncardiac surgery. Nevertheless, careful evaluation of findings on the patient's history, physical examination, and resting electrocardiogram (ECG) constitutes the first step in categorizing risk.

Additional scoring systems have been developed (Table 8–4) to help quantify risk. Such systems are based on observational studies. Many of these scoring systems were developed in the 1980s, when the rule was to wait until 6 months after a myocardial infarction before noncardiac surgery was undertaken. Since then, the cardiologic management and functional assessment of patients have evolved significantly. It appears now that the risk after a previous infarction is related more to the functional status of the ventricles and the amount of myocardium at risk from further ischemia than to the age of the infarction. Modern practice guidelines consider the period within 6 weeks of infarction as a time of high risk for a perioperative event, because this period is the mean healing time of the infarct-related injury.[2] The period from 6 weeks to 3 months is of intermediate risk; this period is extended beyond 3 months in cases with complications such as arrhythmias, ventricular dysfunction, or continued medical therapy.[1] In uncomplicated cases, no benefit can be demonstrated for delaying surgery more than 3 months after an ischemic event.[3]

Probably the most useful measure with regard to ischemic heart disease is the patient's functional ability. Risk is increased in patients who cannot reach a functional workload of 4 metabolic equivalents (METs).[4] One MET is equivalent to the oxygen consumption of a resting 40-year-old 70-kg man. Climbing a flight of stairs, briskly walking on a level surface, mowing the lawn, swimming, and playing a round of golf all are activities rated for at least 4 METs.

Surgery may proceed without further evaluation in patients with minor risk factors and good function who are undergoing low- or intermediate-risk surgery. Patients with intermediate risk factors and poor functional capacity may need further evaluation and optimization before surgery. Exercise ECG testing is widely available but impractical for many high-risk surgical patients. Dobutamine stress echocardiography is the best test to predict perioperative events, according to most studies.[5-7] It has a 100% negative predictive

Table 8–1 ▪ ASA Classification of Disease Severity*

Class	Patient Characteristics
ASA 1	Healthy patient
ASA 2	Patient with mild systemic disease that does not limit function
ASA 3	Patient with moderate systemic disease that limits function
ASA 4	Patient with severe systemic disease that is a constant threat to life
ASA 5	Moribund patient who will not survive 24 hours without surgery

ASA 3E would indicate a patient with disease severity of ASA 3 who is undergoing emergency surgery.

*Mortality increases with class. The ASA classification does not take into account age, smoking, or obesity—factors that also increase risk.
ASA, American Society of Anesthesiologists.

Table 8–2 ▪ Risk of Major Perioperative Cardiac Event with Type of Surgery

Low Risk (<1%)	Intermediate Risk (1-5%)	High Risk (>5%)
Endoscopic procedures	Carotid endarterectomy	Emergency major surgery
Superficial procedures	Head and neck surgery	Aortic/major vascular surgery
Cataract surgery	Intraperitoneal surgery	Peripheral vascular surgery
Breast surgery	Intrathoracic surgery	Prolonged procedure with large fluid shifts or blood loss
	Orthopedic surgery	
	Prostate surgery	

Table 8–3 ▪ Risk of Major Perioperative Cardiac Event with Patient Characteristics

Minor	Intermediate	Major
Advanced age	Mild angina (class 1 or 2)	Unstable coronary syndromes
ECG abnormalities	Previous myocardial infarction (history or ECG evidence)	Recent MI (within 1 month preceding)
Rhythm other than sinus	Compensated or previous heart failure	Unstable or severe angina
Low functional capacity	Diabetes	Decompensated heart failure
History of stroke		Significant arrhythmias
Uncontrolled hypertension		Severe valve disease

ECG, electrocardiogram; MI, myocardial infarction.

Table 8–4 ▪ Goldman's Index of Cardiac Risk in Noncardiac Procedures	
Risk Factor	**Points**
Third heart sound or jugular venous distention	11
Myocardial infarction in the preceding 6 months	10
Rhythm other than sinus or premature atrial beats	7
More than 5 ventricular ectopic beats per minute	7
Abdominal, thoracic, or aortic operation	3
Age older than 70 years	5
Significant aortic stenosis	3
Emergency operation	4
Poor general health	3
Total	53

Scoring:

0-5 points: major cardiac complications 0.3-3%
6-12 points: major cardiac complications 1-10%
13-25 points: major cardiac complications 3-30%
26-53 points: major cardiac complications 19-75%

From Goldman L, Calera DL, Nussbaum SR, et al. Multifactorial index of cardiac risk in non-cardiac surgical procedures. N Engl J Med 1977;297:845.

value and patients with extensive ischemia experience ten times more perioperative cardiac events than those with limited ischemia. Coronary angiography is indicated in appropriate high-risk patients or in intermediate-risk patients after screening.

Several randomized trials have looked at medical therapy to reduce perioperative risk; pharmacologic agents used for this purpose are beta blockers, nitrates, and calcium channel blockers. Some evidence suggests that perioperative beta blockers reduce cardiac complications (ischemic episodes, myocardial infarction, and death).[8] One randomized trial used prophylactic atenolol immediately before and up to 7 days after noncardiac surgery.[9] This strategy reduced the cardiovascular mortality rate at 6, 12, and 24 months. In a study on vascular patients, the cardiac mortality and morbidity rate was reduced by bisoprolol from 34% to 3.4%.[10] Beta blockers are therefore recommended for high-risk patients and patients with hypertension, ischemic heart disease, or risk factors for ischemic heart disease. If preoperative administration is not possible, an intravenous beta blocker given at induction of anesthesia followed by postoperative treatment also is effective. The intraoperative use of nitroglycerin in high-risk patients does not affect outcome despite evidence of reduced ischemia on the ECG.[11]

The diagnosis of myocardial infarction in the perioperative period can be difficult. One half of affected patients do not have typical chest pain. They may present with arrhythmias, pulmonary edema, hypotension, or confusion. ECG changes are common postoperatively and do not necessarily indicate myocardial infarction. Up to 20% of postoperative patients have new ECG abnormalities—usually T wave changes. Creatine kinase rises nonspecifically with surgery, and troponin measurements are more appropriate.

HEART FAILURE

Lack of cardiopulmonary reserve is a more important predictor of perioperative death than is cardiac ischemia. It

has long been observed that high-risk patients who survive surgery have greater compensatory increases in cardiovascular and oxygen transport measurements than patients who die—nonsurvivors are unable to compensate for the added metabolic and cardiorespiratory demands of surgery and die of multiple organ failure. High-risk patients are those who are most critically ill at the time of surgery or who face major surgery.

Echocardiography does not appear to be a useful predictor of perioperative cardiac events, although a reduced ejection fraction correlates with an increased risk of perioperative pulmonary edema.

VALVULAR HEART DISEASE

Severe aortic stenosis poses the greatest perioperative risk because it will complicate correction of hypotension occurring during anesthesia and surgery. Aortic stenosis is a fixed obstruction and limits maximum cardiac output during stress. Patients cannot respond normally to the peripheral dilation associated with anesthesia, and blood pressure can fall dramatically. This drop in pressure causes myocardial ischemia because the myocardial hypertrophy that develops secondary to aortic stenosis is associated with increased oxygen demand. Aortic stenosis may be asymptomatic, and patients with severe stenosis do not necessarily exhibit classic features on examination. According to the Helsinki Ageing Study, 3% of people 75 to 85 years of age have critical aortic stenosis.

Mitral stenosis also is important to recognize because in this condition, control of the heart rate is essential in order to preserve diastole. Preservation of diastole aids filling of the left atrium and generates enough pressure to squeeze through the stenosed valve. The presence of any murmur requires a preoperative echocardiogram. Antibiotic prophylaxis should be given to most patients with valve disease undergoing surgery.

CARDIAC ARRHYTHMIAS, ESPECIALLY ATRIAL FIBRILLATION

Arrythmias following surgery are common, often exacerbated by the abrupt withdrawal of cardiac drugs due to fasting. Such arrhythmias also are caused by hypotension, metabolic derangement, and hypoxemia—all of which are preventable. It is important that patients with heart disease be maintained on their usual drugs, delivered by alternative routes if possible, during the perioperative period. Continued therapy is particularly important for beta blockers, which should be administered on the day of surgery.

Of patients older than 65 years of age, 5% have chronic atrial fibrillation, so that it is a common preoperative finding. Certain procedures are associated with the development of atrial fibrillation—for example, intrathoracic surgery. Patients with chronic lung or cardiac disease are at greater risk for the development of postoperative atrial fibrillation. The main difference in the preoperative period is that beta blockers or calcium channel blockers are considered more effective than is digoxin in controlling the ventricular rate during stress. If the patient is anticoagulated, this needs to be addressed in the perioperative period.

HYPERTENSION

Hypertension is a common finding in Western populations. The risks of preoperative hypertension are unclear, with some studies showing increased cardiovascular complications and others no increased risk. Hypertension alone is therefore considered a borderline risk factor. Uncontrolled and poorly controlled hypertension can be associated with increased intraoperative complications, such as myocardial ischemia, arrhythmias, cerebrovascular accidents, and exaggerated swings in blood pressure. Nevertheless, clear evidence that deferring anesthesia and surgery in such patients reduces perioperative risk is lacking.[12]

PRESENCE OF A PACEMAKER

Patients with pacemakers are not uncommon occurrences on surgical theatre lists and do not generally pose a great problem. ECG and chest x-ray studies should be requested to determine the type and the integrity of the pacemaker. The pacemaker should be checked by the patient's cardiologist before surgery to ensure that it is functioning correctly. Bipolar diathermy ideally should be used, to minimize interference with pacemaker function. Prophylactic cardiac pacing may be required before surgery in patients at risk for the development of complete heart block. These patients include those with bifascicular or trifascicular heart block.

PREVIOUS CARDIAC TRANSPLANTATION

The number of patients with cardiac transplants who present for noncardiac surgical procedures is increasing, both because of the increasing incidence of transplantation and as a result of the increased survival of such patients. The transplanted heart is totally denervated and is therefore unresponsive to autonomic influences. Because of the denervation, any myocardial ischemia or infarction is silent. Cardiac output tends to be low normal and is very dependent on adequate preload. Rises in heart rate and cardiac output depend on an increase in circulating catecholamine. Preoperative evaluation should focus on the functional status of the transplanted heart. Signs and symptoms of heart failure, reduced exercise tolerance, and arrhythmias should be sought and may signal the onset of rejection. Early involvement of the cardiology and anesthetic team is essential.

Assessment of Patients with Lung Disease

Obstructive lung diseases are the most commonly encountered lung dysfunction in anesthetic practice. Use of the Trendelenburg position and establishment of a pneumoperitoneum during surgery can result in severe respiratory embarrassment. At preoperative assessment, presence of dyspnea and wheezing should alert the clinician that the patient's airway disease is not well controlled. Cessation of smoking before surgery should be encouraged for the well-characterized benefits, both immediate and long-term, including reduction in carboxyhemoglobin, decrease in oxygen demand, decrease in airway reactivity, increase in ciliary motility, and decreased risk of postoperative chest infection.

Preoperative lung function tests and arterial blood gases can predict the need for postoperative ventilatory support and quantify the type and degree of respiratory impairment. High-risk patients include those who are breathless at rest or have a $PaCO_2$ greater than 46 mm Hg (6.0 kPa), a forced expiratory volume in 1 minute (FEV_1) less than 1 L, or an FEV_1/forced vital capacity (FVC) ratio of less than 0.5.[13,14]

Other factors that make pulmonary complications more likely include the following:

- High ASA class
- Chronic obstructive pulmonary disease (COPD)
- Smoking within the previous 8 weeks
- Surgery of longer than 3 hours' duration
- Obesity
- Upper abdominal or thoracic surgery (surgical maneuvers closer to the diaphragm carry higher risk)

Certain measures may help to reduce perioperative pulmonary complications: stopping smoking, preoperative use of inhaled beta agonists for patients with COPD or intravenous steroids if needed, the use of regional anesthesia (with or without general anesthesia), and postoperative lung expansion exercises. Morbidly obese patients (body weight greater than 250 lb [115 kg]) and smokers are twice as likely to develop postoperative pneumonia.

Assessment of Patients with Gastrointestinal Disease

Obesity and gastroesophageal reflux can have detrimental effects during endoscopic surgery. Increased intra-abdominal pressure and the Trendelenburg position increase the likelihood of reflux in the anesthetized patient. Contamination of the airway by gastric contents is potentially life-threatening, and measures should be taken to guard against this occurrence. Such measures may include premedication with a proton pump inhibitor and protection of the airway with an endotracheal tube. Obesity alone brings with it multiple systemic problems that are potential risks in anesthesia. Lung volumes normally are reduced during anesthesia and are even more so in obese patients. Adoption of a head-down position and generation of a pneumoperitoneum can further reduce respiratory function, resulting in difficulty with ventilation and subsequent hypoxia and hypercarbia.

Assessment of Patients with Other Problems

Assessment of patients with other problems may be required. Impairment of any organ system leads to an increase in perioperative complications. Endocrine disorders (e.g., diabetes), renal failure, liver disease, and hematologic and neurologic disorders are not discussed here. Other scoring systems have been developed that assist in the assessment of perioperative risk related to such disorders, such as the Child-Pugh classification of liver disease.

Preparation of Patients before Emergency Surgery

Surgery, especially emergency surgery, is a physiologic insult. In some instances, the surgery takes precedence over full resuscitation (e.g., in ruptured aortic aneurysm), but in general there is time to resuscitate the patient. General and spinal anesthesia sometimes involve a drop in blood pressure due to vasodilation; this drop is exaggerated if the patient is volume depleted before induction. Hypovolemia before emergency surgery is common and may be the result of any of several problems:

• Vomiting and diarrhea
• Fasting
• Bleeding
• Fluid loss into an obstructed bowel
• Sepsis or systemic inflammatory response syndrome

Preoperative Optimization of High-Risk Surgical Patients

Resuscitation makes a big difference to outcome—not only in terms of perioperative mortality but also in terms of postoperative morbidity. Preoperative optimization entails two steps: identifying that a patient's status can be improved and then implementing an appropriate management plan. In terms of simple physiology (airway, breathing, circulation), the aim should be to restore functional indices as far as possible toward the patient's baseline values before surgery. Optimal status will allow the patient to mount a successful compensatory response during the perioperative period.

In the preoperative period, high-risk patients have an increased incidence of severe physiologic impairment as measured by pulmonary artery catheter.[15] In many patients, the baseline values can be improved by relatively simple measures, such as giving fluid or inotropes. Several studies have now shown that careful invasive monitoring of high-risk patients in the perioperative period is associated with improved outcome.[16,17] This strategy is not beneficial, however, unless started at an early stage of the acute illness.

In one study, high-risk patients undergoing surgery were randomly assigned to one of three groups.[18] Control subjects received routine perioperative care; patients in the other two groups received preoperative optimization using either epinephrine or dopexamine. The optimization regimen consisted of invasive hemodynamic monitoring, fluid loading to achieve pulmonary artery occlusion pressure of 12 mm Hg, red cell transfusion to a hemoglobin concentration greater than 110 g/L, oxygen therapy to achieve an oxygen saturation (SaO_2) greater than 94%, and either epinephrine or dopexamine to increase oxygen delivery to greater than 600 mL/min per m^2 of body surface. Inotropic support was continued during surgery and for at least 12 hours afterward. Mortality rates were reduced in both the epinephrine and the dopexamine groups (2% and 4%, respectively) compared with the control subjects (17%).

On the basis of this and similar studies, practice is moving in the direction of invasive cardiac monitoring in high-risk patients before major surgery, to permit correction of preexisting physiologic impairment and improvement in compensatory responses. These findings illustrate the general importance of adequate resuscitation before major surgery.

Specific goals of preoperative optimization are as follows:

• Airway secure
• Respiratory rate of 10 to 30 breaths per minute
• PaO_2 greater than 77 mm Hg (10 kPa)
• Well perfused with good cardiac output
• Urine output greater than 1 mL/kg per hour
• Hemoglobin greater than 8 g/dL
• Normal electrolytes (especially K^+ and Mg^{2+})
• Acceptable base excess (less than −5)

INTRAOPERATIVE AND POSTOPERATIVE CONSIDERATIONS

A majority of anesthetic complications related to laparoscopy arise during the establishment and maintenance of pneumoperitoneum and the adoption of the Trendelenburg position. Anesthetic complications during hysteroscopy generally are related to distention media characteristics, the volume of distention medium used, and the duration and extent of surgery.

Laparoscopy

CARDIOVASCULAR CHANGES

Gynecologic laparoscopy involves creation of a pnemoperitoneum with CO_2 gas and positioning of the patient in the lithotomy and Trendelenburg position. Intra-abdominal pressures generated typically are in the region of 15 to 20 mm Hg. The physiologic changes induced by the generation of a pneumoperitoneum are related to the raised intra-abdominal pressures and the effects of hypercarbia secondary to the use of CO_2 gas.

During the initial stages of pnemoperitoneum, cardiac output increases as a result of splanchnic compression occurring with an increase in venous return. Within a few minutes, however, venous return falls owing to an increase in caval compression. A rise in systemic vascular resistance and mean arterial pressure and an increase in afterload are observed as a result of aortic compression and increases in plasma concentration of catecholamine, vasopressin, and renin-angiotensin activity. These factors all contribute to a fall in stroke volume and a fall in cardiac output. Hypercarbia and acidosis resulting from absorption of CO_2 gas have a direct myocardial depressant and a vasodilatory effect; consequently, a further fall in stroke volume and cardiac output also may be observed. Visceral manipulation during surgery may induce vagal stimulation and subsequent bradycardia and hypotension. All of these compensatory changes may endanger patients with myocardial ischemia and dysfunction.[19-22]

RESPIRATORY CHANGES

Abdominal insufflation results in significant changes in lung volumes and lung mechanics. Respiratory compliance falls by 48%, functional residual capacity falls by 24%, and peak airway pressure rises by 50%.[22,23] Diaphragmatic movement is further impaired by the raised intra-abdominal pressure and the adoption of the Trendelenburg position. Basal atelectasis and ventilation-perfusion mismatch ensue, which can result in arterial hypoxemia. Use of positive end-expiratory pressure may be helpful in improving gas exchange during laparoscopy. Peritoneal absorption of CO_2 gas and the ventilatory effects of a pneumoperitoneum result in a raised arterial Pa_{CO_2} and end-expiratory CO_2. The hypercarbia, respiratory acidosis, and hypoxia may be poorly tolerated by patients with respiratory disease, and the surgeon may be forced to terminate the procedure.[24]

GASTROINTESTINAL PROBLEMS

Gastroesophageal reflux is the passive flow of gastric contents across the gastroesophageal sphincter into the esophagus. Presence of refluxed material may result in tracheal aspiration, which is potentially life-threatening. Laparoscopy causes an increase in intra-abdominal pressure, which may result in an increased incidence of reflux. The Trendelenburg position adopted in gynecologic laparoscopy further increases the likelihood of reflux, as do other conditions such as obesity, hiatus hernia, and gastric outlet obstruction. Incidence of reflux during anesthesia generally is low but has been reported to be as high as 40% in laparoscopic cholecystectomy and 53% in gynecologic laparoscopy.[25] Adequate starvation and premedication with proton pump inhibitors and antacids can reduce the incidence and the effects of reflux. Choice of airway control also may have some bearing on the likelihood of reflux. In one study, use of laryngeal masks was suggested to predispose patients to reflux by means of a reflex reduction of lower esophageal barrier pressure.[26] Another, more recent study, however, reported no increase in incidence reflux associated with laryngeal mask use.[27] The "gold standard" modality for airway control is still endotracheal intubation because it prevents tracheal contamination with gastric contents.

GAS EMBOLUS

CO_2 gas is widely used as the distention medium in laparoscopic surgery because it is noncombustible, rapidly absorbed in the blood, cheap, and colorless. CO_2 gas embolus can result as a consequence of direct intravascular injection through the insufflation needle or entry through open venous channels. Clinical signs of an embolus may include hypotension, tachycardia, arrhythmias, a fall in expired CO_2, a mill-wheel heart murmur, and cardiovascular collapse (Fig. 8–1). Paradoxical embolus through a patent foramen ovale can compromise cardiac and cerebral circulation. If an embolus is suspected, the surgeon should evacuate the peritoneal cavity of CO_2; the patient should then be placed in the left lateral position with the head down and a large-bore cannula inserted into the

central venous circulation in order to aspirate gas from the right atrium. Oxygenation should be maintained with 100% oxygen and cardiac output supported with inotropes if necessary. Occasionally, cardiopulmonary resuscitation may be required. Ventilating the patient with an oxygen-air mix, rather than using an oxygen–nitrous oxide mixture, can reduce the effects of a gas embolus. Nitrous oxide diffuses into air-filled cavities and increases the size of these cavities, thereby enlarging the gas embolus and potentiating its effects.

SHOULDER TIP PAIN

Shoulder tip pain following laparoscopy is frequent, with a reported incidence between 35% and 63%.[28] Carbon dioxide under the diaphragm is believed to be responsible for a large component of the pain, although other factors also may play a part. Larger volumes of residual gas left within the abdomen and greater pressures used in laparoscopy have been associated with worsening shoulder pain.[29,30] Care should be taken to use the lowest possible insufflation pressure during surgery, and to release as much gas as possible at the end of the procedure, in order to minimize the frequency of shoulder tip pain.

Hysteroscopy

The reported incidence of anesthetic complications in hysteroscopy is low, ranging from 0.28% to 2.7%.[31,32] Such complications occur with greater frequency in operative hysteroscopy than in diagnostic hysteroscopy. Anesthetic complications in hysteroscopy generally are related to the distention medium, the volume used, and the duration and extent of surgery.

GAS EMBOLUS

With diagnostic hysteroscopy, the most frequently used distention medium is CO_2 gas. CO_2 gas allows good visualization but unlike fluid media is not very effective in removing blood or debris. Distention of the uterus requires generation of a pressure in the range of 75 mm Hg, with a flow of 100 mL/min. Higher pressures and flows are rarely required, and higher flows can increase the likelihood of CO_2 embolus formation. Operative hysteroscopy also constitutes an additional risk, because the presence of multiple open venous sinuses and the head-down position make embolization more likely.

Although a majority of CO_2 emboli probably originate from the distention gas, some unlikely sources of CO_2 emboli also have been reported. CO_2 gas produced as a product of combustion during endometrial ablation and CO_2 gas used to cool the sapphire tip during laser ablation have been implicated.[33,34] The incidence of CO_2 emboli has been reported to be as low as 0.03% and as high as 10% to 50%.[35-37] Death as a result from CO_2 embolus following hysteroscopy is rare, however.

Embolization of room air also is possible during hysteroscopy. The implications of an air embolus and of a CO_2 embolus are quite different. CO_2 gas is highly soluble. Should any gas enter the uterine vessels, much of it will have dissolved before reaching the heart. Air is much less soluble, however,

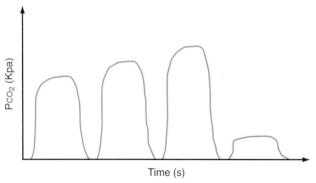

Figure 8–1 ▪ Capnography tracing in gas embolism.

and even small volumes can have deleterious effects. Mechanisms of air embolism during CO_2 hysteroscopy are unclear. Trauma to the cervix followed by insertion of the hysteroscope has been suggested as a likely cause. Risks may be greater during menstruation, when the potential for uterine vessels to be patent is greater. Room air present within the hysteroscope and the gas tubing is another source of potential emboli. Insufflation of the uterus without initially purging the hysteroscopic apparatus can result in entry of as much as 40 mL of air into the uterine cavity. All equipment ideally should be purged with CO_2 gas before insertion.[38] The management of gas emboli is outlined earlier in the chapter.

IDIOSYNCRATIC REACTIONS

Operative hysteroscopy usually is performed in a fluid environment. Selection of the fluid typically is based on the surgeon's preference and the instrument used. Current options available include high-viscosity dextran 70 and low-viscosity electrolyte-free solutions such as glycine 1.5% and sorbitol 3%. The development of newer hysteroscopes that can function in an ionic environment has enabled the use of isotonic electrolyte-containing solutions such as saline or Ringer's lactate.

The major advantage of dextran 70 is that it is immiscible with blood, allowing good visualization. The use of this agent is in decline, however, because it has been associated with a significant number of complications. Idiosyncratic reactions such as noncardiogenic pulmonary edema, coagulopathy, disseminated intravascular coagulation, rhabdomyolysis, and acute renal failure all have been reported after hysteroscopy with dextran solution.[39-41] Allergic reactions including severe anaphylaxis may occur and also have been reported.[42,43] It has been suggested that dextran can directly cause endothelial damage. Changes in alveolar membrane permeability result in flooding of the alveolus with plasma proteins, poor oxygenation, and a reduction in pulmonary compliance. Release of tissue factors after intravasation of dextran could promote fibrinolysis and induce a consumptive coagulopathy. Management of these complications is symptomatic and supportive. Early recognition and liaison with the critical care team are essential.

TOXICITY

Operative hysteroscopy traditionally has required a hypotonic, electrolyte-free, nonconductive solution; otherwise, the electrical energy will be dispersed. Sorbitol 3% and glycine 1.5% are examples of hypotonic electrolyte-free solutions currently available. Absorption of these distention fluids can result in symptoms of cerebral and cardiac toxicity. Hyperglycinemia has been reported following use of 1.5% glycine solution. Glycine is known to be an inhibitory neurotransmitter in the central nervous system and has been implicated in several cases of temporary blindness and central nervous system depression.[44,45] Hyperammonemia, possibly resulting from the breakdown of glycine, may further contribute to these effects. Cardiac arrhythmias also have been reported to follow major glycine poisoning during hysteroscopy.[46] Hyperglycemia from the use of large volumes of sorbitol solution may make glycemic control difficult, especially in patients who are diabetic.

HYPERVOLEMIA, HYPONATREMIA, AND HYPO-OSMOLARITY

Use of large volumes of distention fluid during hysteroscopy potentially allows for systemic absorption of irrigating fluid. Operative hysteroscopy makes the absorption of distention fluid more likely as surgery opens up multiple venous networks within the uterus. Symptoms arising subsequent to absorption of large volumes of fluid are well documented in urologic practice, associated specifically with transurethral resection of the prostate (TURP), and therefore often are referred to as *TURP syndrome*. This syndrome is a complex of clinical complications characterized by dilutional hyponatremia, water intoxication, cerebral edema, and cardiac overload. Similar symptoms also have been reported in patients undergoing operative hysteroscopy. The incidence ranges from 0.4% to 5% of all operative hysteroscopies.[34,47] Symptoms can manifest intraoperatively and in the postoperative period. Complications vary depending on which type of fluid is used. With excessive absorption of large volumes of electrolyte-containing solutions such as Ringer's lactate, symptoms of fluid overload predominate. Absorption of hypotonic electrolyte-free solutions has the added complication of hyponatremia and hypo-osmolarity. Fluid overload may manifest as congestive heart failure, pulmonary edema, and hypertension. Headaches, restlessness, vomiting, confusion, cyanosis, arrhythmias, and seizures herald the development of hyponatremia and plasma hypo-osmolality. Cerebral edema, brain herniation, and death rapidly ensue if prompt treatment is not instituted.

Absorption of small volumes of dextran can precipitate hypervolemia and pulmonary edema. As a result of its hyperosmolarity, dextran solution can act as a plasma expander and draws in fluid from the interstitial compartment into the intravascular compartment. Absorption of 100 mL of dextran solution can expand the plasma volume by 860 mL.[48]

Metabolism of absorbed sorbitol and glycine leaves behind free water that accumulates, resulting in electrolyte imbalance, dilutional hyponatremia, hypervolemia, and plasma hypo-osmolarity. Antidiuretic hormone release also may contribute to the resultant hyponatremia.[49] Signs and symptoms of mental agitation, confusion, nausea, vomiting, visual disturbances, and headache indicate the onset of cerebral edema and raised intracranial pressure. Prompt recognition and co-management with the critical care team are essential to ensure a good outcome.

Management of fluid overload and pulmonary edema involves oxygen therapy and the use of diuretics. Hyponatremic hypervolemia, cerebral edema, and hypo-osmolarity are more difficult to treat. Serum electrolyte measurements, coagulation profile, and determination of arterial blood gases are indicated. Airway control may be required if the patient demonstrates a depressed neurologic state. Measures should be taken to control raised intracranial pressure. Hypervolemia should be managed with diuretics, and any electrolyte imbalance should be corrected. Correction of hyponatremia with normal saline should be done slowly to minimize risks of central pontine myelinolysis.

To avoid absorption of large volumes of distention fluid during hysteroscopy, accurate measurements of fluid deficit must be performed. Fluid deficits should be calculated every 15 minutes by measuring the difference between the amount of fluid that the surgeon instils into the uterus and the amount of fluid returned into the collecting receptacle from the outflow sheath of the hysteroscope. Details of the ongoing deficit should be relayed to the surgical and the anesthetic teams. Intravenous fluids should be kept to a minimum so that the patient does not receive an abundance of intravenous fluid in addition to that received by intrauterine instillation. The point at which surgery should be terminated is unclear. Safe fluid deficit varies in the literature, ranging from as low as 800 mL to as high as 2000 mL for hypotonic and isotonic solutions. For dextran solutions, a limit of 350 to 500 mL is universally accepted.[21,50] Serial measurements of plasma sodium may be helpful if accurate measurements of fluid deficits are not possible. Biochemical assessment of absorbed fluid by the addition of 2% ethanol into the distention medium has been used with moderate success. The concentration of expired alcohol on the patient's breath gives an indication of the volume of distention fluid absorbed and provides an early warning sign of when the safe limit is being approached.[33,51] Limitation of uterine distention pressures to a maximum of 100 mm Hg and of resection time to a maximum of 1 hour also can reduce the amount of distention fluid that is absorbed. A variety of automated pump systems are available that can deliver distention fluid at a constant rate, maintain a constant uterine distention pressure, and accurately calculate fluid deficits. Employment of these systems has demonstrated a decrease in fluid absorption and reduction in morbidity.[52,53]

HYPOTHERMIA

Use of large volumes of distention fluid also can render the patient hypothermic. This is predominantly a problem with low-viscosity fluids, because dextran is not used in sufficient quantity to induce hypothermia. Coagulopathy, confusion, alteration in level of consciousness, shivering, and an increase in myocardial oxygen demand may be present. Some consideration should be given to warming of distention fluid before use.

Monitoring

Use of ECG monitoring, noninvasive blood pressure monitoring, pulse oximetry, temperature probe, airway pressure monitoring, and end-tidal CO_2 monitoring should be part of every routine anesthetic case. Use of invasive arterial monitoring and central venous pressure monitoring should be reserved for patients who have significant cardiorespiratory disease. End-tidal CO_2 monitoring is helpful in detecting the onset of a gas embolus. A sudden fall in end-tidal CO_2 is highly suggestive of an embolic event. Other methods for detecting emboli are available. Transesophageal and transthoracic echocardiography are very sensitive in picking up gas emboli. This modality is expensive, however, and requires training and expertise in its use and interpretation of findings. Thus far, it is not part of routine practice. Esophageal stethoscope and precordial Doppler ultrasound studies may constitute a suitable alternative. Blood loss and fluid deficits should be calculated accurately and frequently. Monitoring serial plasma sodium concentration may be useful when the safe fluid limit has been exceeded. Duration of surgery should be noted and

relayed to the surgeon. Body temperature should be recorded and measures taken to avoid hypothermia. To ensure a good outcome for the patient, monitoring should be instituted in the operating room, carried through into the postanesthetic care unit, and continued after transfer of the patient to the hospital room.

References

1. American College of Physicians. Guidelines for assessing and managing the perioperative risk from coronary artery disease associated with major non-cardiac surgery. Ann Intern Med 1997;127:309.
2. VanBelle E, Lablanche JM, Bauters C. Coronary angioscopic findings in the infracted-related vessel within 1 month of acute myocardial infarction. Natural history and the effect of thrombolysis. Circulation 1998;97:26.
3. Tuman KJ. Perioperative cardiovascular risk: Assessment and management. Anesth Analg 2001;92:S106.
4. Weiner D, Ryan TJ, McCabe CH, et al. Prognostic importance of a clinical profile and exercise test in medically treated patients with coronary heart disease. J Am Coll Cardiol 1984;3:772.
5. Boersma E, Poldermans D, Bax JJ, et al. Predictors of cardiac events after major vascular surgery. Role of clinical characteristics, dobutamine echocardiography, and beta blocker therapy. JAMA 2001;285:1865.
6. Eichelberger JP, Schwartz KQ, Black ER, et al. Predictive value of dobutamine echocardiography just before non-cardiac vascular surgery. Am J Cardiol 1993;72:602.
7. Mantha S. Rational cardiac risk stratification before peripheral vascular surgery: Application of evidence-based medicine and Bayesian analysis. Semin Cardiothorac Vasc Anesth 2000;4:198.
8. Zaugg M, Schaub MC, Pasch T, Spahn DR. Modulation of beta-adrenergic receptor sub-type activities in perioperative medicine: Mechanisms and sites of action. Br J Anaesth 2002;88:101.
9. Mangano DT, Layug EL, Wallace A, Tateo IM. Effects of atenolol on mortality and cardiovascular morbidity after non-cardiac surgery. The multicenter study of Perioperative Ischaemia Research Group. N Engl J Med 1996;335:1713.
10. Poldermans D, Boersma E, Bax JJ, et al. The effect of bisoprolol on perioperative mortality and myocardial infarction in high-risk patients undergoing vascular surgery. N Engl J Med 1999;341:1789.
11. Dodds TM, Stone JG, Coromilas J, et al. Prophylactic nitroglycerin infusion during non-cardiac surgery does not reduce perioperative ischemia. Anesth Analg 1993;76:705.
12. Howell SJ, Sear JW, Foex P. Hypertension, hypertensive heart disease and perioperative risk. Br J Anaesth 2004;92:570.
13. Milledge JS, Nunn JF. Criteria of fitness for anaesthesia in patients with chronic obstructive lung disease. BMJ 1975;3:670.
14. Gass GD, Olsen GN. Preoperative pulmonary function testing to predict postoperative morbidity and mortality. Chest 1986;89:127.
15. Shoemaker WC, Czer LS. Evaluation of the biologic importance of various hemodynamic and oxygen transport variables: which variables should be monitored in post-operative shock? Crit Care Med 1979;7:424.
16. Boyd O, Grounds RM, Bennett ED. A randomised clinical trial of the effect of deliberate perioperative increase of oxygen delivery on mortality in high-risk surgical patients. JAMA 1993;270:2699.
17. Ball J, Rhodes A, Bennett ED. Reducing the morbidity and mortality of high-risk surgical patients. Yearb Intensive Care Emerg Med 2000;331.
18. Wilson J, Woods I, Fawcett J, et al. Reducing the risk of major elective surgery: Randomised control trial of preoperative optimisation of oxygen delivery. BMJ 1999; 318:1099.
19. Sharma KC, Brandstetter RD, Brensilver JM, Jung LD. Cardiopulmonary physiology and pathophysiology as a consequence of laparoscopic surgery. Chest 1996;110:810.
20. Joris JL, Noirot DP, Legrand MJ, et al. Haemodynamic changes during laparoscopic cholecystectomy. Anaesth Analg 1993;76:1067.
21. Coskun F, Salman M. Anaesthesia for operative endoscopy. Curr Opin Obstet Gynaecol 2001;13:371.
22. Puri GD, Singh H. Ventilatory effects of laparoscopy under general anaesthesia. Br J Anaesth 1992;68:211.
23. Pelosi P, Foti G, Cereda M, et al. Effects of carbon dioxide insufflations for laparoscopic cholecystectomy on the respiratory system. Anaesthesia 1996;51:744.

24. Bozkurt P, Kaya G, Yeker Y, et al. The cardio-respiratory effects of laparoscopic procedures in infants. Anaesthesia 1999;54:831.

25. Doyle M, Twomey C, Owens TM, McShane AJ. Gastro-oesophageal reflux and tracheal contamination during laparoscopic cholecystectomy and diagnostic gynaecological laparoscopy. Anesth Analg 1998;86:624.

26. Valentine J, Stakes A, Bellamy MC. Reflux during positive ventilation through a laryngeal mask. Br J Anaesth 1994;73:543.

27. Ho BY, Skinner HJ, Mahajan PR. Gastro-oesophageal reflux during day case gynaecological laparoscopy under positive pressure ventilation: Laryngeal mask vs tracheal intubation. Anaesthesia 1998;53:921.

28. Dobbs FF, Kumar V, Alexander JI, Hull MG. Pain after laparoscopy related to posture and ring versus clip sterilization. Br J Obstet Gynaecol 1987;94:262.

29. Jackson S, Laurence A, Hill J. Does post laparoscopy pain relate to residual carbon dioxide? Anaesthesia 1996;51:485.

30. Sarli L, Costi R, Sansebastiano G. Prospective randomized trial of low-pressure pneumoperitoneum for reduction of shoulder tip pain following laparoscopy. Br J Surg 2000;87:1161.

31. Prospt AM, Liberman RF, Harlow BL. Complications of hysteroscopic surgery: Predicting patients at risk. Obstet Gynaecol 2000;94:517.

32. Jansen FW, Vredevoogd CB, Van Ulzen K, et al. Complications of hysteroscopy: A prospective, multicenter study. Obstet Gynaecol 2000;96:266.

33. O'Connor T. Hyponatremic encephalopathy after endometrial ablation. Letter to the editor. JAMA 1994;271:343.

34. Pasini A, Belloni C. Intraoperative complications of 697 consecutive operative hysteroscopies. Minerva Ginecol 2001;53:13.

35. Brundin J, Thomasson K. Cardiac gas embolism during carbon dioxide hysteroscopy: Risk and management. Eur J Obstet Gynaecol Reprod Biol 1989;33:241.

36. Rythen-Alder E, Brundin J, et al. Detection of carbon dioxide during hysteroscopy. Gynaecol Endosc 1992;1: 207.

37. Brander P, Neis KJ, Ehmer C, et al. The aetiology, frequency and prevention of gas embolus during CO_2 hysteroscopy. J Am Assoc Gynaecol Laparosc 1999;6:421.

38. Neis K, Brander P. Room air as a source of gas embolism in diagnostic CO_2 hysteroscopy. Zentralb Gynakol 2000;122:222.

39. Ellingson T, Aboulafia D. Dextran syndrome: Acute hypotension, non-cardiogenic pulmonary oedema, anaemia and coagulopathy following hysteroscopic surgery using 32% Dextran 70. Chest 1997;111:513.

40. Brandt R, Dunn W. Dextran 70 embolisation. Another case of pulmonary haemorrhage, coagulopathy and rhabdomyolysis. Chest 1993;104:631.

41. Schinco M, Hughes D. Complications of 32% dextran 70. A case report. J Reprod Med 1996;41:455.

42. Users reminded about adverse reactions to Dextran. FDA Drug Bull 1983;13:23.

43. Trimbos-Kemper TCM, Veering BT. Anaphylactic shock from intracavity 32% Dextran 70 during hysteroscopy. Fertil Steril 1989;51:1053.

44. Levin H, Ben-David B. Transient blindness during hysteroscopy: A rare complication. Anaesth Analg 1995;81:880.

45. Karci A, Erkin Y. Transient blindness following hysteroscopy. J Int Med Res 2003;31:152.

46. Gbossou J, Madras M, Roche A, et al. Transient arrhythmia disclosing major glycine poisoning during hysteroscopy. Ann Fr Anesth Reanim 1995;14:370.

47. Agostini A, Bretelle F, Cravello L, et al. [Complications of operative hysteroscopy.] Presse Med (in French) 2003;32:826.

48. Lukascko P. Noncardiogenic pulmonary oedema secondary to intra-uterine instillation of 32% Dextran 70. Fertil Steril 1985;44:560.

49. Agraharkar M, Agraharkar A. Posthysteroscopic hyponatremia: Evidence for a multifactorial cause. Am J Kidney Dis 1997;30:717.

50. Varol N, Maher P, Cooper M, et al. A literature review and update on the prevention and management of fluid overload in endometrial resection and hysteroscopic surgery. Gynaecol Endosc 2002;11:19.

51. Wallwiener D, Aydeniz B, Rimbach S, et al. [Addition of ethanol to the distension medium in surgical hysteroscopy as screening to prevent fluid overload. A prospective randomised comparative study of ablative versus non-ablative surgical hysteroscopy and different ethanol concentration.] Geburts Frauenheilk (in German) 1996;56:462.

52. Tomazevic T, Savnik L, Dintinjana M, et al. Safe and effective management by automated gravitation during hysteroscopy. JSLS 1998; 2:51.

53. Shirk G, Gimpelson R. Control of intrauterine fluid pressure during operative hysteroscopy. J Am Assoc Gynecol Laparosc 1994;2:101.

Reducing Risk and Maximizing Efficacy with Thermal Modalities

9

Andrew I. Brill, Michael P. Traynor, and Resad Pasic

Complications are an inevitable aspect of surgery, whether performed by laparotomy or laparoscopy. Although a significant proportion of complications during laparoscopic surgery can be related to some aspect of peritoneal access, unintended intraoperative thermal injury continues to be a major contributor to medicolegal conflict. Laparotomy presents the surgeon with unfettered visual and manual access to the surgical field, providing immediate tactile feedback during the use of conventional clamps, sutures, and scissors to secure and divide vascular pedicles and to attain hemostasis. By contrast, proprioceptive feedback is comparatively truncated during laparoscopic surgery, requiring the surgeon to employ a modified set of visuospatial skills while using a completely different set of instruments.

For every endoscopic procedure using some type of thermal energy to cut and coagulate tissue, the prospect for unwanted thermal injury can be reduced by adhering to sound anatomic principles, exercising purposeful visiospatial skill, and applying a firm understanding of instrumentation and any particular thermal modality used to produce a desired surgical effect. Knowing "how" and "why," however, constitutes just one aspect of surgery performed with maximum safety and efficacy. Surgery will transcend technique when experience and judgment are coupled with this fundamental knowledge. Only then can science become art in the hands of the endoscopic surgeon.

ELECTROSURGERY

Even though electrosurgery has been widely used since the early 20th century after developments by Bovie were convincingly implemented by Cushing, little, if any, formal training concerning this surgical modality continues to be the rule both in the United States and elsewhere. Quite naturally, electrosurgery rapidly evolved as an indispensable methodology for cutting and hemostasis for the laparoscopic armamentarium, obviating the customary need to clamp, cut, and suture vascular pedicles.

When electrosurgery is aptly employed, it is a safe, effective, and dependable surgical modality for the gynecologic endoscopist. It is used primarily to provide hemostatic incision, coagulate bleeders, and direct thermal destruction of selected tissues. Differences between the intrinsic demands of laparotomy and of laparoscopy (e.g., spatial orientation and hand-eye coordination), however, require a heightened sense of awareness by the gynecologic endoscopist. Although inadvertent electrosurgical injury is not unique to gynecologic endoscopy, it may be more apt to occur because electrosurgical devices are commonly used for ligating, cutting, and focal hemostasis. Any visceral or vascular structure, including the bowel, bladder, and ureter, within the operative field, or which may conduct electrical current outside of this view, may be subject to excessive inadvertent electrosurgical injury. Moreover, despite the seemingly protective effect of the confined uterine environment, electrosurgical complications also can occur with the use of electrosurgery during an operative hysteroscopy.

Although the true incidence of electrosurgical complications is not established, it remains one of the greatest concerns for the laparoscopic surgeon. A survey conducted at a 1995 meeting of the Society of Laparoendoscopic Surgeons revealed that 13% of attending members had one or more laparoscopic electrosurgery–related malpractice cases currently in litigation. During the 1993 meeting of the American College of Surgeons, 54% of the 506 surgeons surveyed reported that they knew of at least one colleague who had encountered a complication related to electrosurgery.

Biophysical Principles

A full understanding of specific behaviors that may contribute to complications associated with electrosurgery requires both familiarity with relevant terminology and comprehension of the biophysical principles that govern the conduction of electrical current in living tissue. Simply defined, *electrosurgery* is accomplished by the generation and delivery of a high-frequency alternating current between an active electrode and a dispersive or return electrode. Resultant thermodynamic phenomena occurring during the intervening tissue conduction ultimately increase tissue temperature, causing a variety of phenomena and tissue effects including cutting (vaporization), fulguration, and desiccation (coagulation).[1,2] Hence, high-frequency alternating current is conducted through a surgical instrument–electrode assembly and then into living tissue, which subsequently is heated at different rates for the desired tissue effect. Electrocautery, however, is not electrosurgery; for this modality, tissue is directly heated by a hot electrode warmed by the passage of direct current.

Given a significant difference in electrical potential, electrons are set in motion in a particular direction within a conductor to carry an *electrical current* (I) that is measured in *amperes* and represents the rate of flow of electrical charge. The electromotive force that pushes the current through the conductor is referred to as the *voltage* (V). *Resistance* (R)—termed *impedance* with high-frequency alternating current—is measured in ohms and represents the property of a conductor that opposes the flow of the current. A "pathway" or completed circuit must exist for electrons to flow. Because energy can be neither created nor destroyed, heat is produced as the moving electrons encounter resistance—so-called resistive heating.

Current is directly proportional to voltage and inversely proportional to resistance, which is expressed by Ohm's law: $V = I \times R$. Greater resistance therefore requires greater voltage. If the resistance is a fixed variable, greater voltage will create a greater current. On the other hand, power (the numerical designation that the operator keys into the electrosurgical unit [ESU]) quantifies the rate of work being done and is expressed in watts (W). Because current is able to flow against resistance, it performs work, which is dissipated as heat (Joule's law)—the raison d'être of electrosurgery. This relation is expressed by the equation $W = I \times V$ or, alternatively, as $W = I^2 \times R$ or $W = V^2/R$. Three important electrosurgical behaviors can be derived from this relationship[3]:

1. When an electrode is applied to tissue with high resistance, such as fat or fascia, the ESU correspondingly outputs greater voltage, provided that the power setting (W) remains the same.
2. Similarly, output voltage will be greater whenever current is conducted through the high-resistance pathways of carbonized tissue—products that inevitably encrust electrode surfaces.
3. Because voltage is the electromotive force that drives the transit of charged particles across a potential difference, greater voltage has the propensity to produce greater lateral and deeper thermal necrosis.

Furthermore, as the surface area of an electrode increases (e.g., needle tip to a spatula electrode, or edge to flat surface), current decreases proportionally to the corresponding decrement in current density. Logically, then, power output is decreased secondary to dispersal of current over a greater surface area (i.e., reduced current density).

The low-frequency alternating current (110 volts at 60 Hz [cycles per second]) from a standard electrical outlet causes neuromuscular contraction, the so-called faradic effect, through sustained nerve depolarization (i.e., you get shocked!). At much higher frequencies (greater than 100 kHz), insufficient time elapses for the current to cause sustained depolarization of the nerves, and the kinetic energy is simply dissipated as heat. The traditional electrosurgical generator (the ESU) converts low-frequency alternating current (60 Hz) to very high radiofrequency (RF) current (range of 300 to 600 kHz). By comparison, the usual RF and television frequencies are within the 550 to 880 kHz range (Fig. 9–1).

Monopolar Electrosurgery

In monopolar electrosurgery, the patient is an integral part of the electrical circuit. The complete monopolar electrosurgical system consists of an electrosurgical generator (the ESU), an active electrode, the patient, and a return or dispersive electrode (often erroneously called the grounding pad). The output current flows out of the active electrode (e.g., scissors, needle tip), through the intended tissue target and a variety of conductive tissues (e.g., muscle, nerve), and then back to the ESU through the return electrode. Despite conducting equivalent amounts of current, the dramatic difference in thermal effects (i.e., heating) between the active and the return electrodes is simply explained by the marked discrepancy in surface areas. Because the rate of heat production and potential for thermal damage (i.e., tissue burning) is determined primarily by the current density (i.e., surface area), heating is maximal at the smaller tip, side, or edge of the active electrode and negligible along the markedly larger surface area of the return electrode.

Waveforms

The alternating current used for electrosurgery has a sinusoidal waveform (constantly changing directions). The typical output settings labeled "cut," "blend," and "coag" on the face of conventional electrosurgical generators are simply variations of current and voltage in relation to time, called *waveforms* (see Fig. 9–1). Three fundamental types of current waveforms (outputs) are used during electrosurgery: *cut*, *blend*, and *coag*. Despite their obvious association with certain tissue effects, they are in fact not necessarily related to any particular tissue end point. A pure cut waveform (also referred to as continuous, uninterrupted, unmodulated, or undamped) is an uninterrupted sine wave of low voltage; being continuously "on," it provides the highest average current.

The pure coag waveform (also referred to as noncontinuous, interrupted, modulated, or damped) is a highly interrupted current with frequent and prolonged gaps. Switched to this mode, the current is in fact "on" only 6% per interval of time. By comparison, the pure cut mode is "on" 100% of the time. In order to maintain the same power output (W), the significantly lower average current of the coag output is automatically balanced by the generation of a higher-output voltage (recall that $W = I \times V$). Thermal damage is consequently more extensive with use of the coagulation waveform with conventional electrosurgical generators.

The blend output should not be misconstrued as being some mixture or blend of other types of waveforms. Correctly speaking, generator settings in this mode (i.e., blend 1, blend 2, and so on) simply produce progressive drops in average current by inserting current interruption of greater duration (i.e., blend 1 is "on" 50% of the time; blend 2, 40%; and blend 3, 25%, respectively) (see Fig. 9–1). As current progressively drops with higher blend settings, the output voltage must progressively increase to conserve energy ($V = I \times R$). Similar to the tissue effects of the coagulation waveform, higher blend settings will generate greater zones of thermal necrosis.

Low Voltage   **High Voltage**

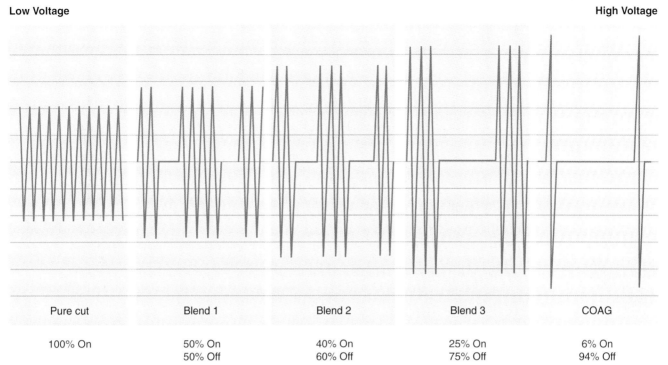

Pure cut	Blend 1	Blend 2	Blend 3	COAG
100% On	50% On 50% Off	40% On 60% Off	25% On 75% Off	6% On 94% Off

Figure 9–1 ▪ **Range of output voltages.** Relative changes in voltage and average current related to "cut," "blend," and "coag" currents. (From Harrell AG, Kercher KW, Heniford BT. Energy sources in laparoscopy. Semin Laparosc Surg 2004;11:201.)

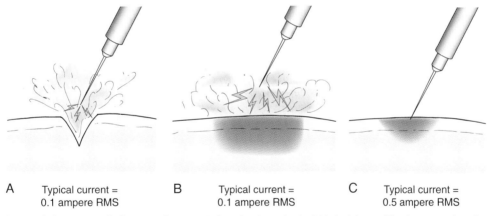

A   Typical current =   B   Typical current =   C   Typical current =
       0.1 ampere RMS   0.1 ampere RMS   0.5 ampere RMS

Figure 9–2 ▪ **Fundamental electrosurgical effects. A,** Electrosurgical cutting (vaporization/ablation) is possible whenever voltage is sufficient to create an electrical spark between an electrode and underlying tissue. **B,** Fulguration is the use of high-voltage sparking produced by "coag" current to coagulate a broad surface with open bleeders. **C,** Desiccation, coagulation. If tissue is heated to 100°C, cellular water completely evaporates (desiccation), and localized hemostasis occurs as a result of contraction of blood vessels and the surrounding tissues (coagulation). (From Harrell AG, Kercher KW, Heniford BT. Energy sources in laparoscopy. Semin Laparosc Surg 2004;11:201.)

CUTTING, FULGURATION, AND DESICCATION

As a phenomenon, electrosurgical cutting (vaporization or electrosection) occurs secondary to high current density created by an electrical spark (Fig. 9–2). Rapid vaporization of cellular water leads to volumetric disruption from steam with consequent tissue separation (cutting). Electrical sparking, the ionization of air between the active electrode and

underlying tissue, requires only 200 V. Because all waveforms are capable of delivering this amount of voltage, tissue cutting can in fact be accomplished with any of the conventional outputs. With use of conventional electrosurgical generators, thermal damage at the margins of an electrosurgical cut is governed by the amount of *voltage* associated with a given current. Because decreases in current from progressive current interruption (cut to blend to coag) lead to greater output voltage, the uninterrupted cutting waveform produces the least amount of thermal damage at the margins of a cut incision. Although all of the typical outputs—cut, blend, and coag—provide sufficient voltage to ionize the air gap and arc to tissue, the higher voltages of blend and coag create progressively wider zones of thermal damage at the margins of the incision (see Fig. 9–2). These effects are amplified by using broad-surface electrodes.

Using blend or coag current to cut in order to provide wider hemostasis can be helpful during myomectomy, as well as in operating down the broad ligament and along the vaginal fornices during hysterectomy, across vascular adhesions, and to clarify the space of Retzius in preparation for colposuspension and paravaginal repair. Higher-voltage currents also facilitate incision of tissues that have greater impedance, such as fatty or desiccated pedicles and adhesions.

On the other hand, it is more prudent to use the lower-voltage cutting current applied with the edge of an electrode for electrosurgical incision whenever lateral thermal spread may pose a higher risk to adjacent tissues, such as the ovarian cortex during cystectomy and the ureter or rectum during incision of mesentery or excision of endometriosis from the lateral pelvic sidewall or cul-de-sac.

Fulguration is the use of high-voltage sparking produced by coag current to coagulate a broad surface with open vessels on end when coaptation is not feasible or desirable. As opposed to the continuous arcing produced by cutting current, the highly interrupted output of coagulation current causes the arcs to strike the tissue surface in a widely dispersed and random fashion. High-voltage sparking results in high-temperature tissue changes including carbonization. This leads to more rapid thermal change, creating a zone of superficial coagulation. Fulguration can be effective to control small bleeders up to 2 mm in diameter, such as along the undersurface of the ovarian cortex during cystectomy, atop the myometrial bed during myomectomy, and alongside Cooper's ligament during colposuspension. If bleeding in the vicinity of the bowel, bladder, or ureter cannot be controlled with pressure alone, carefully directed short bursts of noncontact coag current with a broad-surface electrode can accomplish effective hemostasis with the least possible amount of electrosurgical penetration. Despite the high-voltage output involved, fulguration is useless in a wet, conductive surgical field because of the random diffusion of current.

Regardless of the output setting, *desiccation* and *coagulation* can occur whenever an activated electrode comes into direct contact with tissue for a sufficient amount of time. Depending on the desired effect, this can be accomplished with any particular waveform. Desiccation is fundamentally related to electrode manipulation. The contact of tissue with the surface of any active electrode, regardless of the selected waveform, obliterates any ionizable gap, leading to the diffusion of current with substantially lower current density. Consequently, tissue is heated more slowly, causing cellular dehydration by gradual percolation, rather than by volumetric explosion by superheated steam produced with higher current densities. Because both electrosurgical cutting and fulguration consume energy to ionize the air gap for sparking, contact desiccation heats tissue more efficiently. More energy is available to heat tissue, so thermal damage is predictably deeper and more widespread during contact electrosurgical phenomena. Because the peak voltage of coag current is very high, contact coagulation using this waveform generally is

limited to superficial layers. The high-voltage tissue strikes limit conduction by accelerating the buildup of tissue resistance from rapid desiccation and carbonization. Conversely, electrode contact using the lower-voltage cut waveform heats tissue more gradually, leading to deeper and more effective penetration. Because surface changes associated with deeper-contact electrosurgical burns are relatively bland, it behooves the surgeon to give first attention to white rather than blackened areas of electrosurgical injury (e.g., intestine).

Both contact and coaptive coagulation using monopolar electrosurgery are predictably more effective using cut current. For example, these behaviors can help direct electrosurgical ablation of endometriotic tissue. Because superficial-appearing implants along the peritoneum may extend deeply into the retroperitoneal tissues, these lesions are best ablated using a broad-surface electrode in contact with cut current. By contrast, superficial implants on the ovarian cortex are more prudently treated using coag current to minimize unwanted thermal injury to adjacent follicular tissue.

Coaptive vessel sealing using any type of monopolar current may be ineffective if the blood flow remains uninterrupted. Unless a vessel is sufficiently squeezed before electricity is applied, current density is dramatically reduced by conduction in blood, and luminal temperatures undergo little change because any heat is dissipated by convection. Deceived by the appearance of well-coagulated tissue, a surgeon may discover an alarmingly viable core at the time of incision. Regardless of the selected output current (that is, cut, blend, or coag), coaptive desiccation with monopolar electrosurgery usually is insufficient to reliably secure the uterine or ovarian vessels during hysterectomy and oophorectomy.

In summary, by controlling (1) the configuration or type of electrode (needle, spatula, scissors), (2) the current waveform (cut, blend, or coag), and (3) the degree of contact with the tissue (contact versus no contact), markedly different thermodynamic thermal effects can be produced; therefore, different degrees of thermal damage may occur (Fig. 9–3).

POTENTIAL PROBLEMS WITH MONOPOLAR ELECTROSURGERY AT LAPAROSCOPY

In contrast with the open surgical environment during laparotomy, the bulk of most instruments and nearly all surrounding intra-abdominal structures are not visualized during any laparoscopic procedure. Furthermore, nearly all of the potential conductors during laparoscopic electrosurgery also are out of the surgeon's field of view. Intended and unintended couriers of direct or induced currents include the abdominal wall, metallic trocar sheaths and instruments, the operating laparoscope, contiguous visceral tissues, and the active electrode (which is the only part of the circuit under view!). It comes as no surprise that most accidental electrosurgical burns during laparoscopic surgery are undetected at the time of injury.

Insulation Failure

Insulation failure occurs as a result of development of breaks or holes in the insulation caused by physical abruption during

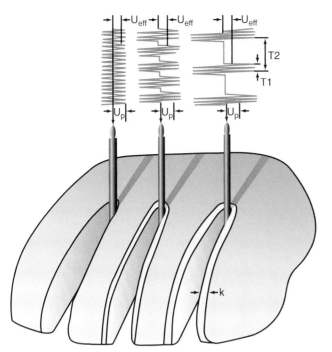

Figure 9–3 ▪ **Zones of thermal damage related to voltage.** Using conventional electrosurgical generator for tissue cutting, the margin of thermal necrosis expands with increasing voltage. (From Vancaillie TG. Electrosurgery at laparoscopy: Guidelines to avoid complications. Gynaecol Endosc 1994;3:1143.)

surgical maneuvers (such as passage through an incompletely engaged trumpet cannula) or during normal reprocessing procedures. Completely intact insulation (especially on disposable instrumentation) can be breached by very high voltage (e.g., during open circuit activation or with use of a modulated coagulation waveform). Any break or breach in insulation may provide an alternate pathway for the flow of current. If the defective portion of insulation contacts tissue during electrode activation, an electric arc will bridge directly from the electrode through the defect to this tissue. Thermal damage will occur if the current density is high enough to heat the tissue to a significant level. Because these defects usually are out of the field of view, this type of injury usually proceeds undetected at the time of insult. Insulation failure can be minimized by periodically inspecting the insulation covering of all laparoscopic electrodes (especially at the distal shoulder) for small cracks and defects. Disposable monopolar electrodes should not be reused. The risk of high voltage can be eliminated by using the unmodulated cutting waveform and by avoiding open circuit activation.

Direct Coupling

Direct coupling of current occurs when an activated electrode makes unintended contact with another metal object in the area of the surgical field. Because rectification (frequency demodulation) can occur during metal-to-metal sparking, sudden neuromuscular twitching may be its first telltale sign. Sparking between the electrode and a titanium staple can cause tremendous heat production by funneling of the current density. Accidental electrode contact with a suction-irrigator probe, the operating laparoscope, or a metal cannula creates

an alternative pathway that normally is conducted up through a metal trocar to the abdominal wall and back to the dispersive electrode. If any of these devices, however, is isolated from direct contact with the abdominal wall by an insulator (e.g., plastic cannula or self-retaining device), the current may take an alternative pathway through a point of contact with adjacent tissue. Again, if the current density is high, thermal damage may occur. Direct coupling can be avoided by ensuring that the generator is never activated when the electrode is touching or in proximity to another metal object in the surgical field.

Capacitive Coupling

Capacitive coupling is the induction of stray current to a surrounding conductor through the intact insulation of an active electrode. In fact, all of the necessary ingredients for the localized genesis of capacitance are provided by an activated monopolar electrode that is passed through a conductive sheath.

Two conductors of differing potentials, the active electrode and the metal sheath (e.g., trocar sheath, working channel of an operating laparoscope, irrigator-aspirator probe), are separated by the insulation of the electrode. On activation, up to 80% of the generator current is induced on the metal sheath by capacitance. Normally this stray current is safely returned to the dispersive electrode by conduction through the large area of contact between the metal trocar sheath and the abdominal wall. The magnitude of capacitance is greater with higher voltage, smaller cannulas, and longer electrodes. Furthermore, the induced charge will persist until the electrode is deactivated or it is conducted through an alternate pathway.

If the metal trocar sheath is attached to the abdominal wall by a nonconductive plastic device (e.g., hybrid trocar [metal plus plastic] or plastic self-retaining screw device), the induced current becomes electrically isolated from the abdominal wall. Contact between the cannula and a visceral structure provides an alternate pathway through which the stray current can discharge. Significant thermal damage will occur if the current density is sufficiently concentrated by a small area of contact. A similar phenomenon of capacitive coupling and isolation of current may occur during activation of an electrode placed through the working port of an operating laparoscope that is isolated from the abdominal wall by an all-plastic cannula. In either case, the thermal injury usually is out of the surgeon's field of view.

Capacitance is minimized by using an unmodulated cutting waveform and avoiding open circuit activation (i.e., minimizing voltage). An all-metal system will suffice for the safe conduction of capacitively coupled current back to the dispersive electrode. Hybrid cannula systems (mixtures of plastic and metal) should not be used to house monopolar electrosurgical devices.

BIPOLAR ELECTROSURGERY

Bipolar electrosurgery consolidates an active electrode and return electrode into an instrument with two small poles. These poles can be the tines of a forceps, blades of a scissors, or an electrode matched to a more proximal conductive collar separated by an insulator. The output typically used is the low-voltage cut current.

Localization of current between the poles offers distinct advantages. Thermal damage generally is limited to a discrete volume of tissue. A bipolar forceps can be used to coapt and thermally weld blood vessels. The concentrated current and small distance between the poles also make it possible to desiccate tissue that is immersed in fluid. This modality is less useful, however, when open blood vessels are retracted or tissue pedicles are very thick.

Although the flow of current and primary thermal effects are restricted to the tissue between the poles, the risk of thermal injury to tissue distant from the site of directed hemostasis is not eliminated. As current is applied between the poles, the intervening tissue gradually desiccates until it becomes thoroughly dehydrated. Desiccation is complete when the tissue whitens and visible steam emission stops. If the application of current continues, the heat spreads well beyond the electrical limits of the instrument. This secondary thermal bloom is caused by the bubbling of steam into the tissue parenchyma as heat is rapidly generated (dry tissue has a high resistance to the flow of electrical current). This phenomenon explains why structures such as the ureter or bowel may suffer irreversible thermal damage despite being at some distance from an operative or bleeding site.

Use of an in-line ammeter, which provides visible and audible signals to monitor the flow of current between the tissue and the jaws of the bipolar grasper, does not prevent this problem. Rather, it tends to promote the flow of energy well beyond desiccation. Consequently, an ammeter should not be used to determine the treatment end point for coagulation of blood vessels in the vicinity of vital tissue.

Because the rate of heat generation is a direct function of the volume of tissue being desiccated, thermal spread also can be reduced by using the sides or tips of a slightly open forceps to press or lift treated tissue, rather than to produce coaptation for hemostasis.

As with contact monopolar coagulation, tissue between the electrodes of a bipolar instrument may become adherent during desiccation. Repeated attempts to shake the tissue free may lead to traumatic avulsion of a key vascular pedicle. A stuck vascular pedicle usually can be "unglued" by energizing the opened device while immersing it in a conductive irrigant, such as saline. Once the solution is boiled by the high-current density between the electrodes, the mechanical action of bubbling usually is sufficient to atraumatically free the pedicle.

The art of surgical hemostasis is preventing vascular trauma while causing the least possible collateral tissue damage. Surgical hemostasis should not be driven by reflex alone. Instead, surgeons should always follow an orderly sequence of steps to minimize risk:

1. Before taking any action, make every effort to accurately determine the source of bleeding and its proximity to vital anatomy. Even in the face of active hemorrhage, the bleeders usually can be identifed by combining mechanical tamponade (using the jaws of a grasper or the side of a simple metallic probe) with active hydrolavage (using an irrigator-aspirator to break up and remove blood and clots).

2. If the bowel, bladder, or ureter is in close proximity to the bleeder, mobilize that structure sufficiently before applying energy. These entities usually can be protected by using a combination of countertraction and incremental tissue dissection.

3. Whenever the peritoneum is involved, a relaxing incision parallel to the structure of concern also may be useful.

This protocol mandates withholding thermal energy until an orderly sequence of anatomic triage is carried out. Whenever a vital structure cannot be adequately mobilized, every effort is made to control hemorrhage by using mechanical tamponade alone for up to 5 minutes. If access to the bleeding site or vessel caliber renders unrealistic the use of pressure alone, either carefully applied thermal energy or a suture ligature should be effective. If the surgeon is uncomfortable using either of these alternatives, conversion to laparotomy may be warranted.

Advances in Bipolar Electrosurgery

The latest advance in bipolar electrosurgery is the introduction of novel ligating-cutting devices that minimize force by delivering electrical energy as high current and low-voltage output. Once tonal feedback from a dedicated generator or accessory confirms complete desiccation of the tissue bundle, the pedicle is cut by advancing a centrally set mechanical blade. By directly responding to incremental increases in tissue resistance during coaptive desiccation, total energy delivery is dramatically less than in conventional bipolar systems. Consequently, carbonization, tissue sticking, smoke, vascular instability, and lateral thermal damage may be significantly reduced.

Relying on the breakthrough finding that vessel wall fusion can be achieved using electrical energy to denature collagen and elastin in vessel walls to re-form into a permanent seal, the LigaSure Vessel Sealing Device (Valleylab, Boulder, Colorado) applies a high coaptive pressure to the tissue bundle during the generation of tissue temperatures under 100°C; hydrogen cross-links first are ruptured and then renature, resulting in a vascular seal that has high tensile strength.

The second device, the Plasmakinetics Cutting Forceps (Gyrus, Minneapolis, Minnesota), uses advanced solid-state generator software to deliver pulsed energy with continuous feedback control. The cycle stops once it senses that tissue response is complete; the cool-down phase ensures that collagen and elastin matrix re-forms without tissue fragmentation.

A third device, the EnSeal Laparoscopic Vessel Fusion System (SurgRx, Inc., Palo Alto, California), is an innovative bipolar instrument that can be retrofitted to most conventional bipolar generators. This "smart electrode" contains a set of plastic jaws embedded with nanometer-sized spheres of nickel that conduct a locally regulated current. Tissue temperatures never exceed 120°C owing to the progressive generation of resistance in the plastic jaws. With this device, desiccation is facilitated by simultaneously advancing a mechanical blade that both cuts and squeezes the tissue bundle to eliminate tissue water.

ULTRASONIC ENERGY

Ultrasonic shears produce mechanical energy to cut and coagulate tissue. Housed in the handpiece of this laparoscopic device is a piezoelectric crystal that vibrates a titanium blade 55,500 times per second over a variable excursion of 50 to 100 μm. As energy is transmitted to tissue, hydrogen bonds of tissue proteins are ruptured, leading to a denatured protein coagulum without significant charring. The tissue cutting that occurs is secondary to mechanical vibration and cavitational fragmentation of tissue parenchyma.

Because ultrasonic energy does not generate the high temperatures created by electrosurgery, it is less predictable for deep-tissue coagulation. Rather, thermal change is gradual, requiring a modicum of patience.

Available instrument configurations include 5-mm curved or hook blades. In addition, 5-mm or 10-mm ligating and cutting shears coaptively desiccate and cut the tissue by securing it between a grooved plastic pad and the vibrating blade.

By using various combinations of blade shapes, blade excursions, and tissue tensions, surgeons can accomplish a variety of specific effects. Cutting velocity is directly proportional to blade excursion, tissue traction, and blade surface area (energy density), and is inversely related to tissue density and elasticity. Thus, the fastest cutting with the least amount of coagulation occurs when tissue is placed on tension and firmly squeezed, lifted, or rotated with the sharpest side of a blade set at maximum excursion. Coagulation is the obverse of cutting: It is inversely related to tissue tension, blade sharpness, blade excursion, and cutting speed. Therefore, coagulation is best achieved by relaxing tension, minimizing blade excursion, and using a blunt edge or flattened blade surface.

The surgeon should be mindful of the potential for premature incision of an incompletely coagulated tissue pedicle when excessive traction or torsion is applied. When used to coaptively desiccate and incise a vascular pedicle, ultrasonic energy should be applied patiently, with great care taken to minimize tissue tension and with use of the broadest blade surface set to the lowest excursion. Hemostatic incision is best ensured by first coagulating several overlapping areas along an untracted pedicle, limiting each application to the point of tissue blanching and initial vapor emission. Only then should the pedicle be incised by gradually lifting, squeezing, or rotating the tissue with the distal device. Following this sequence, ultrasonic energy can be successfully used to secure both the ovarian and the uterine vessels.

FUNDAMENTALS OF LASER SURGERY

Lasers convert electricity to light, which can be further amplified to produce intense beams of light energy. Laser (*l*ight *a*mplification by *s*timulated *e*mission of *r*adiation) technology can be used to cut, vaporize, and coagulate tissue.

Nuclei of a specific material can stimulate within a laser tube so that their electrons jump to a higher state. This excited state is unstable, and as electrons decay back into their resting state, a burst of energy called a *photon* with a specific wavelength is released. Photons then collide with other molecules, causing a cascade effect known as *stimulated emission*.

The spectrum of visible light is determined by its *wavelength* and is measured in nanometers. Specific wavelengths emit characteristic colors of light. Visible light has wavelengths in the range of 385 to 760 nm, with shorter wavelengths (blues) having more energy than longer wavelengths (reds). Lasers usually are named for their active media, because different materials emit characteristic wavelengths (i.e., colors of light).

Three important properties characterize a laser light beam: It is monochromatic, coherent, and collimated. *Monochromatic* means that it is light of a single specific wavelength. If a normal light source is shined through a prism, the prism will break down the light and display the different wavelengths, which will be seen as different colors of the light spectrum. In *coherent* light, all of the photons are exactly in phase, so that the peaks and valleys of one wave occur exactly at the same time as in the other waves. In *collimated* light, all the waves are parallel to each other and do not diverge over distance, allowing the laser to be focused onto very small spots. Laser energy is measured in units of power density, which is related to both the wattage and the area (W/cm^2). The smaller the focus or spot size, the higher the power density.

The four main types of lasers used in gynecologic surgery are the CO_2 laser, the neodymium:yttrium-aluminum-garnet (Nd:YAG) laser, the argon laser, and the potassium titanyl phosphate (KTP) laser. The wavelengths and hence the properties of these lasers differ. The CO_2 laser releases invisible light at a wavelength of 10,600 nm; therefore, addition of a red (helium-neon) beam is required to aim and control the instrument. CO_2 lasers are used primarily for cutting and vaporizing but make poor coagulators and cannot travel through fluids. KTP (532 nm) and argon (488 to 515 nm) lasers are similar in that they both can travel through air and fluids and can be passed through flexible fibers, making them convenient to use with laparoscopy and hysteroscopy. Nd:YAG lasers have a wavelength of 1064 to 1318 nm, can travel through fluids, and are useful for their deep penetration of tissue. Because of these properties, the Nd:YAG was one of the first lasers to be used for endometrial ablation.

OPERATIVE HYSTEROSCOPY AND RESECTOSCOPY

The use of electrical radiofrequency (RF) energy to perform intrauterine surgery can be broken down into three phases: delivery, transmission, and tissue strike. Thermal delivery devices, including monopolar or bipolar electrodes and quartz fibers, transmit energy either directly or indirectly to tissue. Transmission is either unaffected or deterred by the intrauterine distention medium. The final targeted tissue effects represent the complex summation of energy type and concentration, treatment time, tissue constituents and hydration, and the convective currents of tissue vascularity and circulating distention medium. The thoughtful understanding and orchestration of all of these elements are inextricably linked to efficiency, safety, and efficacy.

Electrosurgery in a Fluid Environment

To initiate and sustain a desired electrosurgical effect, a concentration of current density must be maintained between the active electrode and the tissue target. Because electrolyte-containing distention media such as saline are effective conductors, electrosurgery is ineffectual when the active electrode is used in these fluids; the readily conductive nature of the surrounding media acts to enlarge the surface area of the electrode, causing a dramatic reduction of current density. The use of nonconductive water-based distention media such as glycine, sorbitol, and mannitol offers a distinct advantage—they are effective insulators by virtue of their resistance to ionization. Because the current density at the active electrode is unchanged by these solutions, the intended electrosurgical effect remains unaltered.

As with conventional monopolar electrosurgery, electrosurgical sparking occurs once the medium between the active electrode and tissue is ionized to a sufficient degree to facilitate the flow of electrons to the tissue surface. So long as sparking is maintained with a sufficient amount of voltage, both cutting and fulguration are similarly available. Voltage requirements are higher at the outset of this ionization process; therefore, electrosurgical generators designed to deliver higher peak voltage over a broad range of electrode impedances are best suited to electrosurgery in a fluid environment. The best-suited generators have the highest manufacturer-specific "crest factor," determined by the ratio of peak voltage to average voltage. Because contact removes the medium from the electrical circuit, voltage requirements are less crucial for the initiation of tissue desiccation.

Monopolar Resectoscopic Electrodes

With the adaptation of the urologic resectoscope to hysteroscopic surgery, various monopolar electrodes have been designed to accommodate the need to coagulate, resect, and vaporize tissue within the variable confines of the intrauterine environment. The electrosurgical behavior and functional use of each electrode can be predicted by its size, shape, and surface area.

Desiccation Electrodes

A variety of resectoscopic electrodes are available specifically for hemostasis or destruction of large volumes of tissue. Electrode size and shape are best chosen by envisioning anatomic needs and the desired velocity of thermal change. Despite the assortment of different shapes including rollerball, rollerbarrel, ellipsoid, and even a flattened curette, all accomplish the desired electrosurgical effect by contact desiccation by means of resistive heating.

In contrast with the predictable depth of endometrial and superficial myometrial destruction produced by the Nd:YAG laser during endometrial ablation, the thermal depth reached with use of monopolar electrosurgery is far less knowable. In fact, the depth of thermal penetration with electrosurgery is unique to each hysteroscopic stroke, determined by the complex interplay of multiple factors:

- The chosen waveform
- The power setting of the electrosurgical generator
- Tissue exposure time
- Speed and pressure during electrode motion
- The size, shape, and clarity of the electrode
- The degree of endometrial thinning
- The ever-changing resistance of the endometrial tissue during electrosurgical treatment

Although an adequate depth of thermal damage usually is achieved without regard for most of these factors, reduction of menses in the presence of a thickened endometrium or diffuse adenomyosis is more apt to occur when the hysteroscopic technique is fashioned to maximize the summary electrosurgical effect.

Because the transmission of electrical energy causes coagulation by resistive heating, waveform settings that heat tissue more slowly would be expected to result in deeper tissue penetration. Although the cutting waveform has the lowest peak voltage, the uninterrupted delivery yields the highest average voltage. By contrast, despite the higher peak voltage of the coag waveform, maximal interruption limits it to substantially lower average voltage. If higher peak voltage is regarded as a more rapid desiccator, then the cut waveform would be expected to produce comparatively greater penetration. Conversely, the coag waveform would be preferable if the rate of desiccation were related primarily to average voltage. Unfortunately, neither of these presumptions is unilaterally supported by scientific data gathered from in vivo measurements. Although many investigators recommend the use of the cutting waveform to perform endometrial ablation, neither waveform has been conclusively demonstrated to singularly produce a greater reduction of abnormal uterine bleeding.

No matter what combination of desiccation electrode and electrosurgical waveform is used to perform an endometrial ablation, maintaining constant apposition between the electrode and the endometrial surface, with withdrawal of the electrode at a purposeful but slow pace, best ensures thorough destruction of the underlying endometrium and superficial myometrium. Proper electrode velocity is gauged by the symmetrical border of tissue whitening and gas bubbles that precede the advancing electrode.

Cutting and Vaporization Electrodes

The resectoscopic cutting loop can be used to cut and remove tissue by means of vaporization. The fine diameter of a wire electrode is ideally suited for electric arc formation, resulting in extremely high current density. Performed correctly, resectoscopic electrosection can be viewed as a two-stage process. On initial withdrawal of the loop electrode, activation occurs *before* tissue contact. This timing provides several critical seconds to initiate the electric arc. Once the plasma cloud reaches a steady state, the electrode then sinks effortlessly into the tissue by electrosective rather than mechanical force. Electrosection may cease altogether if the electrode is withdrawn too rapidly; tissue contact terminates the plasma cloud, thereby converting vaporization to contact desiccation.

The cutting waveform customarily is used for resectoscopic electrosection. Using the higher peak voltage of blend waveforms, however, can better satisfy the need for hemostasis at the incisional edges. These waveforms produce ample energy for electrosection and create predictably wider zones of thermal penetration. Exemplary applications for electrosection with a blend waveform include submucous myomectomy and endomyometrial resection.

Hysteroscopic visualization frequently is hampered by the adherence of electrosected tissue strips to the cutting loop. Stickiness between tissue and electrode occur secondary to the conversion of collagen to glucose and tissue char from higher temperatures. Rather than attempting to dislodge a resected fragment by mechanically shaking the electrode, it can be easily released by gently rubbing the chip against an adjacent endometrial surface with a side-to-side motion while simultaneously activating a short burst of coag current; the tissue fragment is freed by the onrush of gaseous bubbles that are instantly generated by the high peak voltage of this modulated waveform.

A newer generation of resectoscopic electrodes that vaporize, rather than "electrosect," take advantage of the electrosurgical phenomenon known as *edge density*—by nature, electrosurgical current is concentrated at the edge of any electrode. A deeply grooved barrel electrode presents a number of such edges, each capable of developing a current density high enough to vaporize rather than desiccate as it is rolled over the surface of tissue. The multiple vaporization tracts created on withdrawal ultimately blend together, creating a large furrow from vaporized tissue. Because high current densities must be produced at each edge for spark generation, power requirements are significantly higher for this type of electrode. Greater power potentiates greater risk by producing faster and deeper thermal penetration; thus, the use of high-power vaporization electrodes should be avoided at the cornua and the isthmus.

Bipolar Technology

Departing entirely from monopolar electrosurgery, a new family of instrumentation has been introduced that uses bona fide bipolar technology to attain the desired electrosurgical effect. The primary advantage of bipolar electrosurgery stems from the isolation of the electrical circuit between a set of closely separated active electrodes.

The Versapoint system consists of a dedicated electrosurgical generator and a variety of flexible electrodes that are accommodated by the 5F working channel of an operating hysteroscope. The patient contact end of the electrode consists of two poles separated by a ceramic insulator, referred to as the *return tip* and the *active tip*. The active tip electrode is fabricated in a range of configurations to produce different tissue effects. The footswitch has two activation pedals: a yellow pedal to activate the vaporizing or blend output modality and a blue pedal to activate the desiccate output. Hence, both vaporization and desiccation are possible with this system. Normal saline must be used as the distention medium within the uterine cavity.

Although in a bipolar system the relative potentials on each pole will alternate, the return electrode is not intended for tissue contact. To function, however, both electrodes have to be simultaneously immersed in isotonic saline. When the output voltage is applied between the active tip and the return electrode, a migration of Na^+ and Cl^- ions occurs to complete the electrical circuit. Because saline constitutes part of the electrical circuit, the electrodes may be placed further apart than with conventional bipolar instruments. In fact, this separation is a key parameter in deriving tissue effect because the electromagnetic field pattern created dictates the depth of thermal action.

MEASURES TO REDUCE THERMAL INJURY

Minimizing Risk and Managing Injuries to Bowel

Inadvertent thermal injury to the bowel is best averted by choosing mechanical dissection for enterolysis, minimizing the use of electrosurgery in its vicinity, using a rectal probe during cul-de-sac dissection, and the creation of relaxing incisions to mobilize it out of harm's way. Rectal defects too small to visualize may be detected by performing proctoscopy under laparoscopic view to look for air bubbles or by retrograde filling with methylene blue, with use of a large balloon catheter to seal the rectum.

The treatment of thermal injury to the bowel depends on when it is discovered, as well as on the depth of thermal penetration. Despite the more ominous appearance of blackened tissue from electrosurgical carbonization, bland-appearing thermal injuries tend to be substantially deeper and are associated with more widespread thermal necrosis. Because many partial-thickness injuries will commonly result in full-thickness necrosis after several days, such injuries should be appropriately repaired at the time of surgery. Whenever possible, intraoperative consultation with a general or colorectal surgeon is recommended. Depending on the skill and experience of the surgeon, these injuries can be repaired using either laparoscopy or laparotomy to place interrupted stitches through the seromucosal layers of the bowel using delayed absorbable suture, typically 3-0 Vicryl or Dexon. The sutures should be placed transverse to the lumen of the bowel, to avoid the possibility of luminal narrowing. Management of partial-thickness injury is the same for small bowel and for large bowel. Any area of thermal insult of short duration and superficial penetration can simply be reinforced using interrupted 3-0 delayed absorbable or silk sutures placed in an imbricating fashion.

If the full-thickness small bowel injury is discovered, immediate repair should follow. The injury can be repaired by laparoscopy or laparotomy, or a combination of both. One of the port incisions can be expanded to 2 to 3 cm, allowing the injured bowel to be exteriorized for repair and then pushed back into the abdomen after suturing is completed. Full-thickness small bowel injury is repaired by suturing in two layers using a delayed absorbable suture. The first layer typically is repaired using full-thickness interrupted sutures of 3-0 chromic suture material, whereas the second layer is closed in an imbricating seromuscular fashion using interrupted sutures of 3-0 Vicryl. As with partial-thickness repair, the suture line is placed transversely.

Generally speaking, full-thickness injury to the large bowel can be treated in the same manner, so long as the injury does not encompass more than one third of the intestinal circumference. Management is not necessarily affected by the presence or absence of bowel preparation. Regardless, copious irrigation of the field is recommended. If the extent of injury approximates 50% or more of the large bowel circumference, it is prudent to repair by segmental resection and reanastomosis or segmental resection and colostomy.

If thermal injury to the bowel is not recognized at the time of surgery, symptoms usually become apparent at least 2 to 3 days postoperatively. Symptoms commonly are less apparent after laparotomy than after the laparoscopic approach. Accordingly, it behooves the laparoscopic surgeon to be exceptionally vigilant to recognize any signs or symptoms indicative of underlying bowel injury and to act expeditiously whenever the postoperative course is not marked by continuous improvement.

Important signs and symptoms of underlying bowel injury include the following:

- Increasing abdominal pain
- Increasing abdominal distention
- Vomiting (with or without nausea)
- Abdominal tenderness (with or without rebound)
- Leukocytosis *or* leukopenia with a left shift and increased bands
- Elevated serum creatinine
- Persistent and otherwise unexplained fever (temperature greater than 101°F)
- X-ray findings suggesting ileus or air under the diaphragm (after 36 hours)
- Unexplained tachycardia (heart rate greater than 120 beats per minute)

Unfortunately, these features are not always present. The signs of small bowel injury often are subtler, and abdominal pain and distention may be minimal. The white blood count may be normal during the early postoperative period. Leukopenia with a left shift in the white blood cell count and tachycardia are ominous signs indicating impending septic shock, however. Septic shock after unrecognized bowel injury carries a mortality rate as high as 30%.

Quite consistently, after laparoscopic surgery patients remain afebrile and do not suffer from progressive abdominal pain, ileus, or abdominal distention. If any of these symptoms are encountered, assessment for the presence of unrecognized bowel injury must be of the highest priority. Carbon dioxide usually is absorbed from the abdominal cavity by 24 to 36 hours after laparoscopy. If radiographic evidence of air under the diaphragm persists beyond 36 hours, a follow-up computed tomography (CT) scan or repeat study should be ordered depending on the severity and progression of signs and symptoms. If the patient's condition continues to deteriorate, no other justification is needed to return to surgery.

Minimizing Risk and Managing Injuries to Bladder

Inadvertent thermal injury to the bladder is more apt to occur after previous surgical disruption of the vesicouterine fold and when excisional procedures are performed in adjacent peritoneal and retroperitoneal tissue. The bladder must be clearly identified before an energy modality is used to ablate or excise contiguous tissue and prior to dissection off the lower uterine segment. Mobilization of especially dense adhesions is facilitated by starting the dissection atop identified pubocervical

fascia just medial to the uterine vessels and by retrograde bladder inflation with dilute methylene blue. Focal ablative or excisional procedures of the bladder peritoneum may be assisted by first lifting the target tissue from the underlying bladder muscle using hydrodissection.

Surgical repair of thermal bladder injury depends on the perceived depth of penetration and the proximity of the injury to the trigone and ureteral orifices. Important telltale signs of full-thickness bladder injury during laparoscopy include sudden hematuria and inflation of the urinary drainage bag with carbon dioxide. The emergence of blood in the urinary drainage bag mandates methodical evaluation for lower urinary tract injury. Superficial injuries outside the trigone that are confined to the peritoneum and outer muscular layer of the bladder usually will heal without subsequent disability. On the other hand, deeper and also full-thickness injuries should be repaired intraoperatively. Injury near or in the trigone is best managed using the intraoperative judgment of a consulting urologist to determine the risk for ureteral compromise. Any repair near a ureteral orifice usually requires intraoperative ureteral stenting to detect obstruction by sutures and to maintain patency during the inevitable postoperative edema. Depending on the skill and experience of the surgeon, repair of the bladder can be accomplished using laparoscopy or laparotomy. With full-thickness or through-and-through incisional-type burns, all visually apparent as well as potentially devitalized tissue must be completely excised to unaffected and well-vascularized margins. If such devascularized tissue is left unexcised, the risk of breakdown of the repair, as well as of fistula formation, increases.

Once damaged tissue is excised to healthy margins, full-thickness bladder injury can be successfully repaired using a standard two-layer repair with delayed absorbable suture. Closure of the first layer, including both the muscular and the mucosal portions of the bladder, typically is accomplished with continuous or interrupted nonlocking stitches of 3-0 delayed absorbable suture. A second layer, including the muscular and the serosal portions of the bladder, is then closed continuously using 2-0 or 3-0 delayed absorbable suture.

The integrity of any full-thickness repair should be visually tested by distending the bladder with either blue dye (i.e., methylene blue) or sterile infant milk. If ureteral stenting was not used during the repair, ureteral patency can be ascertained by cystoscopy performed at least 5 minutes after intravenous administration of indigo carmine. Postoperative healing is best ensured by continuous decompression with a urinary catheter for 7 to 10 days. The catheter is subsequently removed only after the integrity of the entire bladder wall is confirmed by an interval cystogram.

Minimizing Risk and Managing Injuries to Ureter

The relative avascularity and anatomic course of the pelvic ureter predispose it to accidental thermal injury by virtue of its superficial locale, close relationship to key vascular structures such as the uterine and ovarian vessels, and frequent involvement with fibrosis and scarring from endometriosis along the lateral pelvic sidewall and the uterosacral ligament. The ureter must be protected during thermal ligation of vascular pedicles by visualization, traction, and, when needed, creating a linear relaxing incision. In cases in which its path is tracted by peritoneal or retroperitoneal endometriosis, the ureter should be surgically mobilized in a cephalocaudal direction before thermal modalities are applied to either ablate or excise tissue involved in periureteral disease. Whenever a bipolar electrosurgical instrument is used for hemostasis along the lateral pelvic sidewall, the ureter is best protected by using its tips in an opened position to lightly tamponade while energy is applied in a pulsatile fashion during intermittent lavage with a suction-irrigator.

Early recognition followed by definitive repair of ureteral injury yields the best long-term results. Hence, whenever thermal injury to the ureter is identified or seriously suspected, intravenous indigo carmine should be used to determine ureteral integrity and patency on both laparoscopic and cystoscopic views. If on cystoscopic examination dye is not seen to exit from one or both of the ureteral orifices, intraoperative consultation with a urologist is warranted to further elucidate the nature of the injury, by means of retrograde stenting and imaging. Ureteral stenting alone without resection and reanastomosis may constitute adequate management, provided that the ureteral wall has not been abrogated and the thermal injury is focal and superficial in nature.

Postoperatively, signs and symptoms of ureteral injury may include an elevation in serum creatinine, flank pain, fever, chills, hematuria, increasing abdominal pain, or prolonged ileus. If ureteral injury is suspected, an intravenous pyelography (IVP) or CT urogram should be performed. Extravasation of contrast from the ureter or nonfilling of a distal segment constitutes an indication for immediate evaluation by a urologist or surgeon skilled at ureteral repair. Renal injury may occur within 24 hours of obstruction and can progress to failure within 1 to 6 weeks. Unfortunately, management of ureteral injury is often complicated by delay in diagnosis. Corrective options with late diagnosis include drainage if urinoma is present, interval antegrade or retrograde stent placement, nephrostomy, and ultimate surgical repair.

The type of surgical repair will depend on the exact location and extent of the thermal injury. If the injury is in close proximity to the bladder (less than 5 cm from the ureterovesical junction), a ureteroneocystostomy with or without a psoas hitch may be performed. For an injury along the pelvic sidewall or at the pelvic brim (greater than 5 cm from the ureterovesical junction), a ureteral end-to-end anastomosis may be performed provided that the injury is not extensive and adequate mobilization of the ureter is possible. With exquisite suturing skills, this can be performed laparoscopically. The site of injury must first be precisely identified. Under cystoscopic view, a ureteral stent is passed in retrograde fashion to the point of obstruction. The use of a stent also will help outline the course of the ureter and facilitate its dissection. Once the ureter is appropriately mobilized, any damaged tissue is excised. The ureter is transected and then spatulated at an angle, to increase the circumference for the site of reanastomosis. The two opposing ends are then carefully reapproximated with a 4-0 or 5-0 delayed absorbable suture.

To facilitate healing, adequate mobilization of the ureter along its course (both proximal and distal to the site of injury and repair) is necessary so as not to place the repair site on undue tension. Furthermore, a Jackson-Pratt drain should be placed close to the site of anastomosis (but not touching it) to assist with any possible drainage. A double-J ureteral stent typically is left in place for a period of 4 to 6 weeks. Follow-up IVP studies or CT urogram should be performed before removal of the Jackson-Pratt drain and the double-J stent, to ensure ureteral patency and healing.

Measures to Reduce Thermal Injury

Most thermal injury is the result of direct contact between the active electrode and an adjacent tissue (bowel, bladder, and ureter) after either electrosurgical or mechanical perforation of the uterus. As such, it may be viewed as a thermal complication secondary to a mechanical complication. This injury typically occurs during an endometrial ablation or resection of an intracavitary fibroid when the surgeon erroneously extends the active electrode away from the hysteroscope rather than retracting the instrument back toward the surgeon.

Thermal injury has been reported to occur in the lower genital tract in women undergoing resectoscopic surgery. Mechanisms by which such injuries occur remain undefined, but as Munro[4] and others suggest could include the diversion of current secondary to direct and/or capacitive coupling to the resectoscope outer sheath. At hysteroscopy, capacitive coupling can theoretically be promulgated by one or a number of variables including surgical technique, uterine distention medium, damaged electrodes, waveform, and specific output characteristics of the electrosurgical generator. Reports of lower genital tract burns associated with monopolar resectoscopic surgery are relatively rare. This finding may relate to the fact that the contact between the cervix and the external sheath of the resectoscope is quite broad, effectively diffusing current in a fashion similar to that of the dispersive electrode. However, if contact between cervix and sheath is significantly reduced or lost, current induced on the sheath could divert and/or concentrate at other sites in the genital tract, resulting in thermal injury. Given the typical operative positions of the resectoscope, this is most likely to occur at the cervix, posterior vagina, and anterior perineum, which in fact are common locations described in the literature. Munro experimentally established that the risk of potentially clinically significant capacitive induction of current on the external sheath is lowest if low-voltage or cutting current is used regardless of electrode insulation status. The picture for high-voltage output is less clear, but under these conditions risk seems to be low provided that electrode insulation remains intact. However, if a break in insulation occurs, the risk may in fact escalate.

References

1. Odell RC. Pearls, pitfalls, and advancement in the delivery of electrosurgical energy during laparoscopy. Prob Gen Surg 2002;19:5.
2. Brill AI. Energy systems for operative laparoscopy. J Am Assoc Gynecol Laparosc 1998;5:333.
3. Harrell AG, Kercher KW, Heniford BT. Energy sources in laparoscopy. Semin Laparosc Surg 2004;11:201.
4. Munro MG. Factors affecting capacitive current diversion with a uterine resectoscope: An in vitro study. J Am Assoc Gynecol Laparosc 2003;10:450.

Additional Reading

Angioli R, Penalver MA. Urinary tract injuries. In: Hurt WG, ed. Urogynecologic surgery, 2nd ed. Philadelphia: Lippincott Williams & Wilkins, 2000.

Brill AI: Energy-based techniques to ensure hemostasis during laparoscopy. Obstet Gynecol Manag 2003;15:27.

Feste JR. Physics and clinical application of laser surgery. In: Liu CY, ed. Laparoscopic hysterectomy and pelvic floor reconstruction. New York: Blackwell Science, 1996.

Harkki-Siren P, Sjoberg J, Kurki T. Major complications of laparoscopy: A follow-up Finnish study. Obstet Gynecol 1999;94:94.

Landman J, Kerbl K, Rehman J, et al. Evaluation of a vessel sealing system, bipolar electrosurgery, harmonic scalpel, titanium clips, endoscopic gastrointestinal anastomosis vascular staples and sutures for arterial and venous ligation in a porcine model. J Urol 2003;169:697.

Liu CY. Complications of laparoscopic hysterectomy: Prevention, recognition, and management. In: Liu CY, ed. Laparoscopic hysterectomy and pelvic floor reconstruction. New York: Blackwell Science, 1996.

Munro MG. Capacitive coupling: A comparison of measurements in four resectoscopes. J Am Assoc Gynecol Laparosc 2004;11:379.

Nezhat CR, Nezhat FR, Luciano AA, et al. Operative gynecologic laparoscopy: Principles and practice. New York: McGraw-Hill, 1995.

Odell RC. Physics and clinical application of electrosugery. In: Liu CY, ed. Laparoscopic hysterectomy and pelvic floor reconstruction. New York: Blackwell Science, 1996.

Soderstrom RM. Electrosurgical injuries during laparoscopy: Prevention and management. Curr Opin Obstet Gynecol 1994;6:248.

Vancaillie TG. Electrosurgery at laparoscopy: Guidelines to avoid complications. Gynaecol Endosc 1994;3:1143.

Vilos GA, Brown S, Graham G, et al. Genital tract burns during hysteroscopic endometrial ablation: Report of 13 cases in the United States and Canada. J Am Assoc Gynecol Laparosc 2000;7:141.

Vilos GA, McCulloch S, Borg P, et al. Intended and stray radiofrequency electrical currents during resectoscopic surgery. J Am Assoc Gynecol Laparosc 2000;7:55.

Wu MP, Ou CS, Chen SL, et al. Complications and recommended practices for electrosurgery in laparoscopy. Am J Surg 2000;179:67.

Perioperative and Postoperative Infection

Sandra Abadie Kemmerly

10

BACKGROUND

Overall, it is estimated that surgical site infections (SSIs) occur in 2% to 5% of clean extra-abdominal surgical procedures and in up to 20% of intra-abdominal procedures. The Centers for Disease Control and Prevention (CDC) estimates that approximately 500,000 SSIs occur annually in the United States.[1] It has been demonstrated that surgical infections prolong hospital stays, increase the costs of care, and constitute a significant cause of morbidity and mortality.[2-8]

Catheter-associated urinary tract infections are the most frequent and account for approximately 35% of nosocomial or hospital-acquired infections. They also are associated with the lowest mortality rate and the lowest costs of all infectious complications. The risk of acquiring a urinary tract infection depends on the method and duration of catheterization. The incidence of infection ranges from 1% to 5% after a single brief catheterization to virtually 100% in patients with catheters draining into an open system for longer than 4 days.[9]

SSIs are ranked second among nosocomially acquired infections.[10-12] SSI rates following laparoscopic surgery are not well known because of the lack of well-defined and reported surveillance systems. National Nosocomial Infection Surveillance (NNIS) reports rates for vaginal (1.22) and abdominal hysterectomies (1.37 to 5.34) but does not report laparoscopic gynecologic procedure rates. NNIS does track laparoscopic infection rates for four other operative procedures: cholecystectomy, colon, appendectomy, and gastric procedures, with infection rates ranging from 0.44 to 2.55. The highest laparoscopic infection rate is associated with laparoscopic colon procedures. Overall, the laparoscopic infection rates were lower than those for conventional procedures; however, some differences in patient risk factors, American Society of Anesthesiologists (ASA) scores, and other factors may have influenced the selection of operative procedure.[12,13] For gynecologic procedures, an early study indicated a complication rate of 3 to 4 per 1000 operations, and 320 cases of infection were reported out of 117,705 laparoscopies.[14]

A large-scale, observational study of 10,110 hysterectomies in Finland demonstrated that infections were the most common complication of the types of hysterectomies performed—abdominal, vaginal, and laparoscopic. The laparoscopic infection rate was 9%, compared with 10.5% for abdominal and 13.0% for vaginal procedures. The rate of postoperative wound and urinary tract infections was statistically lower for the laparoscopic hysterectomies than for the abdominal hysterectomies, but the laparoscopy-associated rate of intra-abdominal and vaginal infections was statistically higher than for the abdominal procedures. The overall infection rates were not statistically different for the three procedures.[15]

The CDC classifies wound infection risks in the categories shown in Table 10–1.[5]

In a review of early complications in 34 publications, Harris and Daniell[16] identified 2412 patients who underwent hysterectomy by one of three different surgical approaches. Infection rates were 8.4% for the traditional approach, 3.3% for the vaginal approach, and 1.27% for the laparoscopic approach.

PREVENTION

To keep postoperative infections in laparoscopic surgery to a minimum, the CDC guidelines for prevention of surgical site infections are recommended. This approach involves attention to the principles of asepsis and excellent surgical technique. It is assumed that standard surgical technique and operating room procedures are followed regarding skin preparation, surgical scrub, barrier devices, masks, caps, gowns, drapes, and shoe covers.[5] Urinary cathethers should be used only when necessary and removed as soon as possible. Simple measures such as hand hygiene can be effective in reducing cross-contamination of infections by the hands of health care workers. The use of waterless antiseptic hand rubs has been shown to be more effective than standard hand washing alone and has improved adherence to hand hygiene programs in non–operating room settings.[17,18]

Preoperative Antibiotics

No data are available to support the use of antibiotic prophylaxis in clean abdominal surgery that does not involve the vagina or intestines. Additionally, antibiotic prophylaxis is not

Table 10–1 ▪ Classification of Wound Infection Risk

Class I: Clean	Class II: Clean-Contaminated	Class III: Contaminated	Class IV: Dirty-Infected
Uninfected operative wound with no inflammation Respiratory, alimentary, genital, or uninfected urinary tract not entered Clean wounds primarily closed and, if necessary, drained with closed drainage	Respiratory, alimentary, genital, or urinary tract entered under controlled conditions and without unusual contamination Includes operations involving biliary tract, appendix, vagina, and oropharynx without evidence of infection or major break in technique	Open, fresh, accidental wounds Major breaks in sterile technique or gross spillage from gastrointestinal tract Includes incisions that reveal acute, nonpurulent inflammation	Old traumatic wounds with retained devitalized tissue and those involving existing clinical infection or perforated viscera Suggests that organisms causing postoperative infection were present in operative field before surgery

recommended in patients undergoing diagnostic laparoscopy or hysteroscopy. Antibiotic prophylaxis is, however, recommended in patients undergoing hysterectomy by all techniques.[19-21] Surgical site infections that develop after a hysterectomy result from the ascending spread of the microorganisms that inhabit the upper vagina, endocervix, vaginal cuff, and paravaginal tissues dissected during the procedure.[22]

Despite impeccable aseptic technique, bacterial contamination of the operative site may be inevitable. Systemic antibiotic prophylaxis is distributed within the host tissue and is believed to augment the natural immune defense mechanisms and help kill the bacteria that are inoculated into the surgical wound.

The antibiotics chosen for gynecologic surgery should have activity against the pathogens most often recovered from infection occurring after the specific procedure and against the endogenous flora of the anatomic operative region. These gynecologic pathogens include gram-negative bacilli, anaerobic bacteria, streptococci, and enterococci. The selected agent for surgical prophylaxis should be of low toxicity, be relatively easy to administer, and penetrate tissue in concentrations that are effective against microorganisms. The duration of therapy should be short (usually one dose is sufficient), and most experts recommend that the antibiotics be discontinued within 24 hours of surgery. The timing of antimicrobial prophylaxis should allow the drug to achieve serum and tissue drug levels that exceed, for the duration of the operation, the mean inhibitory concentrations of the organisms. For antibiotics to be available in the tissues at the time of bacterial inoculation, they must be administered before the incision is made. In general, administration 30 to 60 minutes before the surgical procedure is considered adequate to ensure tissue levels of the antibiotic administered. The risk of infection increases when prophylaxis is given too early (more than 2 hours before incision) or too late (after the incision is made). Incorrect timing of the surgical prophylaxis is associated with increases by a factor of 2 to 6 in the rates of SSI for operative procedures in which prophylaxis generally is recommended.[23] If the surgical procedure is prolonged (e.g., duration greater than 4 hours) or excessive blood loss occurs, a subsequent dose of the prophylactic antibiotic is recommended so that adequate levels are maintained throughout the operation. Delaying the administration by even a few hours negates the benefit of prophylactic antibiotics.[24-27]

Surgical Infection Prevention Project Guidelines

The Centers for Medicare and Medicaid Services (CMS), along with the CDC, implemented a National Surgical Infection Prevention project (SIP) to decrease postoperative infection–associated morbidity and mortality rates in the Medicare patient population. The SIP Guidelines Writers Workgroup included an American College of Obstetricians and Gynecologists (ACOG) representative. The SIP group revalidated the following principles:

- Give antibiotics within 1 hour before the surgical incision is made.
- Give prophylactic antibiotics consistent with current recommendations.
- Discontinue prophylactic antibiotics within 24 hours after surgery.
- Because of the longer infusion time required for vancomycin, it is acceptable to start this antibiotic (when indicated for beta-lactam allergy) within 2 hours before incision.[37]

More than 25 prospective, randomized studies and 2 meta-analyses support the use of perioperative antibiotics for patients undergoing abdominal hysterectomy.[21,28] No specific antibiotic appears to be superior to all others. For abdominal or vaginal hysterectomy, cefotetan is preferred, but reasonable alternatives include cefazolin and cefoxitin.[24,26] In one study in women undergoing abdominal hysterectomy, cefotetan was superior to cefazolin, and the latter was associated with a greater number of and more serious infections. These findings may reflect the activity of cefotetan against a wider spectrum of gram-negative and anaerobic bacteria and its longer serum half-life. An agent with a longer half-life has the theoretical advantage over shorter-acting agents because of the potentially decreased need for redosing in prolonged procedures.[29]

Adverse Reactions to Antibiotics

Adverse effects of antibiotics can range from minor skin rashes to severe anaphylaxis. Additionally, the risk of *Clostridium difficile* colitis is increasing in the United States, although it is still only a rare complication from preoperative antibiotic administration.[30] Prolonged antibiotic use has been associated with superinfection with *C. difficile* and may have an impact on the development of resistant strains of bacteria.[31]

Perhaps the single greatest challenge in selecting the antibiotic is a patient history of an adverse reaction to penicillin that may or may not be substantiated. A beta-lactam antibiotic often is the drug of choice for antimicrobial prophylaxis, and the medical history should ascertain whether the patient probably experienced a true allergy such as anaphylaxis, angioedema, bronchospasm or asthma, or urticaria and whether the reaction was a significant adverse event. Allergic reactions occur in 0.7% to 4% of penicillin treatment courses.[32] All four types of immunopathologic reactions may be seen with beta-lactam antibiotics[33]:

- Type 1: IgE-mediated reactions (immediate hypersensitivity reaction)
- Type 2: antibody-mediated reactions
- Type 3: immune complex–mediated reactions
- Type 4: T lymphocyte–mediated reactions

IgE-mediated penicillin reactions can be identified by penicillin skin testing, usually performed by an allergist or immunologist. Such testing can help determine if a patient with a penicillin allergy can safely be given penicillin or a penicillin derivative.[33]

Although the incidence of clinically relevant cross-reactivity between the penicillins and cephalosporins is low, anaphylactic reactions, including death, have occurred.[34] The overall incidence of severe cephalosporin reactions in patients with documented IgE-mediated penicillin hypersensitivity is most recently estimated to be between 2% and 4.5%.[35-37] Before 1980, the cross-reactivity rate between cephalosporins and penicillins was estimated to be approximately 10% to 20%. This decrease is thought to be due to improved purity of cephalosporin preparations. Cephalosporin antibiotics may be used in those patients with a history of penicillin allergy not manifested by an immediate hypersensitivity reaction; however, patients with a history of immediate hypersensitivity reaction to penicillin should not receive cephalosporins, in view of the availability of alternative agents.[38,39] Alternative agents include metronidazole, doxycycline, clindamycin, and the quinolones.[19]

The SIP Workgroup has suggested additional combination therapies in beta-lactam–allergic patients: clindamycin plus gentamicin; clindamycin plus aztreonam; clindamycin plus ciprofloxacin; metronidazole plus gentamicin; metronidazole plus ciprofloxacin; clindamycin monotherapy; and levofloxacin 750 mg substituted for ciprofloxacin.

Vancomycin may be used in patients who are truly beta-lactam antibiotic allergic, but this agent lacks activity against gram-negative bacilli, which are present in areas where gynecologic surgery is performed. Consequently, an additional agent with gram-negative activity, such as aztreonam or gentamicin, should be added to the vancomycin regimen. Li and associates recently reported a decrease in prophylactic use of vancomycin after a negative penicillin skin test result for elective surgery in orthopedic patients with a history of penicillin allergy.[40] Whether avoiding prophylactic vancomycin is practical for gynecologic surgery remains uncertain, but this precaution may be wise in the patient who reports multiple drug allergies.

Table 10–2 illustrates commonly used gynecologic prophylactic antibiotics, the standard dosing, and rates of both intravenous injection and infusions. A reasonable time for administration of these agents is during the induction of anesthesia; however, some centers use a preoperative holding area for administration of antibiotics.

RECOGNITION AND MANAGEMENT

Recognition, diagnosis, and management of surgically associated infections vary in complexity. Diagnosis of such infection in a patient who has fever, dysuria, and other signs or symptoms of a urinary tract infection may be straightforward, whereas a deep organ space infection that is well contained may be harder to recognize.

Superficial wound infections are characterized by a localized area of erythema, induration, and possible drainage around the wound site. Treatment requires removal of the suture or staples, with local drainage of the infection. In most circumstances, antibiotics are not required unless cellulitis surrounds the wound.

Deep wound infections generally demonstrate extensive induration and erythema, with or without purulent discharge. The patient usually is febrile, has an elevated white blood cell count, and may be toxic. Blood culture results are rarely positive, but attempts to culture material from the wound are recommended to guide specific antibiotic therapy.

Organ space infections are those in which the fascia and the muscle may be involved. They appear to be similar to deep

Table 10–2 ▪ Commonly Used Gynecologic Prophylactic Antibiotics

Antibacterial	Standard Dose	Rate of Intravenous Injection	Rate of Intravenous Infusion
Aztreonam	1-2 g	3-5 min	20-60 min
Cefazolin	1-2 g	3-5 min	20-60 min
Cefotetan	1-2 g	3-5 min	20-60 min
Cefoxitin	1-2 g	3-5 min	20-60 min
Ciprofloxacin	400 mg	Not recommended	60 min
Clindamycin	900 mg	Not recommended	30 min (not to exceed 30 mg/min)
Gentamicin	1.5 mg/kg	Not recommended	30-120 min
Metronidazole	500 mg	Not recommended	60 min
Vancomycin	1 g	Not recommended	60-90 min (not to exceed 10 mg/min)

Adapted from Trissel LA. Handbook of injectable drugs, 12th ed. Bethesda, Md: American Society of Health Systems Pharmacists, 2003.

wound infections, with the deeper infection progression to fascial separation. Cultures and operating room débridement are advisable. Rare cases of catastrophic infections, such as necrotizing fasciitis, have been reported.[41]

Management of postoperative infection involves prompt recognition and diagnosis, incision and drainage when appropriate, and antimicrobial therapy if warranted for significant infections. Organism-specific therapy is ideal; however, broad-spectrum therapy may be used if an organism is not recovered.

Development of a standardized approach to postprocedure surveillance for SSIs is recommended, because it is estimated that 10% to 85% of infections manifest after discharge from the hospital.[5,42] Shorter hospitalizations, use of outpatient surgical centers, and office procedures continue to increase in today's health care systems. Voluntary reporting of postoperative wound infections by surgeons has, in general, not been predictably successful. Health care organizations are tasked with having to develop solutions that identify cases by trained personnel and consideration of automated detection systems.[43] At this time, no consensus exists on which postdischarge surveillance methods would be applicable to all surgical procedures in general or for laparoscopic gynecologic procedures.

References

1. Wong ES. Surgical site infection. In: Mayhall DG, ed. Hospital epidemiology and infection control, 2nd ed. Philadelphia: Lippincott Williams & Wilkins, 1999;189.
2. Fraser VJ. Starting to learn about the costs of nosocomial infections in the new millennium: Where do we go from here? [Editorial]. Infect Control Hosp Epidemiol 2002;23:174.
3. Hollenbeak CS, Murphy D, Dungan WC, et al. Nonrandom selection and the attributable cost of surgical-site infections. Infect Control Hosp Epidemiol 2002;23:177.
4. Kirkland KB, Briggs JP, Trivette SL, et al. The impact of surgical-site infections in the 1990s: Attributable mortality, excess length of hospitalization, and extra costs. Infect Control Hosp Epidemiol 1999;20:725.
5. Mangram AJ, Horan TC, Pearson ML, et al. Guideline for prevention of surgical site infection, 1999. Infect Control Hosp Epidemiol 1999;20:250.
6. Orsi GB, Di Stefano L, Noah N. Hospital-acquired, laboratory-confirmed bloodstream infection: increased hospital stay and direct costs. Infect Control Hosp Epidemiol 2002;23:190.
7. Surgical Infection Protection Project. Available at http://www.medquic.org/sip.
8. Whitehouse JD, Friedman ND, Kirkland KB, et al. The impact of surgical-site infections following orthopedic surgery at a community hospital and a university hospital: Adverse quality of life, excess length of stay, and extra cost. Infect Control Hosp Epidemiol 2002;23:183.
9. Wong ES (in consultation with Hooten TM). Guideline for prevention of catheter-associated urinary tract infections. Available at http://www.cdc.gov/ncidod/hip/GUIDE/uritract.htm.
10. Burke JP. Infection control—a problem for patient safety. N Engl J Med 2003;348:651.
11. Leape LL, Brennan TA, Laird N, et al. The nature of adverse events in hospitalized patients: Results of the Harvard Medical Practice Study II. N Engl J Med 1991;324:377.
12. National Nosocomial Infections Surveillance (NNIS) Report, data summary from October 1986–April 1996, issued May 1996: A report from the National Nosocomial Infections Surveillance (NNIS) System. Am J Infect Control 1996;24:380.
13. National Nosocomial Infections Surveillance (NNIS) System Report, data summary from January 1992 through June 2003, issued August 2003. Am J Infect Control 2003;31:481.
14. Phillips J, Hulka B, Hulka J, et al. Laparoscopic procedures: The American Association of Gynecologic Laparoscopists' Membership Survey for 1975. J Reprod Med 1977;18:227.
15. Mäkinen J, Johansson J, Tomás C, et al. Morbidity of 10,110 hysterectomies by type of approach. Hum Reprod 2001;16:1473.
16. Harris WJ, Daniell JF. Early complications of laparoscopic hysterectomy. Obstet Gynecol Surv 1996;51:559.
17. Boyce JM, Pittet D. Guideline for hand hygiene in health-care settings: Recommendations of the Healthcare Infection Control Practices Advisory Committee and the HICPAC/SHEA/APIC/IDSA Hand Hygiene Task Force. MMWR Morb Mortal Wkly Rep 2002;51(RR-16):1. (Also available at http://www.cdc.gov/ncidod/hip/default.html.)
18. Pittet D, Hugonnet S, Harbarth S, et al. Effectiveness of a hospital-wide programme to improve compliance with hand hygiene. Lancet 2000;356:1307.
19. ACOG Practice Bulletin. Antibiotic prophylaxis for gynecologic procedures. Clinical Management Guidelines for Obstetrician-Gynecologists 2001: Jan, No. 23.
20. Kamat AA, Brancazio L, Gibson M. Wound infection in gynecologic surgery. Infect Dis Obstet Gynecol 2000;8:230.
21. Tanos V, Rojansky N. Prophylactic antibiotics in abdominal hysterectomy. J Am Coll Surg 1994;179:593.
22. Hemsell DL. Gynecologic postoperative infections. In: Pastorek JG II, ed. Obstetric and gynecologic infectious disease. New York: Raven Press, 1994;141.
23. Classen DC, Evans RS, Pestotnik SL, et al. The timing of prophylactic administration of antibiotics and the risk of surgical-wound infection. N Engl J Med 1992;326:281.
24. Antimicrobial prophylaxis in surgery. Med Lett Drugs Ther 2001;43:92.
25. Bratzler DW, Houck P, for the Surgical Infection Prevention Guidelines Writers Workgroup. Antimicrobial prophylaxis for surgery: An advisory statement from the National Surgical Infection Prevention Project. Clin Infect Dis 2004; June 15:38.
26. Dellinger EP, Gross PA, Barrett TL, et al. Quality standard for antimicrobial prophylaxis in surgical procedures. Clin Infect Dis 1994;18:422.
27. Page CP, Bohnen JMA, Fletcher JR, et al. Antimicrobial prophylaxis for surgical wounds: Guidelines for clinical care. Arch Surg 1993;128:79.
28. Hemsell DL. Prophylactic antibodies in gynecologic and obstetric surgery. Rev Infect Dis 1991;13:S821.
29. Hemsell DL, Johnson ER, Hemsell PG, et al. Cefazolin is inferior to cefotetan as single-dose prophylaxis for women undergoing elective total abdominal hysterectomy. Clin Infect Dis 1995;20:677.
30. Thomas C, Stevenson M, Riley TV. Antibiotics and hospital-acquired *Clostridium difficile*–associated diarrhoea: A systematic review. J Antimicrob Chemother 2003;51:1339.
31. Scher KS. Studies on the duration of antibiotic administration for surgical prophylaxis. Am Surg 1997;63:59.
32. Parker CW. Drug allergy (first of three parts). N Engl J Med 1975;292:511.
33. Arroliga ME, Pien L. Penicillin allergy: Consider trying penicillin again. Cleve Clin J Med 2003;70:313.
34. Weiss ME, Adkinson NF Jr. β-Lactam allergy. In: Mandell GL, Bennett JE, Dolin R, eds. Mandell, Douglas, and Bennett's principles and practice of infectious diseases, 5th ed. Philadelphia: Churchill Livingstone, 2000;299.
35. Bernstein IL, Gruchalla RS, Lee RE, et al. Disease management of drug hypersensitivity: A practice parameter. Ann Allergy Asthma Immunol 1999;83:665.
36. Martin JA, Igea JM, Fraj J, et al. Allergy to amoxicillin in patients who tolerated benzylpenicillin, aztreonam, and ceftazidime. Clin Infect Dis 1992;14:592.
37. Romano A, Guéant-Rodriguez R-M, Viola M, et al. Cross-reactivity and tolerability of cephalosporins in patients with immediate hypersensitivity to penicillins. Ann Intern Med 2004;141:16.
38. Anne S, Reisman RE. Risk of administering cephalosporin antibiotics to patients with histories of penicillin allergy. Ann Allergy Asthma Immunol 1995;74:167.
39. Robinson JL, Hameed T, Carr S. Practical aspects of choosing an antibiotic for patients with a reported allergy to an antibiotic. Clin Infect Dis 2002;35:26.
40. Li JT, Markus PJ, Osmon DR, et al. Reduction of vancomycin use in orthopedic patients with a history of antibiotic allergy. Mayo Clin Proc 2000;75:902.
41. Golshani S, Simons AJ, Der R, et al. Necrotizing fasciitis following laparoscopic surgery: Case report and review of the literature. Surg Endosc 1996;10:751.
42. Mayhall CG, ed. Hospital epidemiology and infection control, 2nd ed. Philadelphia: Lippincott Williams & Wilkins 1999;207.
43. Platt R. Progress in surgical-site infection surveillance. Infect Control Hosp Epidemiol 2002;23:361.

Pelvic Adhesions

Roger J. Ferland

11

Pelvic surgery often causes unavoidable tissue injury that can lead to the formation of postsurgical adhesions in 55% to 100% of surgical patients.[1-3] Such injuries include mechanical trauma from retractors and tissue handling, ischemia at suture sites and with electrocautery use, foreign bodies, tissue desiccation, and infection. These stimuli of adhesion formation occur with both open and laparoscopic approaches.

The complications resulting from adhesion formation are a common cause for readmission due to small bowel obstruction, reoperation for pelvic pain, and an estimated 15% to 20% of female infertility cases. In addition to these adverse clinical sequelae, the economic impact is significant. A review of the MedPARS database of hospital utilization for adhesion complication diagnostic-related groups (DRGs) indicates the use of 861,244 hospital days at total cost of more than 2.4 billion dollars for the year 2002 (Table 11–1).

Additionally, Ellis and colleagues[4] followed a group of patients who had undergone abdominal or pelvic surgery in the United Kingdom for 10 years in an effort to assess the likelihood of complications from adhesion formation. The readmission rate for adhesion-related complications was 5.7%, and reoperation rate was 3.8%. These investigators concluded that nearly 35% of 30,000 patients who underwent abdominal or pelvic surgery were readmitted for reoperation or complications possibly related to adhesions. Although 22% of readmissions occurred in the first year following the primary surgery, admissions continued steadily over a 10-year period of observation.

PERITONEAL HEALING AND ADHESION FORMATION

Hertzler[5] was the first to publish that minimally damaged peritoneum heals rapidly without adhesions across the entire surface at the site of injury. This mode of healing is unlike the centripetal pattern seen in skin healing. He described the process as follows: "[T]he entire surface becomes endothelialised simultaneously and not gradually from the border as in epidermitization of skin wounds . . . . That the endothe-

lium of the surrounding surface of the peritoneum [defect] has any direct part in covering these surfaces cannot be demonstrated."

Rafferty[6] concluded, on the basis of light microscopy studies, that "(1) peritoneal defects heal rapidly; (2) large defects heal as rapidly as small ones; (3) healing occurs for the most part without adhesion formation; (4) centripetal growth from the wound margin contributes little to the healing process; and (5) mesothelium is derived from the metaplasia of subperitoneal connective tissue cells . . . ."

Tissue injury by trauma from instrumentation, desiccation, energy sources, or sutures first leads to cellular and vascular disruption at the site of injury. Outpouring of blood and fibrin immediately follows. After hemostasis and the associated fibrin deposition, tissue repair cells, primarily macrophages and fibroblasts, populate the defect in response to various cytokines, including platelet-derived growth factor (PDGF), transforming growth factor-β1 (TGF-β1), TGF-β2, and fibroblast growth factor (FGF), among others.[7] At peritoneal defects without ischemia due to excessive vascular or cellular damage by cautery or sutures, the formation of a permanent fibrin structure is prevented by tissue thromboplastin activity that breaks down the initial fibrin structure.[8]

With minimal injury and preservation of tissue plasminogen activator (tPA) activity, healing progresses rapidly across the entire surface area simultaneously. New mesothelium appears to be generated by subperitoneal perivascular mesenchymal cells at the site of the defect.[6] These cells possess fibrinolytic activity to promote dissolution of the fibrin resulting from the injury.

The next phase of healing, at days 2 to 3, involves the recruitment or attraction of cells that will form the new mesothelium. It is unclear if these cells arise from the margins of the defect, are free in the peritoneal fluid, or are recruited and undergo metaplasia from perivascular stem cells in the base of the defect. Within 7 to 8 days of the injury, a new layer of mesothelium is formed, and healing is complete barring infection or other adverse conditions.

Figure 11–1 shows the peritoneum of the porcine pelvic sidewall with a wide area of electrocautery damage of the underlying muscle at the time of injury (time zero). Figure

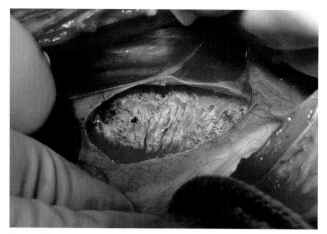

Figure 11–1 ■ At time of injury ("time zero"): Cautery injury across base of pelvic sidewall defect. (Courtesy of Confluent Surgical, Waltham, Massachusetts.)

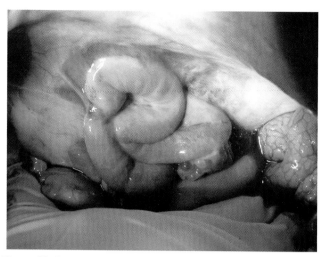

Figure 11–2 ■ At 10 days after laparoscopy: Uterine horn adherent to sidewall defect at cautery injury site. (Courtesy of Confluent Surgical, Waltham, Massachusetts.)

11–2 shows the same defect at 10 days with adherent uterine horn at the injury site. Figure 11–3, by comparison, shows the same type of defect without the cautery injury at 10 days, which has healed without adhesions.

When the tPA activity of the injured tissue is reduced or absent, the fibrin structure persists. Subsequently, under the influence of chemotactic factors and integrins, fibroblasts will populate the fibrin scaffolding. These fibroblasts are stimulated by various growth factors such as TGF-β and PDGF to elaborate collagen, transforming the initial thin, filmy adhesions due to fibrin, seen within the first days after injury, to more dense, collagen-rich adhesions. Over time, blood vessels develop to culminate in the formation of thick vascular adhesions, which have the potential to cause more severe complications. Although a complete discussion of the humoral agents that mediate peritoneal healing is beyond the scope of this chapter, a balance between mediators that stimulate and inhibit tissue healing appears likely.

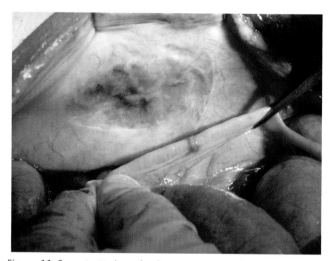

Figure 11–3 ■ At 10 days after laparoscopy: Complete healing without adhesions in absence of cautery injury. (Courtesy of Confluent Surgical, Waltham, Massachusetts.)

INCIDENCE OF ADHESIONS

The incidence of postoperative adhesions is difficult to estimate in the absence of second-look evaluations. Multiple authors, however, have identified an incidence ranging from 55% to 100% after open pelvic surgery procedures at second-look laparoscopy performed 4 to 12 weeks after the initial surgery.[1-3,9,10]

It has been widely held that laparoscopy results in fewer adhesions than those observed after laparotomy, presumably owing to the lack of desiccation, introduction of foreign

Table 11–1 ■ Inpatient Hospital Utilization for Adhesion-Related Complications for Fiscal Year 2002*						
DRG	Total Charges	Covered Charges	Medicare	Total Days	No. of Cases	Ave. Days
150	$868,585,854	$863,819,102	$335,485,256	241,789	21,370	11.3
151	$96,038,398	$95,555,607	$31,840,521	28,958	5,222	5.5
180	$1,249,983,451	$1,240,275,997	$415,354,031	497,705	91,497	5.4
181	$208,066,576	$206,682,411	$56,542,994	92,792	27,500	3.4
Total	**$2,422,674,279**	**$2,406,333,117**	**$839,222,802**	**861,244**	**145,589**	**5.9**

*Based on diagnosis-related groups (DRGs), as follows: 150, peritoneal adhesiolysis with complication or co-morbidity; 151, peritoneal adhesiolysis without complications or co-morbidity; 180, gastrointestinal obstruction with complications or co-morbidity; 181, gastrointestinal obstruction without complications or co-morbidity. See http://new.cms.hns.gov.
From MEDPAR database, Center for Medicare Services, and modified from Moscowitz I, Wexner S. Contributions of adhesions to cost of healthcare. In: diZerega G, ed. Peritoneal surgery. New York: Springer, 1999.

materials such as talc and cotton fibers, and reduction of tissue handling. The evidence to support this dogma, however, is lacking.

In 1991, the Operative Laparoscopy Study group headed by Diamond[2] reported findings at second-look laparoscopy performed after laparoscopic adhesiolysis by sharp dissection with either laser or electrocautery. In this multicenter study, 68 reproductive-age women had a significant decrease in adhesion scores at second-look laparoscopy; however, adhesion re-formation occurred at initial operative sites in 97%. The rate of re-formation at ovariolysis sites was 80%, compared with 67% at tubal sites. The rate for de novo adhesions at sites not initially operated on, however, was only 18%. This compares favorably with an incidence of 50% for postoperative de novo adhesions after laparotomy, largely attributable to de novo adhesions at the laparotomy incision site.

Furthermore, the most current reliable data confirm that the potential for reduction in adhesion re-formation with laparoscopy versus laparotomy has not been realized. These data show a similar rate of re-formation of adhesions in both laparotomy and laparoscopy treatment groups.[3,11,12]

Wiseman and associates[13] completed a meta-analysis of 22 reports with evaluable second-look data to assess adhesion formation after laparotomy and laparoscopy, with or without the use of crystalloid instillation. These investigators found no significant differences in incidence of both re-formed and de novo adhesions between the laparoscopy and the laparotomy treatment groups reviewed. A surprising finding was a lower percentage of patients free of re-formed adhesions in the laparoscopy group (Table 11–2).

Other investigators have found a reduced incidence of re-formed adhesions and an absence of de novo adhesions in their study of laparoscopic cases. Nezhat and colleagues[14] reported on 157 patients undergoing laser laparoscopy for endometriosis-related infertility. They noted significantly lower adhesion scores at second-look procedures among 22 patients who subsequently conceived, compared with the 135 who did not, and an absence of de novo adhesions in both groups.

When abdominal surgery was considered, the incidence of adhesion-related small bowel obstruction after laparoscopic abdominal surgery was similar to that seen after cholecystectomy, appendectomy, and transperitoneal herniorrhaphy by laparotomy. This is further evidence that laparoscopic surgery may not result in a lower rate of adhesion formation than that observed for open surgery.[15,16]

The preponderance of data in the literature supports the hypothesis that laparoscopy is not superior to laparotomy regarding re-formation of adhesions but may be superior in avoiding de novo adhesions.

In addition to the recognized adhesiogenic injuries of tissue handling, ischemia, presence of blood clot, and sutures, laparoscopic cases may expose the peritoneum to smoke, particulates, barotrauma, and chemical changes from the CO_2 pneumoperitoneum that could promote adhesion formation. Ott[17,18] described a rapid cooling of up to 20°C and desiccation with resultant peritoneal cell damage due to evaporation of peritoneal fluid from insufflation of dry, cool CO_2. These problems presumably may be avoided by use of warm, humidified insufflation gas, but data to support this hypothesis are lacking.

CLASSIFICATION OF ADHESIONS

Classification of adhesions is valuable not only for comparison of data from clinical investigations but also for accurate recording of findings for individual patients. Furthermore, with data permitting prognosis for future pregnancy based on the adhesion scores, patients may then be appropriately triaged to surgical therapy versus in vitro fertilization for best outcomes. For example, Nezhat and colleagues[14] reported successful pregnancy in 22 of 156 patients after laser ablation of endometriosis with lower adhesion scores at second-look laparoscopy. At present, however, reliable data on pregnancy rates by adhesion score defining a threshold for surgical therapy or in vitro fertilization are lacking.

The extent and character of adnexal adhesions are well defined by the American Society of Reproductive Medicine (ASRM) scheme documenting the area involved and the consistency of the adhesions. This scoring system is commonly used in clinical studies (Table 11–3).

In an effort to further characterize outcomes after surgery and efficacy of adhesion barriers, Diamond and co-workers[1] classified adhesions as "re-formed" at sites with adhesions at the time of the primary procedure or "de novo" when they occurred at sites that were adhesion free before surgery. This category is further classified according to "no operative" versus "operative" procedure performed at the site (Table 11–4).

Many other classification systems exist that describe the location, extent, and tenacity of adhesions. All seem to measure the common characteristics of surface area and distinguish between thin, filmy adhesions and thick, vascular adhesions. The best example of an alternative scoring system is the More Comprehensive Adhesion Scoring Method (MCASM) developed by the Adhesion Scoring Group (Table 11–5).

PREVENTION OF ADHESION FORMATION

The avoidance of complications from adhesion formation is based on prevention. Surgical technique that avoids conditions favoring adhesion formation is the cornerstone of prevention.

Minimal tissue handling, limiting trauma from retraction, and avoiding desiccation or ischemia will help prevent

Table 11–2 ▪ Frequency of Adhesions at Second-Look Evaluation		
	Percent of Patients Adhesion Free	
Adhesion Type	**After Laparotomy**	**After Laparoscopy**
De novo	45.2%	37.2%
Re-formed	26.6%	14.3%

Adapted from Wiseman DM, Trout JR, Diamond MP. The rates of adhesion development and the effects of crystalloid solutions on adhesion development in pelvic surgery. Fertil Steril 1998;70:702.

Table 11–3 ▪ ASRM Adhesion Scoring System

	Extent of Enclosure by Adhesion		
Adhesions	<1/3	1/3 to 2/3	>2/3
Ovary			
Right			
Filmy	1	2	4
Dense	4	8	16
Left			
Filmy	1	2	4
Dense	4	8	16
Tube			
Right			
Filmy	1	2	4
Dense	4*	8*	16
Left			
Filmy	1	2	4
Dense	4*	8*	16

*If the fimbriated end of the fallopian tube is completely enclosed, change the point assignment to 16.

ASRM, American Society for Reproductive Medicine.

Prognostic Classification for Adnexal Adhesions

	Left	Right
A, Minimal 0-5		
B, Mild 6-10		
C, Moderate 11-20		
D, Severe 21-32		

Prognosis for Conception and Subsequent Viable Infant†

_____ Excellent (>75%)   _____ Good (50%-75%)

_____ Fair (25%-50%)   _____ Poor (<5%)

†Physician's judgment based on adnexa with least amount of pathologic change.

From American Fertility Society. The AFS classification of adnexal adhesions, distal tubal occlusion, tubal occlusion secondary to tubal ligation, tubal pregnancies, mullerian anomalies and intrauterine adhesions. Fertil Steril 1988;49:444.

Table 11–4 ▪ Classification of Postoperative Adhesion Formation

Type	Description
1	De novo adhesion formation: development of adhesions at sites that did not have adhesion initially
	A. No operative procedure at site of adhesion formation
	B. Operative procedure performed at site of adhesion formation (other than adhesiolysis)
2	Adhesion re-formation: redevelopment of adhesions at sites at which adhesiolysis was performed.
	A. No operative procedure at site of adhesion re-formation (other than adhesiolysis)
	B. Operative procedure performed at site of adhesion re-formation (in addition to adhesiolysis)

This classification is especially useful to assess clinical efficacy of adhesion barriers by distinguishing between re-formed and de novo adhesions.

From Diamond MP, Nezhat F. Adhesions after resection of ovarian endometriomas. Letter to the editor. Fertil Steril 1993;59:934.

such conditions. The microsurgical techniques advocated by Gomel[19] incorporate these features. The use of atraumatic instruments and reduction of tissue manipulation and handling both are important. Maintaining a moist operative field with electrolyte solutions or warm, humidified CO_2 pneumoperitoneum will avoid desiccation.[20] The judicious use of energy sources with minimal lateral thermal spread also may reduce zones of ischemia and reduce adhesion incidence. Use of sutures of smaller diameter and in minimal number also will avoid tissue ischemia and maintain the tPA activity needed to prevent adhesions. Use of large numbers of sutures of larger caliber, such as in myomectomy, will inevitably lead to adhesion formation rates approaching 100%.[10]

Early second-look laparoscopy, defined by a time window of 8 to 28 days after the primary procedure, has been advocated as therapeutic because the adhesions are easily lysed in this early stage of development. Although this procedure is technically easy to perform, the evidence does not support better reproductive outcomes. Farquhar and associates' review of two randomized controlled studies concluded that the studies were underpowered.[21] Although the studies suggested better pregnancy rates with second-look laparoscopy, the findings did not constitute sufficient evidence to validate the practice of routine second-look laparoscopy. Alborzi and colleagues' study of 92 infertile patients who were randomized to receive second-look laparoscopy or observation after initial salpingo-ovariolysis showed no significant improvement in pregnancy rates between the two groups after 1 year of follow-up.[12]

Second-look laparoscopy may have an advantage in prevention of pelvic pain or bowel obstruction, although this question has not been studied. Additionally, third-look laparoscopy would be necessary to assess change in adhesion scores, which is impractical and difficult to study.

Adhesion Prevention Barriers and Adjuvants

Historically, crystalloid solutions or high-molecular-weight Dextran 70 (Hyskon, Pharmacia, Piscataway, New Jersey) instilled at the conclusion of procedures were used to prevent adhesions. This approach has largely been abandoned owing to lack of efficacy. The failure of these agents probably is related to their absorption from the peritoneal cavity well before peritoneal healing is complete.[22,23] Additionally, they may dilute or remove the necessary tissue repair cells that promote adhesion-free peritoneal healing.[23] Pharmacologic agents including corticosteroids and antihistamines also have been used in the past but failed to demonstrate clinical benefit, presumably also because of limited time of effect at the operative site.

Adjuvants that are used *before* surgery were theorized to protect tissues from desiccation and injury, thereby preventing adhesions. Sepracoat, or HAL-C (Gynezyme, Cambridge, Massachusetts), is a dilute solution of sodium hyaluronate, a high-molecular-weight polysaccharide present in synovial fluid and amniotic fluid. It has been shown to prevent de novo adhesions when applied before and during adhesiolysis, although animal studies showed no benefit in preventing re-formation of adhesions. In a randomized clinical trial by Diamond, 13.1% of patients in the treatment group were free of de novo adhesions, compared with 4.6% of control

Table 11–5 ▪ More Comprehensive Adhesion Scoring Method (MCASM)			
Severity	**Location**	**Severity**	**Extent**
0 = no adhesions present	Anterior abdominal wall (1-4)		
1 = filmy, avascular	(1) Left side to		
2 = am = vascularity and/or dense	(2) Right side to		
3a = cohesive, falls apart on touch	(3) Incision line to		
3b = cohesive, visible, dissectable planes; can be separated with minimal dissection	(4) Above incision to		
3c = cohesive, no visible dissectable planes; requires extensive dissection for separation	Anterior cul-de-sac (5-8)		
	(5) Over uterus to		
Extent	(6) Over bladder to		
0 = no adhesions present	(7) Left side to		
1 = mild (covering 25% total area/length)	(8) Right side to		
2 = moderate (covering 26% to 50% total area/length)	(9) Posterior uterus to		
3 = severe (covering >51% of total area/length)	*(10) Posterior cul-de-sac to		
*Modified MCASM locations	*(11) Pelvic sidewall-left to		
	*(12) Pelvic sidewall-right to		
	*(13) Posterior broad ligament-left to		
	*(14) Posterior broad ligament-right to		
	*(15) Round ligament to tube-left to		
	*(16) Round ligament to tube-right to		
	*(17) Ovary-left to		
	*(18) Ovary-right to		
	*(19) Tube-left to		
	(20) Tube-right to		
	(21) Small bowel to		
	(22) Large bowel to		
	*(23) Omentum to		

*Indicates 13 of 23 sites that correspond to the area of the pelvis that is likely to be involved with tubal and ovarian adhesions.
From Adhesion Scoring Group. Improvement in interobserver reproducibility of adhesion scoring system. Fertil Steril 1994;62:984.

subjects. Although this difference was statistically significant, the clinical benefit appears marginal.[24]

Cross-linking sodium hyaluronate with ferric ions increases the duration of persistence within the peritoneum postoperatively and increases the viscosity of the solution. This product, Intergel (Lifecore Biomedical Inc., Chaska, Minnesota), was shown to be effective in reducing both de novo and re-formed adhesions in both U.S. and European studies.[25,26] Johns and the Intergel Adhesion Prevention Group[25] randomized 265 patients to receive treatment with Intergel or crystalloid after a variety of gynecologic procedures including myomectomy, adhesiolysis, ovarian procedures, and tubal procedures. The treatment group had a 59% reduction overall in American Fertility Society (AFS) adnexal adhesion scores compared with controls, although the reduction in ovarian sites was the least, at 39%. Lundorff and co-workers[26] reported a significant reduction in AFS adnexal adhesion scores at sites of adhesiolysis and ovarian procedures, but score reduction did not reach significance at myomectomy or tubal sites using Intergel. The overall reduction in AFS adhesion scores was 69% relative to control subject scores. The safety profile in both pilot and multicenter pivotal trials was well established; however, postmarketing reports of abdominal pain and reoperation after use of Intergel have led to its voluntary withdrawal from commercial sales by the manufacturer, although it remains Food and Drug Administration (FDA) approved. The possible causal link is under study.

More efforts have been directed at development of physical barriers that separate operative sites during the reperitonealization process. Two FDA-approved absorbable materials and one nonabsorbable material are available: Interceed (Ethicon, Inc., Somerville, New Jersey) and Seprafilm (Gynezyme Inc., Cambridge, Massachusetts), and Preclude (WH Gore, Flagstaff, Arizona).

Interceed is a woven mesh of oxidized, regenerated cellulose that becomes a gelatinous coating if applied to an operative site and irrigated with crystalloid solution. The material is hydrolyzed and reabsorbed by 28 days.

Interceed is perhaps the best-studied adhesion barrier in gynecologic surgery. Thirteen different studies found efficacy of various degrees for ovarian, adhesiolysis, and myomectomy cases.[27]

Sekiba[28] in Japan found significant efficacy for Interceed in the prevention of pelvic sidewall lesions after endometriosis treatment through an open approach. Approximately 41% of patients in the treatment group were found to have adhesions, compared with 76% of controls. Franklin[27] reported results for the largest series of patients (55) undergoing laparoscopic ovariolysis. In this study, the patients had bilateral ovarian disease and underwent adhesiolysis and treatment of endometriosis if present. Fifty-five patients then had one ovary treated with Interceed; the contralateral ovary was left untreated. At second-look laparoscopy performed up to 14 weeks postoperatively, 47% of treated ovaries were adhesion free, compared with 25% of untreated ovaries. A significant reduction in AFS adhesion scores on the treated sides also was observed, reflecting a reduction in extent and severity of re-formed adhesions.

Mais and co-workers[29,30] also demonstrated efficacy with Interceed in laparoscopic myomectomy and endometriosis cases. Up to 75% of treated endometriosis and 60% of myomectomy patients were adhesion free, compared with 12.5% and 12% of control patients, respectively.

Interceed must be applied only when complete hemostasis has been achieved and all irrigation fluid is removed from the abdomen. Failure to do so invites the trapping of blood clot at the operative site, which may serve as a nidus for adhesion formation. Residual irrigation fluid may float the material off the operative site, rendering it ineffective. In a manufacturer-sponsored randomized multicenter trial in the United States, the investigators found a significant increase in adhesions at sites treated laparoscopically ($P < .05$). The current labeled indications for Interceed are as follows: "Interceed barrier is indicated as an adjuvant in open (laparotomy) gynecologic pelvic surgery . . . ." The conditions for Interceed use, however, are difficult or impossible to achieve at laparoscopic procedures (i.e., complete hemostasis and removal of all irrigation fluid); therefore, the efficacy of this barrier material, even for its off-label use, appears to be of questionable value in laparoscopic surgery.

Seprafilm is an adhesion barrier membrane composed of sodium hyaluronate and carboxymethylcellulose. It is supplied in a sheet backed by paper and is somewhat difficult to handle because it is not flexible and is likely to break if bent or distorted. It also absorbs water and becomes adherent to moist surfaces. It is indicated for use at laparotomy according to the label indications. The material persists at the operative site for 7 to 8 days and is cleared by 28 days.

Most reports in the general surgery literature show efficacy in laparotomy for bowel resections. The Seprafilm Adhesion Study Group[31] reported on a group of 127 myomectomy patients by laparotomy in 1996. The patients were randomly assigned to a treatment group or a no treatment group and underwent second-look laparoscopy at 7 to 70 days. Anterior uterine incision sites were adhesion free in 39% of the patients in the treatment group, compared with 6% of control patients. Posterior uterine incision sites were not significantly improved between the two groups.

Khaitan and co-workers[32] treated chronic abdominal pain in 19 patients by laparoscopic adhesiolysis with Seprafilm application accomplished after rolling the material within its sheath and passing it through a trocar. Postoperatively, 14 of the 19 patients (73%) reported subjective improvement with decrease in pain symptoms, but second-look assessment was not done. In view of the similarity of these results to those reported by Swank and colleagues[33] for adhesiolysis without use of barriers, it is not likely that Seprafilm is efficacious in treatment of chronic abdominal pain from adhesions.

Expanded polytetrafluoroethylene (PTFE), or Preclude (WH Gore, Flagstaff, Arizona), is a nonabsorbable material used for adhesion prevention that shows efficacy as well. The Myomectomy Adhesion Multicenter Study Group[34] reported that 55.7% of treated uterine incisions were adhesion free at second-look laparoscopy versus 7.4% of untreated control incisions. Haney and colleagues[35] compared PTFE membrane

with Interceed in sidewall laparotomy cases and showed better adhesion scores with the former at second-look laparoscopy.

The disadvantage of Preclude is the need for secondary removal. The material is applied and anchored by sutures to the operative site. As with most foreign bodies in the peritoneal cavity, new mesothelium will overgrow the material after 10 days. The difficulty of laparoscopic placement and suturing, along with the need for secondary removal, limits the clinical utility of Preclude.

Future Developments

Although the ultimate solution to this problem probably will result from an increased understanding of the humoral agents and cellular events that control adhesion formation, current clinical needs can be met by an effective adhesion barrier that is easy to apply, prevents both de novo and re-formed adhesions, and is cost-effective.

Several promising materials are now in pilot and early pivotal trials. Spraygel (Confluent Surgical, Waltham, Massachusetts) is a hydrophilic polymer of polyethylene glycol that polymerizes from two liquid precursors as it is sprayed on the operative site. The material is hydrolyzed over the next 7 to 10 days and has been shown to be efficacious in a pilot trial.[35] Oxiplex (FzioMed, San Luis Obispo, California) is a viscous liquid material of polyethylene oxide and carboxymethylcellulose that effectively coats the operative site and shows promise in early pilot trials also.

Various pharmacologic agents and allografts are currently under study as well.

RECOGNITION OF ADHESION-RELATED DISEASE

Patients present with a spectrum of signs and symptoms related to adhesive disease. The diagnosis must be suspected in patients with chronic abdominal pain, infertility, and bowel obstruction when a risk factor such as previous surgery, Crohn's disease, or pelvic inflammatory disease also is present.

The evaluation of such patients should be based on the presenting symptoms. Careful history and physical examination should allow the clinician to differentiate those patients with chronic abdominal pain suggesting a gastrointestinal origin from those with infertility or chronic pelvic pain related to adhesions or pelvic endometriosis.

Patients who appear to have gastrointestinal problems are best evaluated by routine complete blood count and chemistry profiles, along with an abdominal computed tomography (CT) scan with contrast. Colonoscopy, upper endoscopy, upper gastrointestinal barium studies and barium enema, stool culture, stool for ova and parasites, and thyroid function studies would be indicated only in cases with associated hematochezia, weight loss, or leukocytosis with fever.

In addition to the routine laboratory investigation, cultures to rule out gonorrhea and chlamydial infection or *Chlamydia* serologic studies should be included for patients presenting with infertility or chronic pelvic pain. Hysterosalpingogram and pelvic sonogram should be considered as indicated by the clinical circumstances. Pelvic CT is of less use in assessment for the presence of endometriomas or uterine or adnexal pathologic conditions.

Intestinal Adhesions

Multiple authors have consistently found that adhesions are the primary cause of small bowel obstruction, followed by Crohn's disease, hernias, and malignancy.[36-39] Gynecologic surgery appears to be nearly equal in frequency to colorectal surgery as the inciting procedure (22% versus 24%).[37] Al-Took and Tulandi found that adhesions after open gynecologic surgery accounted for 37% of small bowel obstruction cases in a retrospective 10-year review.[40]

Those patients with bowel adhesions may suffer from symptoms ranging from intermittent colic-like abdominal pain to symptoms of partial or complete bowel obstruction. Large bowel adhesions of the rectosigmoid colon may produce constipation, obstipation, and painful defecation.

Adhesions of the liver to anterior abdominal wall or diaphragm can cause pain in the phrenic nerve distribution, producing shoulder pain on deep inspiration. Fitz-Hugh–Curtis syndrome (infectious perihepatitis) may manifest as acute right upper quadrant pain and is sometimes mistaken for acute cholecystitis.

Intermittent, crampy abdominal pain that is sometimes linked to a high-residue diet and is not well localized by the patient typically is present. Other symptoms may include nausea and vomiting of variable severity, depending on the degree of stenosis of the gastrointestinal tract caused by adhesions. Fever usually is not a feature. Acholic or melanotic stool would suggest cholecystitis or gastritis. Hematochezia, diarrhea, weight loss, and fever may suggest underlying diverticulitis, Crohn's disease, or ulcerative colitis. Acute onset of symptoms also may indicate infectious colitis such as in *Clostridium difficile* infection or parasitic diseases. Malabsorption syndromes may be identified by determinations of stool fat and total stool weight over 24 hours.

Irritable bowel syndrome is a common condition, with a 2 : 1 female-to-male ratio of incidence. The presenting symptoms of abdominal pain and altered bowel habits may overlap the symptoms of adhesions short of causing obstruction, making the distinction very difficult clinically. No laboratory or imaging studies are specific for diagnosis of irritable bowel syndrome; rather, it is based on diagnostic criteria[41] of pain lasting for longer than 12 weeks in combination with two of the three following features: (1) relief with defecation, (2) onset associated with a change in frequency of stool, and (3) onset associated with a change in the form of stool. Additional features that support the diagnosis are passage of mucus with stool, bloating, straining, urgency, and a subjective feeling of incomplete emptying on defecation.

The associated signs of abdominal distention, tympany, and high-pitched bowel sounds, or absence of bowel sounds with advanced complete obstruction, are commonly present. Patients may have localized tenderness but more commonly complain of diffuse abdominal pain in the splanchnic distribution.

Laboratory evaluation of adhesion-related abdominal pain is useful in cases of partial or complete bowel obstruction but is unrevealing otherwise. Electrolyte imbalances, hemoconcentration related to dehydration, and possible hyperamylasemia from incarcerated or compromised bowel may be identified on routine laboratory work.

Radiographs obtained with the patient flat and in the upright position are useful in the diagnosis of bowel obstruction; however, they may have limited utility for patients with adhesions causing decreased peristalsis and pain but not causing obstruction. CT scan with contrast or upper gastrointestinal series with small bowel follow-through are better studies to identify areas of narrowed or kinked small bowel. Typical CT findings include prestenotic dilatation of bowel loops, edema of bowel wall, and vascular engorgement of the mesenteric vessels (Figs. 11–4 and 11–5A and B).

In the absence of clear radiographic signs of adhesion-related bowel obstruction, the diagnosis of intestinal adhesions remains one of exclusion and may require diagnostic laparoscopy to distinguish from irritable bowel syndrome.

Pelvic Adhesions and Infertility

The correlation between pregnancy rates and presence of adhesions is similarly well established.

Maruyama and co-workers[38] noted a pregnancy rate of only 18% among a group of patients with bilateral adnexal adhesions, compared with a rate of 45.7% among another group of patients with only unilateral adhesions, at 18-month follow-up evaluation. Alborzi and associates[12] reported similar findings with their observation that none of the 14 patients described as having severe adhesions conceived after adhesiolysis, whereas those with "mild" adhesions achieved a term pregnancy rate of 42%.

Infertility caused by distal tubal obstruction related to adhesions may be identified by absence of or delayed spill of contrast material or hydrosalpinx on hysterosalpingogram. Diagnostic laparoscopy with chromopertubation is a more accurate diagnostic method that excludes the false-positive results of hysterosalpingogram due to tubal spasm. Sonohysterogram can reliably demonstrate tubal patency and identify intrauterine lesions, especially when performed using

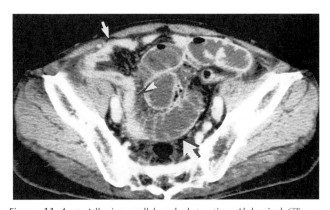

Figure 11–4 ▪ Adhesive small bowel obstruction. Abdominal CT scan shows the transition zone *(arrowhead)*, distended proximal bowel loops *(thick arrow)*, and collapsed distal bowel loops *(thin arrow)*. No adhesive band is actually seen at the transition zone; however, no other specific cause of obstruction is identified either, which suggests the diagnosis of adhesive bowel obstruction. (From Furukawa A, Yamasaki M, Furuichi K, et al. Helical CT in the diagnosis of small bowel obstruction. Radiographics 2001;21:341.)

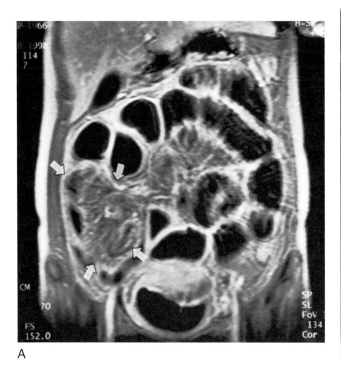
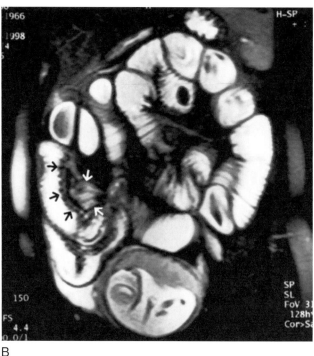

A   B

Figure 11–5 ■ Strangulated bowel obstruction due to bands and adhesions in a 25-year-old pregnant woman. **A,** Coronal contrast-enhanced magnetic resonance (MR) image shows diffuse small bowel dilatation and poor enhancement *(arrows)* in the strangulated segment. **B,** Coronal half-Fourier single-shot fast spin-echo MR image shows bowel wall thickening with a target appearance *(black arrows)* and regional mesenteric vascular engorgement *(white arrows)*. (From Rha SE, Ha HK, Lee SH, et al. CT and MR imaging findings of bowel ischemia from various primary causes. Radiographics 2000;20:29.)

air/water contrast. Patients may or may not have a history of previous salpingitis or surgery.

Adnexal adhesions that alter tubal fimbria function and ovulation also may cause infertility in the absence of tubal obstruction. Ultrasonography has limited utility—it may identify endometriomas, ovarian masses, or torsion, but it cannot image adhesions with adequate specificity. Borzellino and colleagues[42] reported a specificity of 31.8% in diagnosis of adhesions of the anterior abdominal wall by ultrasound examination in 130 patients. Patients with adhesions in this location can be reliably diagnosed only by diagnostic laparoscopy.

Pelvic Adhesions and Chronic Pelvic Pain

Although it is well known that adhesions are a common cause for bowel obstruction and infertility, the causal link to chronic pelvic pain is less clear. Studies reporting laparoscopic findings in patients who had chronic pelvic pain show a high incidence (35% to 90%) of adhesions in these populations.[12,43,44]

Although it is probable that dense adhesions interfering with bowel motility or periovarian adhesions with symptoms that are exacerbated by ovulation cause pain, a placebo effect of laparoscopic adhesiolysis argues against a strong cause-and-effect relationship. The presence of adhesions may be suspected after exclusion of other organic causes for the symptoms and after consideration of irritable bowel syndrome; however, the diagnosis is made or ruled out by laparoscopy.

MANAGEMENT OF SYMPTOMATIC ADHESIONS

Adhesions causing bowel dysfunction or obstruction are best treated surgically if the problem does not resolve with management by conservative means. After initial stabilization of the patient by correction of dehydration and electrolyte imbalances, along with nasogastric drainage if obstruction is present, failure to resolve the problem by conservative means should be corrected surgically by adhesiolysis and resection if indicated.

A large series of laparoscopically managed cases of intestinal obstruction by Franklin and associates[45] consisted of 167 patients. Small bowel obstruction accounted for 70% of the procedures; adhesions were the most common cause, followed by hernias and malignancies. 92.2% of cases were successfully managed laparoscopically. Conversion to laparotomy was most commonly related to inadequate exposure due to massively dilated loops of bowel. Six inadvertent enterotomies and four perioperative deaths from sepsis were reported. Levard and co-workers[46] performed a retrospective analysis of results in 308 patients in France. The laparoscopic approach was successful in 54% of the patients. Complication and mortality rates were not significantly different between laparotomy and laparoscopy treatment groups.

Wullstein and Gross[47] reported a similar rate of success with laparoscopic management of small bowel obstruction in 25 of 52 patients. The intraoperative complication rate was higher than that in a similar cohort of patients managed by laparotomy, but the hospital stay was shorter. These investigators concluded that a laparoscopic approach is feasible.

Most investigators found higher rates of conversion to laparotomy among patients who have had two or more previous laparotomies.

In summary, it would seem prudent to base the approach on the patient's individual history and clinical presentation. Women with multiple previous laparotomies or markedly dilated loops of bowel should be considered for laparotomy. Alternatively, those with less complicated histories in whom adhesions are suspected could be managed laparoscopically. These patients also should be managed by practitioners with the training and experience to perform enterotomy repair or bowel resection, because these techniques may be required for optimal management, as described in the published series.

Tubal Factor Infertility

Management of adhesion-related infertility has been well studied. Schmidt and associates[48] followed 154 patients for 14 months after laparoscopic salpingostomy or fimbrioplasty and noted an inverse relationship between the presence and extent of adnexal adhesions and subsequent pregnancy rates (Fig. 11–6).

Distal tubal occlusion accounts for 85% of the cases of tubal factor infertility.[49] Laparoscopic adhesiolysis, fimbrioplasty, and salpingostomy have become common procedures, with successful pregnancy rates directly proportional to the extent of adhesions. Salpingostomy in patients who are classified as having mild, moderate, or severe disease results in corresponding pregnancy rates of 81%, 31%, or 16%, respectively.[50] These rates compare favorably with the success rates of in vitro fertilization programs among the patients with moderate or severe disease, rendering the surgical approach less advantageous.

Similarly, fimbrioplasty to restore normal fimbrial function and anatomy with respect to the ovary improves pregnancy rates to 60%.[49] Ectopic pregnancy rates may be as high as 14% in laparoscopically managed cases.[51]

The diagnosis and assessment of extent of adhesions or tubal obstruction can be accomplished reliably only at diagnostic laparoscopy. In view of the current understanding,

patients with mild to moderate adhesions causing distal tubal obstruction or dysfunction are best managed with adhesiolysis, salpingostomy, or fimbrioplasty, depending on the findings at laparoscopy. Those with extensive adhesive disease may be better served by in vitro fertilization.

Chronic Pelvic Pain

Several authors report clinical improvement with decrease in pain symptoms after laparoscopic adhesiolysis in a majority of patients. Nezhat and colleagues[43] followed 48 patients for up to 5 years after laparoscopic enterolysis. These investigators found that 64% of patients were pain free or significantly improved at 6 to 12 months. Malik and co-workers[37] followed 187 patients for 18 months after laparoscopic adhesiolysis. Complete relief was demonstrated in 30%, with a majority of the patients experiencing a decrease in pain.

Swank and associates[52] retrospectively reviewed results in 265 patients with chronic abdominal pain treated by laparoscopic adhesiolysis. After exclusion of 65, the 200 remaining patients were categorized as having a good result (disappearance of pain or less pain) or a bad result (pain unchanged or worse). Of these patients, 74% had a good result and 26% a bad result at 3-month follow-up evaluation by subjective questioning. These investigators also reported a 10% major complication rate, with 11 bowel perforations, 40% of which were not recognized or did not exist at the time of surgery, and a mortality rate of 1% from sepsis. The factors associated with improvement that reached significance were age and female gender with previous gynecologic surgery. Analysis of the energy source used showed a lower rate of bad results with agron beam coagulator and ultrasonic scalpel than with electrosurgery, but this finding did not reach significance. Bowel perforation and conversion to laparotomy were associated with a bad result at a level of significance ($P = .03$).

The question regarding the association between presence of adhesions and pain symptoms remains, however. Some level I evidence suggests that laparoscopic adhesiolysis does not produce better results than those achieved with diagnostic laparoscopy alone.

Swank and associates[33] also published an interesting prospective study of chronic pain treated by laparoscopy in the Netherlands in 2003. In this study, 116 patients with chronic pain underwent laparoscopy. Of the 100 patients who had adhesions and met the inclusion criteria, 52 were randomized to receive laparoscopic adhesiolysis and 48 to receive diagnostic laparoscopy alone without adhesiolysis. The patients and the evaluators were blinded to the findings and procedure. Visual Analogue Scores (VASs) were kept to assess pain after the procedure for 12 months. Both groups of patients reported substantial pain relief and improvement in quality of life, but no significant difference ($P = .53$) in VAS was observed between the groups. Peters and colleagues[53] reported findings in 48 patients with known pelvic adhesions on previous laparoscopy who were randomized to receive adhesiolysis by laparotomy or observation. At 12-month follow-up evaluation, no significant difference in pain symptoms was found between the groups, except for those with thick vascular adhesions. The patients in the treatment group reported decreased symptoms by McGill Pain Questionnaire.[54]

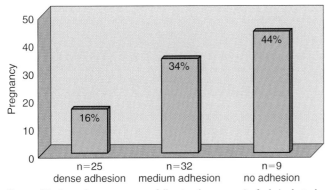

Figure 11–6 ▪ Pregnancy rates following laparoscopic fimbrioplasty by degree of adnexal adhesions. (From Schmidt S, Wagner U, Krebs D, Swolin K. Predicting the outcome of infertility surgery. Arch Gynecol Obstet 2000; 264:116.)

Little evidence is available to support surgical adhesiolysis as a treatment for chronic pelvic pain, except in patients with thick, vascular adhesions involving bowel adherent to peritoneum.[55] Adhesiolysis does not appear to increase pelvic pain, however, and may improve fertility, reduce chances of bowel obstruction, and increase pregnancy rates if done in a manner that does not result in de novo or more extensive recurrent adhesions.

SUMMARY

Postoperative adhesions occur at a high rate and represent significant cost and morbidity. Adhesions constitute a leading cause of postoperative intestinal obstruction and infertility. Surgical correction is warranted in the case of obstruction or mild to moderate tubal adhesions. Patients with adhesions who have chronic pelvic pain may expect improvement only if the adhesions are of advanced stage involving bowel adherent to peritoneum.

Good surgical techniques and use of effective adhesion prevention adjuvants or barriers improve outcomes, but the problem still remains in at least 30% to 50% of patients after pelvic surgery. Clinical research is under way to find more effective techniques and agents to minimize this complication.

References

1. Diamond MP, Daniell JF, Feste J, et al. Adhesion reformation and de novo adhesion formation following reproductive pelvic surgery. Fertil Steril 1987;47:864.
2. Diamond MP, Daniell JF, Johns DA, et al. Postoperative adhesion development following operative laparoscopy: Evaluation at early second-look procedures. Fertil Steril 1991;55:700.
3. Diamond MP, DeCherney AH. Pathogenesis of adhesion formation/reformation: Application to reproductive pelvic surgery. Microsurgery 1987;8:103.
4. Ellis H, Moran BJ, Thompson JN, et al. Adhesion-related hospital readmissions after abdominal and pelvic surgery: A retrospective cohort study. Lancet 1999;353:1476.
5. Hertzler A. Wound healing. In: Hertzler A. The peritoneum, vol 1. St Louis: Mosby, 1919.
6. Rafferty A. In: diZerega G, DeChurny A, Diamond M, et al. Pelvic surgery. New York: Springer-Verlag, 1996.
7. Rodgers K. In: diZerega G, ed. Peritoneal surgery. New York: Springer, 1999.
8. Ellis H. The cause and prevention of post-operative intraperitoneal adhesions. Surg Gynecol Obstet 1971;133:497.
9. Trimbos-Kemper TCM, Trimbos JB, vanHall EV. Adhesion formation after tubal surgery: Results of the eighth-day laparoscopy in 188 patients. Fertil Steril 1985;43:395.
10. Tulandi T, Murray C, Guralnick M. Adhesion formation and reproductive outcome after myomectomy and second look laparoscopy. Obstet Gynecol 1993;82:123.
11. Dubuisson JB, Fauconnier A, Chapron C, et al. Second look after laparoscopic myomectomy. Hum Reprod 1998;13:2102.
12. Alborzi S, Motazedian S, Parsanezhad ME. Chance of adhesion formation after laparoscopic salpingo-ovariolysis: Is there a place for second-look laparoscopy? J Am Assoc Gynecol Laparosc 2003;10:172.
13. Wiseman DM, Trout JR, Diamond MP. The rates of adhesion development and the effects of crystalloid solutions on adhesion development in pelvic surgery. Fertil Steril 1998;70:702.
14. Nezhat CR, Nezhat FR, Metzger DA, Luciano AA. Adhesion reformation after reproductive surgery by videolaseroscopy. Fertil Steril 1990;53:1008.
15. Duron JJ, Hay JM, Msika S, et al. Prevalence and mechanisms of small intestinal obstruction following laparoscopic abdominal surgery: A retrospective multicenter study. Arch Surg 2000;135:208.
16. Polymeneas G, Theodosopoulos T, Stamatiadis A, Kourias E. A comparative study of postoperative adhesion formation after laparoscopic vs open cholecystectomy. Surg Endosc 2001;15:41.
17. Ott DE. Desertification of the peritoneum by thin-film evaporation during laparoscopy. JSLS 2003;7:189.
18. Ott DE. Laparoscopy and tribology: The effect of laparoscopic gas on peritoneal fluid. J Am Assoc Gynecol Laparosc 2001;8:117.
19. Gomel V. Principles of infertility surgery. In: Microsurgery in female infertility. Boston: Little, Brown, 1983.
20. Pellicano M, Bramante S, Cirillo D, et al. Effectiveness of autocrosslinked hyaluronic acid gel after laparoscopic myomectomy in infertile patients: A prospective, randomized, controlled study. Fertil Steril 2003;80:441.
21. Farquhar C, Vandekerckhove P, Watson A, et al. Barrier agents for preventing adhesions after surgery for subfertility. Cochrane Database Syst Rev 2000;2:CD000475.
22. Shear L, Swartz C, Shinaberger J, et al. Kinetics of peritoneal fluid absorption in adult man. N Engl J Med 1965;272:123.
23. Sites CK, Jensen BA, Jacob BS, et al. Transvaginal ultrasonographic assessment of Hyskon or lactated Ringer's solution instillation after laparoscopy: Randomized, controlled study. J. Ultrasound Med 1997;16:195.
24. Diamond MP. Reduction of de novo postsurgical adhesions by intraoperative precoating with Sepracoat (HAL-C) solution: A prospective, randomized, blinded, placebo-controlled multicenter study. The Sepracoat Adhesion Study Group. Fertil Steril 1998;69:1067.
25. Johns DB, Keyport GM, Hoehler F, diZerega GS, for the Intergel Adhesion Prevention Study Group. Reduction of postsurgical adhesions with Intergel adhesion prevention solution: A multicenter study of safety and efficacy after conservative gynecologic surgery. Fertil Steril 2001;76:595.
26. Lundorff P, van Geldorp H, Tronstad SE, et al. Reduction of postsurgical adhesions with ferric hyaluronate gel: A European study. Hum Reprod 2001;16:1982.
27. Franklin RR. Reduction of ovarian adhesions by the use of Interceed. Ovarian Adhesion Study Group. Obstet Gynecol 1995;86:335.
28. Sekiba K. Use of Interceed (TC7) absorbable adhesion barrier to reduce postoperative adhesion reformation in infertility and endometriosis surgery. The Obstetrics and Gynecology Adhesion Prevention Committee. Obstet Gynecol 1992;79:518.
29. Mais V, Ajossa S, Marongiu D, et al. Reduction of adhesion reformation after laparoscopic endometriosis surgery: A randomized trial with an oxidized regenerated cellulose absorbable barrier. Obstet Gynecol 1995;86(4 Pt 1):512.
30. Mais V, Ajossa S, Piras B, et al. Prevention of de-novo adhesion formation after laparoscopic myomectomy: A randomized trial to evaluate the effectiveness of an oxidized regenerated cellulose absorbable barrier. Hum Reprod 1995;10:3133.
31. Diamond MP. Reduction of adhesions after uterine myomectomy by Seprafilm membrane (HAL-F): A blinded, prospective, randomized, multicenter clinical study. Seprafilm Adhesion Study Group. Fertil Steril 1996;66:904.
32. Khaitan L, Scholz S, Houston HL, Richards WO. Results after laparoscopic lysis of adhesions and placement of seprafilm for intractable abdominal pain. Surg Endosc 2003;17:247. Epub 2002;Oct 29.
33. Swank DJ, Swank-Bordewijk SC, Hop WC, et al. Laparoscopic adhesiolysis in patients with chronic abdominal pain: A blinded randomised controlled multi-centre trial. Lancet 2003;361:1247.
34. Myomectomy Adhesion Multicenter Study Group. An expanded polytetrafluoroethylene barrier (Gore-Tex Surgical Membrane) reduces post-myomectomy adhesion formation. Fertil Steril 1995;63:491.
35. Haney AF, Hesla J, Hurst BS, et al Expanded polytetrafluoroethylene (Gore-Tex Surgical Membrane) is superior to oxidized regenerated cellulose (Interceed TC7+) in preventing adhesions. Fertil Steril 1995;63:1021. [Erratum appears in Fertil Steril 1995;64:668.]
36. Johnson NP, Watson A. Cochrane review: Post-operative procedures for improving fertility following pelvic reproductive surgery. Hum Reprod Update 2000;6:259.
37. Malik E, Berg C, Meyhofer-Malik A, et al. Subjective evaluation of the therapeutic value of laparoscopic adhesiolysis: A retrospective analysis. Surg Endosc 2000;14:79.
38. Maruyama M, Osuga Y, Momoeda M, et al. Pregnancy rates after laparoscopic treatment. Differences related to tubal status and presence of endometriosis. J Reprod Med 2000;45:89.

39. Menzies D, Parker M, Hoare R, Knight A. Small bowel obstruction due to postoperative adhesions: Treatment patterns and associated costs in 110 hospital admissions. Ann R Coll Surg Engl 2001;83:40.

40. Al-Took S, Platt R, Tulandi T. Adhesion-related small-bowel obstruction after gynecologic operations. Am J Obstet Gynecol 1999;180(2 Pt 1):313.

41. Drossman DA, Corazziari E, Tally NJ, et al, eds. In: Rome II, ed. The functional gastrointestinal disorders, 2nd ed. MacLean, VA: Degnon Associates, 2000;355.

42. Borzellino G, De Manzoni G, Ricci F. Detection of abdominal adhesions in laparoscopic surgery. A controlled study of 130 cases. Surg Laparosc Endosc 1998;8:273.

43. Nezhat FR, Crystal RA, Nezhat CH, Nezhat CR. Laparoscopic adhesiolysis and relief of chronic pelvic pain. JSLS 2000;4:281.

44. Onders RP, Mittendorf EA. Utility of laparoscopy in chronic abdominal pain. Surgery 2003;134:549.

45. Franklin ME, Gonzalez JJ, Miter DB, et al. Laparoscopic diagnosis and treatment of intestinal obstruction. Surg Endosc 2004;18:26.

46. Levard H, Boudet MJ, Msika S, et al. Laparoscopic treatment of acute small bowel obstruction: A multicentre retrospective study. Aust N Z J Surg 2001;71:641.

47. Wullstein C, Gross E. Laparoscopic compared with conventional treatment of acute adhesive small bowel obstruction. Br J Surg 2003;90:1147.

48. Schmidt S, Wagner U, Krebs D, Swolin K. Predicting the outcome of infertility surgery. Arch Gynecol Obstet 2000;264:116.

49. Mishell D. Infertility. In: Stevencher MA, Droegenmueller W, Herbest AL, Mishell DR. Comprehensive gynecology, 4th ed. St. Louis: Mosby, 2001.

50. Schlaff WD, Hassiakos DK, Damewood MD. Neosalpingostomy for distal tubal obstruction: Prognostic factors and impact of surgical technique. Fertil Steril 1990;54:984.

51. Kodaman PH, Arici A, Seli E: Evidence-based diagnosis and management of tubal factor infertility. Curr Opin Obstet Gynecol 2004;16:221.

52. Swank DJ, Van Erp WF, Repelaer Van Driel OJ, et al. A prospective analysis of predictive factors on the results of laparoscopic adhesiolysis in patients with chronic abdominal pain. Surg Laparosc Endosc Percutan Tech 2003;13:88.

53. Peters AA, Trimbos-Kemper GC, Admiraal C, et al. A randomized clinical trial on the benefit of adhesiolysis in patients with intraperitoneal adhesions and chronic pelvic pain. Br J Obstet Gynaecol 1992;99:59.

54. Reading AE. The internal structure of the McGill pain questionnaire in dysmenorrhea patients. Pain 1979;7:353.

55. Stones RW, Mountfield J. Interventions for treating chronic pelvic pain in women. Cochrane Database Syst Rev 2000;4:CD000387.

Additional Reading

Beck DE, Cohen Z, Fleshman JW, et al for the Adhesion Study Group Steering Committee. A prospective, randomized, multicenter, controlled study of the safety of Seprafilm adhesion barrier in abdominopelvic surgery of the intestine. Dis Colon Rectum 2003;46:1310.

Bremers AJ, Ringers J, Vijn A, et al. Laparoscopic adhesiolysis for chronic abdominal pain: An objective assessment. J Laparoendosc Adv Surg Tech A 2000;10:199.

Chapron C, Guibert J, Fauconnier A, et al. Adhesion formation after laparoscopic resection of uterosacral ligaments in women with endometriosis. J Am Assoc Gynecol Laparosc 2001;8:368.

Diamond MP, Luciano A, Johns DA, et al. Reduction of postoperative adhesions by *N,O*-carboxymethylchitosan: A pilot study. Fertil Steril 2003;80:631.

diZerega GS, Verco SJ, Young P, et al. A randomized, controlled pilot study of the safety and efficacy of 4% icodextrin solution in the reduction of adhesions following laparoscopic gynaecological surgery. Hum Reprod 2002;17:1031.

Gomel V. Salpingo-ovariolysis by laparoscopy in infertility. Fertil Steril 1983;40:607.

Kossi J, Salminen P, Laato M. The epidemiology and treatment patterns of postoperative adhesion induced intestinal obstruction in Varsinais-Suomi Hospital District. Scand J Surg 2004;93:68.

Levrant SG, Bieber EJ, Barnes RB. Anterior abdominal wall adhesions after laparotomy or laparoscopy. J Am Assoc Gynecol Laparosc 1997;4:353.

Liu SI, Siewert B, Raptopoulos V, Hodin RA. Factors associated with conversion to laparotomy in patients undergoing laparoscopic appendectomy. J Am Coll Surg 2002;194:298.

The Myomectomy Adhesion Multicenter Study Group. An expanded polytetrafluoroethylene barrier (Gore-Tex Surgical Membrane) reduces postmyomectomy adhesion formation. Fertil Steril 1995;63:491.

Pelosi MA 2nd, Pelosi MA 3rd. A new nonabsorbable adhesion barrier for myomectomy. Am J Surg 2002;184:428.

Saravelos HG, Li TC, Cooke ID. An analysis of the outcome of microsurgical and laparoscopic adhesiolysis for chronic pelvic pain. Hum Reprod 1995;10:2895.

Sokol AI, Chuang K, Milad MP. Risk factors for conversion to laparotomy during gynecologic laparoscopy. J Am Assoc Gynecol Laparosc 2003;10:469.

Swank DJ, van Erp WF, Repelaer van Driel OJ, et al. Complications and feasibility of laparoscopic adhesiolysis in patients with chronic abdominal pain. A retrospective study. Surg Endosc 2002;16:1468. (Epub 2002;Jun 20.)

Taskin O, Sadik S, Onoglu A, et al. Role of endometrial suppression in the frequency of intrauterine adhesions after resectoscopic surgery. J Am Assoc Gynecol Laparosc 2000;7:351.

Tsapanos VS, Stathopoulou LP, Papathanassopoulou VS, Tzingounis VA. The role of Seprafilm bioresorbable membrane in the prevention and therapy of endometrial synechiae. J Biomed Mater Res 2002;63:10.

Vrijland WW, Tseng LN, Eijkman HJ, et al. Fewer intraperitoneal adhesions with use of hyaluronic acid–carboxymethylcellulose membrane: A randomized clinical trial. Ann Surg 2002;235:193.

Complications of Laparoscopic Surgery in Gynecologic Oncology

12

Farr Nezhat and Ali Mahdavi

Advanced operative laparoscopy in gynecologic oncology developed after advances in laparoscopic retroperitoneal surgery, particularly pelvic and para-aortic lymphadenectomy. Historically, the performance of these retroperitoneal dissections opened the door for more advanced oncologic operations, including revival of radical vaginal surgery, and complete laparoscopic management and staging for a variety of gynecologic malignancies.

Although laparoscopic techniques generally follow the same principles of open surgical techniques, the use of laparoscopy in patients with cancer has introduced unique complications and risks in these patients. For example, an increasing number of reports in the literature describe postoperative tumor growth at the specific puncture sites associated with trocar placement.

This chapter reviews current applications of laparoscopy in evaluation and treatment of gynecologic cancers and then provides guidelines for prevention, recognition, and management of laparoscopic complications in gynecologic cancers.

APPLICATIONS OF LAPAROSCOPY IN GYNECOLOGIC ONCOLOGY

Ideally, the role of laparoscopic surgery in gynecologic oncology should be defined by randomized clinical trials, such as the ongoing Gynecologic Oncology Group (GOG) LAP2 trial. On the basis of the available data, the applications of laparoscopy in gynecologic cancers can be categorized as follows.

Laparoscopic Lymphadenectomy

Since the initial report by Dargent and Salvat[1] in the late 1980s, laparoscopic lymphadenectomy has been utilized in the management of gynecologic and urologic malignancies as well as in some lymphomas. Nezhat and colleagues[2,3] were the first to describe para-aortic lymphadenectomy performed laparoscopically for cancer of the uterine cervix. Over the recent years, an expanding literature has evolved regarding outcomes and complications of laparoscopic lymphadenectomy.

Lymph node status is the most important prognostic factor in gynecologic cancer, and surgical removal of pelvic and para-aortic lymph nodes for histologic assessment is an integral part of staging for gynecologic malignancies. Additionally, removal of the bulky lymph nodes may have therapeutic benefit.

Transperitoneal pelvic lymphadenectomy begins with identification of the ureter, coagulation and cutting of the round ligament, and opening of the posterior peritoneum and the pelvic sidewall. The common iliac and external iliac nodes are dissected, with care taken to avoid the genitofemoral nerve, which lies medial on the psoas muscle. The nodes are dissected from the common iliac artery bifurcation to the circumflex iliac vein caudally. After development of paravesical space between the obliterated hypogastric artery and external iliac artery and vein, the obturator space is opened and the obturator nerve and vessels are identified. Although in a majority of patients both the obturator artery and vein lie dorsal to the obturator nerve, an aberrant obturator vein arising from the external iliac vein is seen in 10% of patients. The obturator lymph nodes are grasped just under the external iliac vein, and traction is applied medially. The node chain is thereby separated from the obturator nerve and vessels, and the nodes are dissected cephalad to the hypogastric artery. Finally, the hypogastric lymph nodes are removed up to the common iliac artery, with care taken to avoid injury to the hypogastric vein. For the para-aortic dissection, the peritoneum is excised over the sacral promontory or right common iliac artery, with the right ureter in view. This incision is extended up to the inferior mesenteric artery or up to the left renal vein in cases of ovarian or fallopian tube carcinoma. The lymph node packages are retrieved along the common iliac vessels and along the aorta and vena cava, with careful attention given to the ovarian vessels, the ureters, the renal vessels, and the inferior mesenteric artery.

An alternative to the transperitoneal laparoscopic lymphadenectomy is the extraperitoneal endoscopic lymphadenectomy, which was first described by Vasilev and McGonigle[4] in 1996 and by Dargent and Salvat.[1] The extraperitoneal endoscopic lymphadenectomy combines the benefits of laparoscopy with those of extraperitoneal dissection. In comparison with the transperitoneal approach, the advantages include operative feasibility and decreased risk of direct bowel injury and bowel adhesion formation, which can result in a reduced incidence of post-radiation enteritis. A complication specific to extraperitoneal endoscopic lymphadenectomy is the potential for creating defects in the peritoneum requiring conversion to a laparoscopic transperitoneal approach. An alternative solution, however, is to reduce any remaining pneumoperitoneum, thereby facilitating further extraperitoneal dissection. In cases of larger peritoneal defects, clips or sutures may be applied to reapproximate the peritoneal edges, thereby maintaining the extraperitoneal insufflation. In the early experience with this technique, formation of symptomatic lymphoceles constituted a majority of the postoperative problems. The frequency of this complication has been reduced by creating a peritoneal window in the paracolic gutter on completion of the procedure.

Laparoscopically Assisted Radical Vaginal Hysterectomy with Laparoscopic Pelvic Lymphadenectomy

With the popularization of complete pelvic lymphadenectomy in the 1940s as an important component of the surgical management of cervical cancer, laparoscopically assisted radical vaginal hysterectomy (LARVH) became less popular because the lymphadenectomy could not be performed through the vaginal route. Dargent and Salvat[1] revived this procedure through a combined laparoscopic retroperitoneal lymphadenectomy and radical vaginal hysterectomy. The current literature contains 11 reports on 382 patients who underwent this procedure for stage IA2 or IIB cervical cancer.[5] The surgical complications included cystotomy (in 4% to 5%), ureteral injuries (in 1% to 2%), vascular injuries (in 1% to 2%), abscess formation (in 1% to 2%), hematoma (in 1% to 2%), and transfusion (in 6% to 7%).

Total Laparoscopic Radical Hysterectomy

A laparoscopic radical hysterectomy with pelvic and para-aortic lymph node dissection was first reported by Nezhat and colleagues[2] in 1992. No randomized trials are yet available comparing total laparoscopic radical hysterectomy (TLRH) and abdominal radical hysterectomy; however, data for greater than 150 patients have so far been reported, with encouraging results. Abu-Rustum[5] recently reviewed eight reports on 146 patient who underwent TLRH with pelvic and para-aortic lymphadenectomy. The mean operative time was 300 minutes, with mean hospital stay of 4 days. Complications included conversion to laparotomy in 3% to 4% of patients, cystotomy in 2% to 3%, ureteral injury in 2% to 3%, and transfusion in 1% to 2%. It appears that the overall complication rate is acceptable, with no compromise in the oncologic outcome.

Laparoscopic Staging and Second-Look Surgery in Ovarian Cancer

The role of laparoscopy in ovarian cancer surgery may be divided in four categories: laparoscopic staging of apparent early ovarian cancer; laparoscopic assessment of disease extent and potential for resectability; hand-assisted laparoscopy for resection of selected cases of advanced ovarian cancer; and second-look laparoscopy to rule out recurrence.

The safety of the laparoscopic approach for ovarian cancer has been documented, with minimal intraoperative and postoperative complications, in recent reports. With advanced laparoscopic techniques, adhesions usually can be released to improve visualization of peritoneal surfaces, allowing suspicious lesions to be biopsied and areas of tumor persistence, including pelvic and para-aortic lymph nodes, to be sampled. Peritoneal washings can be obtained and intraperitoneal catheters can be inserted under direct visualization. Potential limitations to laparoscopy have been recognized—mainly, the inability to palpate unvisualized areas and possible limited exposure to the posterior diaphragm, mainly behind the liver, where disease may be missed. In addition, an increasing number of reports describe port site metastasis after laparoscopy in patients with ovarian cancer.

COMPLICATIONS: PREVENTION, RECOGNITION, AND MANAGEMENT

Complications of laparoscopic surgery can affect different organ systems. Although most of these complications are inherent to the laparoscopic approach and can occur with other laparoscopic procedures, others occur more often in patients with gynecologic cancers. Some complications, such as port site metastasis, are seen exclusively in this patient population.

Vascular Complications

Vascular injuries related to lymphadenectomy are potentially life-threatening complications. Perhaps the most common vascular injury in general, and with laparoscopic lymphadenectomy in particular, is injury to the inferior epigastric and other superficial anterior abdominal wall vessels. In a series of laparoscopic lymphadenectomies,[6] seven of nine reported that vascular complications occurred as a result of trocar injury to the anterior abdominal wall vasculature. Potential vasculature compromise specific to pelvic lymphadenectomy includes injury to the obturator, internal iliac, external iliac, and common iliac vessels. Vessels at risk for injury during a para-aortic lymphadenectomy include the aorta and vena cava, as well as the common iliac, inferior mesenteric, lumbar, ovarian, and renal vessels.

Prevention of anterior abdominal wall vessel injury during trocar insertion is discussed in detail in previous chapters. Prevention of pelvic vasculature injury requires paying close attention to the anatomy. Cautious dissection of the obturator space is of paramount importance, because aberrant obturator vein was the most commonly injured pelvic vessel during pelvic lymphadenectomy in one study.[7] As mentioned earlier, this aberrant vessel usually travels anterior to the obturator nerve and can be a ready target for an unanticipated vascular injury.

Laparoscopic management of vascular injuries varies according to the type (artery or vein) and size of the injured vessel. The modalities utilized in managing these vascular injuries include pressure, monopolar and bipolar electrocautery, clips, and sutures. Depending on the caliber of the injured vessel, any one of these modalities may achieve hemostasis satisfactorily.

When a vessel is injured, it is important to control the bleeding as quickly as possible. This usually can be accomplished by using a laparoscopic grasper to occlude the bleeding vessel or by applying gentle pressure with a suction-irrigator cannula. If visualization is obscured, or if the vessel is a large vein and grasping may result in further laceration, pressure should be applied. Laparoscopic instruments, lymph node pads, a 4 × 4-inch gauze, or a mini-laparotomy pad can be placed through a 10- to 12-mm port before the lymph node dissection is begun.

Small venous bleeders can be controlled with pressure alone. A laparotomy pad can be packed into the retroperitoneal space while the procedure is continued in another part of the surgical field. Later during the procedure, the packing can be removed and the area inspected for hemostasis. Placing pads into the abdomen laparoscopically can be a helpful technique; however, care should be taken to avoid the problem of retained laparotomy pads.

Arterial bleeders should be quickly controlled, because the blood loss can be rapid. Care should be taken to avoid arterial pumping of blood onto the laparoscope. When this occurs, visualization of the field is obscured, and the laparoscope must be removed for cleaning, which spends valuable time and increases blood loss. Another common pitfall occurs during the aspiration of pooled blood. While the pooled blood is being suctioned, the pneumoperitoneum frequently is suctioned as well if the suction tip is not completely submerged. Loss of the pneumoperitoneum can result in poor exposure of the operative field and can create a cascade of time-consuming events.

To achieve hemostasis, monopolar electrocautery or ultrasonic harmonic coagulation can be used for small arterial and venous bleeders. The bipolar electrocautery device is especially useful to control venous and arterial bleeders of a large caliber. The bipolar can be used to coapt vessels or can be applied along the length of the instrument, to provide surface cauterization over a friable area. Bipolar electrocautery, however, is an unacceptable form of vascular injury control in vessels that should not be sacrificed or in vessels of extremely large caliber, such as the iliac vessels and the vena cava. For control of bleeding in these situations, clips or suturing techniques should be used. Laparoscopically applied clips can control large venous bleeders adequately. Prefabricated slip-knots can be used to control moderate-sized arterial bleeders. With this technique, a grasper is placed through the prefabricated loop and affixed to the injured vessel. The loop is slipped over the grasper and onto the vessel. Suturing techniques using needles may require laparotomy; in such instances, consideration should be given to intraoperative consultation with a vascular surgeon. In our experience with 100 consecutive laparoscopic pelvic and para-aortic lymphadenectomies using harmonic scalpel,[8] two vascular injuries occurred. One injury was to the hypogastric vein during pelvic lymphadenectomy, and the other injury was to a branch of inferior mesenteric artery during para-aortic lymphadenectomy. Bleeding in both cases was controlled laparoscopically by application of vascular clips, and neither of the patients required transfusion or experienced any complications.

Genitourinary Complications

Laparoscopic injury to the urinary tract is well described in the literature. Cystotomy during trocar insertion, adhesiolysis, or dissection with endoscopic scissors, with or without electrocautery, has been delineated as a complication of laparoscopic lymphadenectomy, although one not specific to this procedure. Cystotomy can occur during the development of bladder flap and vesicovaginal space in a laparoscopic radical hysterectomy, or when the paravesical and pararectal spaces are opened, if obliterated umbilical artery is not retracted medially.

To prevent injuries to the bladder, a Foley catheter is placed for urine drainage. The position of the bladder should be assessed during the initial examination with the laparoscope. If the boundaries of the bladder are not clear, particularly when the pelvic anatomy is distorted, the bladder should be filled with 200 to 300 mL of normal saline to delineate its position. During laparoscopic radical hysterectomy, the assistant should push up the uterus during bladder dissection and development of the vesicocervical space.

Signs of intraoperative bladder injury include visualization of the Foley catheter bulb, presence of air in the urinary catheter, hematuria, urine drainage from the accessory trocar incision, intraperitoneal leakage of indigo carmine if this has been used, suprapubic bruising, and abdominal wall or pelvic mass.

Trocar injuries to the bladder dome require closure followed by urinary drainage for 5 to 7 days. Nezhat and colleagues[9] described the closure of intentional and unintentional bladder lacerations during operative laparoscopy in 19 women. The defect was repaired laparoscopically in one layer using interrupted polyglycolic suture (in 17 patients) or polydioxanone suture (in 2 patients), with 7 to 14 days of transurethral drainage after the repair. Complications were limited to one vesicovaginal fistula, which required reoperation. In a study on mongrel dogs, Sokol and associates[10] concluded that double-layer bladder closure appeared to be superior to single-layer repair for prevention of vesicovaginal fistula after monopolar cystotomy.

Knowledge of the ureter's course through the pelvis and of vulnerable points is key to preventing injuries. The intrapelvic segment of the ureter is near the broad, infundibulopelvic, and uterosacral ligaments. To prevent injuries, the ureter must be identified before irreversible action is taken. Methods to prevent ureteral injury include hydrodissection and resection of affected peritoneum. A small opening is made in the peritoneum, and 50 to 100 mL of lactated Ringer's solution is injected along the course of the ureter. This displaces it laterally, providing a plane for lysis of adhesions or resecting the involved peritoneum. Before the bipolar forceps is used during an adnexectomy, the infundibulopelvic ligament is put under traction to identify the ureter and avoid thermal damage. If the ureter is not clearly identified through the peritoneum, it must be located by retroperitoneal dissection. Using hydrodissection, a horizontal incision is made in the peritoneum midway between the ovary and the uterosacral ligament.[11] The lower edge of the peritoneum is grasped and pulled medially. Blunt dissection with the suction-irrigator helps locate the ureter lateral to the peritoneum.

Intraoperative early recognition is critical to successful treatment. Intraoperative ureteral damage is suspected if urine leakage or blood-tinged urine is noted or indigo carmine dye is seen intraperitoneally after intravenous administration. When surgical procedures involve the ureter, postoperative ureteral patency is evaluated by cystoscopy, ureteral catheterization, an intravenous pyelogram, or a CT urogram. Unfortunately, diagnosis of ureteral injury usually is made postoperatively by intravenous pyelogram. Fever, flank pain, peritonitis, and abdominal distention developing within 48 to 72 hours postoperatively should alert the physician to pos-sible ureteral injury. Leukocytosis and hematuria may be present.

Specific to the laparoscopic lymphadenectomy is the possibility of a ureteral injury. Pelvic lymphadenectomy places the ureter at risk for sharp, crush, or thermal injury. The lumbar portion of the ureter is at risk during para-aortic lymphadenectomy, especially on the left side. Injury in this location is possible if the lateral dissection overlying the psoas muscle is carried out above the ureter, instead of in the correct plane. A portion of the ureter can thereby be included with the nodal bundle for resection. Such an injury, if recognized intraoperatively, can be managed laparoscopically. A trans-ureteral stent should be placed, the ureteral defect oversewn, and a retroperitoneal drain placed laparoscopically. Although it is an area of current investigation, no proven role for prophylactic ureteral stent placement before laparoscopic lymphadenectomy has been recognized.

Whether the discovery of postoperative ureteral complications is immediate or delayed, a urologist should be consulted. Initial therapy should involve attempts at retrograde or antegrade stenting. Therapeutic options include uretero-ureterostomy and ureteroneocystostomy, by either laparotomy or laparoscopy. Both require stenting and drainage with a ureteral catheter.

Ureterovaginal and vesicovaginal fistulas, as well as injury to a patent urachus, are other potential complications. Vesicovaginal fistulas usually manifest 7 to 21 days after surgery. Most patients have urinary incontinence or persistent vaginal discharge. If the fistula is very small, leakage may be intermittent, occurring only at maximum bladder capacity or with a particular body position. Other signs and symptoms include unexplained fever; hematuria; recurrent cystitis or pyelonephritis; vaginal, suprapubic, or flank pain; and abnormal urinary stream.

Office testing often can distinguish between fistulas involving the bladder or ureters. Instillation of methylene blue or sterile milk into the bladder stains vaginal swabs or tampons in the presence of vesicovaginal fistula. If this test is not diagnostic, a transurethral Foley catheter should be placed to prevent any staining of the distal tampon from the urethral meatus. Unstained but wet swabs may indicate a ureterovaginal fistula. If leakage is not demonstrated, the bladder is filled to maximum capacity, and provocative maneuvers such as Valsalva maneuver or manual pressure over the bladder are used to reproduce and confirm the patient's symptoms. Intravenous indigo carmine can be given to rule out ureterovaginal fistula. Further evaluations, such as cystoureteroscopy and intravenous urogram, permit the physician to localize the fistula, determine adequacy of renal function, and exclude or identify other types of urinary tract injury.

In operative laparoscopy, meticulous dissection of vesicovaginal space and good hemostasis are essential for prevention of vesicovaginal fistula. Based on a study in mongrel dogs by Cogan and colleagues,[12] cystotomy induced by electrosurgery during laparoscopic hysterectomy can be a risk factor for formation of vesicovaginal fistulas. Cautious use of electrosurgery in the vicinity of the bladder is recommended. The benefit of electrosurgical burn margin excision or omental flap interposition remains unclear, but both are accomplished easily with little risk and may play a role in fistula prevention. As mentioned earlier, Sokol and associates[10] concluded that double-layer bladder closure appeared to be superior to single-layer repair for prevention of vesicovaginal fistula after monopolar cystotomy. Meticulous suture placement and avoidance of tissue strangulation are also essential for prevention of vesicovaginal fistula.

Vesicovaginal fistulas are treated with different surgical techniques, depending on their cause and location. Small vesicovaginal fistulas that are not responsive to nonsurgical management usually are repaired easily. The edges of the fistula are resected, and the defect is closed. Latzko's technique commonly is used for fistulas that are surrounded by severe fibrosis and located close to the bladder neck or urethral meatus. Lee and coworkers[13] recommend an abdominal approach for fistulas in the upper part of a narrow vagina, multiple fistulas, those associated with other pelvic abnormalities, and fistulas close to the ureter. A combined abdominal and vaginal approach is used in some instances. Laparoscopy can be an alternative to laparotomy for managing vesicovaginal fistula. Proposed advantages include magnification during the procedure, better hemostasis, shorter hospital stay, and more rapid postoperative recovery.

A total of seven patients with laparoscopic vesicovaginal fistula repair have been reported in the literature.[14-17] Despite minor differences in surgical techniques, fistula repair was successful in all seven cases 3 to 6 months postoperatively. All cases were treated by surgeons with extensive experience and interest in advanced operative laparoscopy.

Gastrointestinal Injuries

Bowel injury is a potential complication of any laparoscopic procedure. Bowel can easily be damaged at trocar insertion, adhesiolysis, or thermal injury during dissection. Prevention of this complication begins with appropriate patient selection and preoperative preparation. Adhesions between the small bowel and the anterior abdominal wall are associated with the risk of trocar injury, especially in patients with a history of bowel resection or previous omentectomy and debulking for ovarian cancer. Complete mechanical bowel preparation and intraoperative placement of an orogastric or nasogastric tube are essential. The net effect is to keep the bowel flat and empty, resulting in easier "packing" of the bowel into the upper abdomen.

Intestinal inspection after sharp dissection that shows bleeding or hematoma should alert the operator to potential intestinal injury. Manipulation of the bowel from the pelvis with a blunt metal probe should be done cautiously, and blunt dissection should be avoided.

Delayed bowel motility can occur throughout the post-operative period. Bowel herniation can result if fascial closure of the trocar defects is not accomplished or if such closure is inadequate. Nezhat and colleagues[18] reported 11 incisional hernias in their series of 5300 laparoscopic surgical procedures, for an incidence of approximately 0.2%. The hernia occurred through a 5-mm trocar incision site in five cases. Six patients required laparoscopic surgery to retract the entrapped omentum or bowel. These investigators concluded that the underlying fascia and peritoneum should be closed not only when 10-mm or larger trocars are used but also when extensive manipulation is performed through a 5-mm trocar port, causing extension of the incision. Although not reported, bowel obstruction can occur as a result of post-laparoscopy adhesion formation. At Mount Sinai Medical Center, we have managed a case of partial small bowel obstruction occurring after a laparoscopic lymphadenectomy for endometrial cancer, which resolved with conservative management.

Laparoscopic management of gastrointestinal injuries is discussed elsewhere in this book (see Chapters 4 and 6). Laparoscopic hernia reduction has been accomplished and reported in the literature.[19] Large and small bowel injuries can be repaired intracorporeally or extracorporeally through a slightly enlarged port site. These techniques are discussed in detail in other chapters.

Port Site Metastasis

Recently, an increasing number of reports in the literature have described postoperative tumor growth at the specific puncture sites associated with trocar placement. In fact, cases of port site metastasis have been reported involving cancers of ovary, cervix, endometrium, fallopian tube, and vagina, as well as nongynecologic cancers including those of the stomach, large bowel, liver, pancreas, and urinary tract.[20] The true incidence of this phenomenon, however, has not been clearly defined. For example, three studies that specifically addressed this issue have demonstrated a wide range in reported incidence. Childers and co-workers[21] reported port site metastases in 1 of 88 patients undergoing a laparoscopic procedure for ovarian cancer, for a rate of 1.4%, whereas Kruitwagen and colleagues[22] reported the incidence of port site metastases to be 16% in patients with ovarian cancer undergoing laparoscopic procedures 9 to 35 days before the initial debulking procedure. In a retrospective study of 83 patients at Mount Sinai Medical Center with gynecologic cancer,[20] the overall incidence rate of port site metastasis was 2.3%. The incidence of port site metastasis per procedure for cancers of the ovary, peritoneum, and fallopian tube was 6.25%. These investigators found the presence of ascites and recurrent ovarian cancer to be independent risk factors for port site metastasis.

The mechanism by which wound metastasis occurs is still not completely understood. Several factors related to the surgery have been implemented in causing spread of cancer cells. These include accidental incision of the tumor, transection of lymphatic channels that contain cancer, direct dissemination of surface tumors, and even the biologic conditions created by the trauma of surgery itself. The tumor cell entrapment hypothesis suggests that free cancer cells are able to implant on raw tissue surfaces, including damaged peritoneal surfaces. Postoperatively, these areas become covered by a fibrinous exudate, which could serve to protect the tumor cells from destruction by the normal defense mechanisms. Hypotheses specific to laparoscopy include exfoliation and spread of tumor cells by laparoscopic instruments; direct implantation at the trocar site by frequent changes of instruments; direct implantation from the passage of the specimen; the presence of the pneumoperitoneum, which can create a "chimney effect" that causes an increase in the passage of tumor cells at port sites; and preferential growth of malignant cells at areas of laparoscopic peritoneal perforation.

Several measures have been proposed to prevent port site metastasis; however, they remain controversial, and further research is needed in this area. The use of intraperitoneal cytotoxic agents at the time of laparoscopy, early onset of postoperative chemotherapy, irrigation of the port sites, securing the port to the abdominal wall, avoiding gas leakage and trauma to the trocar site incision, removing all malignant or suspicious tissue with an Endo bag, removing the ports after reduction of the pneumoperitoneum, closure of all trocar sites, and possible irradiation of high-risk trocar sites are among these measures. Other suggestions include avoiding diagnostic or palliative laparoscopic procedures for recurrent ovarian cancer, especially in the presence of ascites, and performing a comprehensive cytoreductive procedure whenever possible.

Although port site or wound site recurrences may be disfiguring and difficult to treat, prospective evidence indicating that port site metastasis worsens prognosis is lacking. Treatment options include surgical excision and primary irradiation of the recurrence site, with or without systemic chemotherapy. Long-term outcomes with these therapeutic measures have not been compared; however, therapy should be individualized according to the extent, location, and other characteristics of recurrent disease.

Neurologic Injury

Operative nerve injury can complicate any surgical procedure in the pelvis. Concerns that are particular to gynecologic oncologic procedures, however, have been recognized. Genitofemoral nerve injury is most likely to occur during removal of the lateral pelvic lymph nodes. Such an injury results in medial thigh numbness but is otherwise of limited clinical consequence. It is arguably the most common injury encountered by the gynecologic oncologist.

Injury of the obturator nerve is a more concerning although extremely rare complication of laparoscopic lymph node dissection. In the division of gynecologic oncology at the Mount Sinai Medical Center, we have not experienced this complication since the early 1990s when first performing laparoscopic lymphadenectomies. This complication occurs only if the obturator nerve is not reliably identified before resection of the obturator lymph node package. It manifests as adductor weakness and decreased sensation of the anteromedial thigh.

Theoretically, the femoral nerve, which lies within the body of the psoas muscle in the pelvis, also is at risk during pelvic lymphadenectomy. Risk is particularly high if the nerve is superficial in the belly of the muscle and is exposed to extensive electrocautery during the dissection. Femoral nerve injury manifests as numbness over the anteromedial thigh, knee joint instability, absence of patellar reflex, and the patient's inability to raise the thigh while supine.

Other peripheral neuropathies also can occur secondary to poor patient positioning for operative laparoscopy.

Complications Requiring Laparotomy

Complications that can require conversion to laparotomy include damage to the ureter, bladder, or bowel and vascular injury. Kavoussi and associates[6] reported a 4% incidence of laparotomy with laparoscopic pelvic lymphadenectomy. Reasons for conversion to laparotomy included transection of the ureter (in two patients), cystotomy (in two patients), bowel injuries or obstruction (in four patients), and vascular injuries (in four patients). In another study by Boitke and colleagues,[23] laparotomy was required in 10% (3 of 29) of patients undergoing laparoscopic pelvic or para-aortic lymphadenectomy, or both, for endometrial cancer. Other authors have reported a lower incidence of laparotomy consequent to laparoscopy for gynecologic cancers. None of the 39 patients who underwent laparoscopic surgery for cervical cancer in the study reported by Querleu and co-workers[24] required laparotomy. In a review of four large series of 449 patients with gynecologic cancers, the mean conversion rate to laparotomy was 9.3%.[25]

Adequacy of Laparoscopic Surgery for Management of Gynecologic Cancers

Lymphadenectomy is performed primarily to evaluate for micrometastasis in the setting of a malignancy. It is therefore essential that the lymph node dissection achieve an adequate node retrieval by laparotomy or laparoscopy. Schlaerth and colleagues studied the adequacy of laparoscopic para-aortic lymph node sampling and therapeutic pelvic lymphadenectomy in women with stage IA, IB, and IIA cervical cancers.[27] In 69 patients, across seven institutions, the average number of lymph nodes retrieved was up to 70 (mean of 32) for pelvic nodes and up to 37 (mean of 12) for para-aortic nodes. The complication rate was 10% for vascular injury and 1.4% for ureteral injury. The investigators concluded that laparoscopic approach is a feasible alternative for retroperitoneal lymphadenectomy by laparotomy.

Other Complications

Various other complications can result as a consequence of laparoscopic surgery in patients with gynecologic cancer. As with laparotomy, both lymphoceles and lymphedema have been reported to occur after laparoscopic lymphadenectomy. In Childer and co-workers' experience with more than 300 pelvic lymphadenectomies, two symptomatic lymphoceles were reported.[7] In our report of 100 retroperitoneal lymphadenectomies using the harmonic scalpel, no lymphoceles were noted.[8] As might be expected with any operative procedure, infectious complications also have been reported, including infected pelvic hematomas, *Clostridium difficile* infection, and wound complications. Likewise, retained foreign bodies and equipment failure can preclude a safe and effective surgical exercise.

Thromboembolic events can complicate any major operative procedure in the pelvis, especially in patients with cancer. In a series of 40 patients who underwent bilateral pelvic and para-aortic lymphadenectomy for endometrial and ovarian cancer, the procedure was completed laparoscopically in 35 patients. Deep vein thrombosis developed in 2 of the patients (5.7%) during the postoperative period.

Complications and the Learning Curve

Most surgeons report a decrease in the number and severity of complications and a reduced operative time as they gain experience with advanced laparoscopic procedures. Of the aborted laparoscopic lymphadenectomies reported by Kavoussi and associates,[6] 88% occurred during the initial dissections at each contributing institution. Lang and co-workers[26] reported a significantly higher complication rate for the first 50 laparoscopic lymphadenectomies (14%) than for the next 50 such procedures (4%). It appears that with increasing experience, laparoscopic gynecologic oncologic procedures become safer and more efficient.

CONCLUSIONS

Laparoscopy is an evolving technique that plays an increasingly important role in the management of gynecologic malignancies. Laparoscopic radical hysterectomy, pelvic and para-aortic lymphadenectomy, and staging of early ovarian cancer all appear to be safe, adequate, and feasible procedures with low complication rates. The risks include those traditionally attributed to laparoscopy, as well as those inherent to open gynecologic oncologic procedures. The use of simple preventive measures allows the patient to benefit from this technique while diminishing the likelihood of complications.

References

1. Dargent D, Salvat J. L'envahissement ganglionnaire pelvien: Place de la pelviscopie retroperitoneale. Medsi, Paris: McGraw-Hill, 1989.
2. Nezhat CR, Burrell MO, Nezhat FR, et al. Laparoscopic radical hysterectomy with para-aortic and pelvic node dissection. Am J Obstet Gynecol 1992;166:864.
3. Nezhat CR, Nezhat FR, Ramirez CE, et al. Laparoscopic radical hysterectomy and laparoscopic assisted vaginal radical hysterectomy with pelvic and paraaortic node dissection. J Gynecol Surg 1993;9:105.
4. Vasilev SA, McGonigle KF. Extraperitoneal laparoscopic para-aortic lymph node dissection. Gynecol Oncol 1996;61:315.
5. Abu-Rustum NR. Laparoscopy 2003: Oncologic perspective. Clin Obstet Gynecol 2003;46:61.
6. Kavoussi LR, Sosa E, Chandhoke P, et al. Complications of laparoscopic pelvic lymph node dissection. J Urol 1993;149:322.
7. Childers JM, Hatch KD, Surwit EA. Laparoscopic para-aortic lymphadenectomy in gynecologic malignancies. Obstet Gynecol 1993;82:741.
8. Nezhat F, Yadav J, Rahaman J. Laparoscopic lymphadenectomy using ultrasound activated shears: Analysis of first 100 cases. 10th Biennial Meeting of the International Gynecologic Cancer Society, Edinburgh, Scotland, October 2004.
9. Nezhat CH, Seidman DS, Nezhat F, et al. Laparoscopic management of intentional and unintentional cystotomy. J Urol 1996;156:1400.
10. Sokol AI, Paraiso MF, Cogan SL, et al. Prevention of vesicovaginal fistulas after laparoscopic hysterectomy with electrosurgical cystotomy in female mongrel dogs. Am J Obstet Gynecol 2004;190:628.
11. Nezhat CR, Siegler AM, Nezhat FR, et al. Complications. In: Nezhat CR, Siegler AM, Nezhat FR, et al., eds. Operative gynecologic laparoscopy: Principles and techniques, 2nd ed. New York: McGraw-Hill; 2000;365.

12. Cogan SL, Paraiso MF, Bedaiwy MA. Formation of vesicovaginal fistulas in laparoscopic hysterectomy with electrosurgically induced cystotomy in female mongrel dogs. Am J Obstet Gynecol 2002;187:1510.

13. Lee RA, Symmonds RE, William TJ. Current status of genitourinary fistula. Obstet Gynecol 1988;72:313.

14. Nezhat CH, Nezhat F, Nezhat C, Rottenberg H. Laparoscopic repair of a vesicovaginal fistula: A case report. Obstet Gynecol 1994;83:899.

15. Ou CS, Huang UC, Tsuang M, Rowbotham R. Laparoscopic repair of vesicovaginal fistula. J Laparoendosc Adv Surg Tech 2004;14:17.

16. Nabi G, Hemal AK. Laparoscopic repair of vesicovaginal fistula and right nephrectomy for nonfunctioning kidney in a single session. J Endourol 2001;15:801.

17. Miklos JR, Sobolewski C, Lucente V. Laparoscopic management of recurrent vesicovaginal fistula. Int Urogynecol J Pelvic Floor Dysfunct 1999;10:116.

18. Nezhat C, Nezhat F, Seidman DS, Nezhat C. Incisional hernias after operative laparoscopy. J Laparoendosc Adv Surg Tech 1997;7:111.

19. Nezhat C, Nezhat F, Ambroze W, Pennington E. Laparoscopic repair of small bowel and colon. Surg Endosc 1993;7:88.

20. Nagarsheth NP, Rahaman J, Cohen CJ, et al. The incidence of port-site metastasis in gynecologic cancers. JSLS 2004;8:133.

21. Childers JM, Aqua KA, Surwit EA, et al. Abdominal-wall tumor implantation after laparoscopy for malignant conditions. Obstet Gynecol 1994;84:765.

22. Kruitwagen R, Swinkels BM, Keyser K, et al. Incidence and effect on survival of abdominal wall metastases at trocar or puncture sites following laparoscopy or paracentesis in women with ovarian cancer. Gynecol Oncol 1996;60:233.

23. Boitke GM, Lurain JR, Burk JJ. A comparison of laparoscopic management of endometrial cancer with traditional laparotomy. Society of Gynecologic Oncologists, Orlando, FL, February 1994.

24. Querleu D, Le Blanc E, Castelain B. Laparoscopic pelvic lymphadenectomy in the staging of early carcinoma of the cervix. Am J Obstet Gynecol 1991;164:579.

25. Scribner DR, Walker JL, Johnson GA. Laparoscopic pelvic and para-aortic lymph node dissection: Analysis of the first 100 cases. Gynecol Oncol 2001;82:498.

26. Lang GS, Ruckle HC, Hadley HR. 100 consecutive laparoscopic lymph node dissections: Comparing complications of the first 50 cases to the second 50 cases. Urology 1994;44:221.

27. Schlaerth JB, Spirtos NM, Carsow LF, et al. Laparoscopic retroperitoneal lymphadenectomy followed by immediate laparotomy in women with cervical cancer: A gynecologic oncology group study. Gynecol Oncol 2002;85:81.

Complications of Minimally Invasive Urogynecologic Surgery

Neeraj Kohli, John R. Miklos, and Rob Moore

The last decade has seen significant advances in minimally invasive treatment options for pelvic prolapse and stress urinary incontinence using the vaginal approach. Many of the recently introduced minimally invasive techniques for treatment of prolapse and incontinence are associated with blind needle passage through the retropubic, transobturator, and ischiorectal spaces and incorporation of mesh materials in order to minimize incision size, reduce postoperative pain, and improve long-term surgical outcomes. With rapid proliferation of these minimally invasive techniques, it is imperative that the gynecologic surgeon have a strong knowledge of the relevant pelvic anatomy and proper surgical technique and be able to recognize and manage common postoperative complications.

PROCEDURAL OVERVIEW

To provide a basic foundation for a discussion of recognition, prevention, and management of postoperative complications associated with minimally invasive prolapse and incontinence procedures, a basic procedural overview of the commonly employed surgical techniques for prolapse and incontinence is beneficial.

Anterior/Posterior Colporrhaphy

Traditional colporrhaphy techniques for surgical correction of cystocele and rectocele, first introduced in 1914 by Kelly and Dunn,[1] have long been the mainstay for anterior and posterior vaginal segment prolapse and continue to be the most commonly performed surgical procedures for cystocele and rectocele, respectively. A key concept in these repairs is general weakness or laxity of the endopelvic fascia resulting in descent of the bladder or rectum. For anterior colporrhaphy, the vaginal mucosa is incised in the midline from the bladder neck to the bladder base and then dissected off the underlying pubocervical fascia by means of a combination of blunt and sharp techniques. This dissection is carried out laterally to the pubic ramus on each side to assess for paravaginal defects. The repair is then performed by plicating the pubocervical fascia in the midline using a series of interrupted, delayed,

absorbable, or permanent sutures (Fig. 13–1). Excess vaginal mucosa is excised and the incision closed. An analogous procedure can be performed for the posterior vaginal segment for surgical correction of rectocele. In this case, the rectovaginal fascia is plicated from the apex of the rectocele to the perineal body, and corresponding perineoplasty is then performed (Fig. 13–2).

Site-specific defect repair implicates discrete breaks in the endopelvic fascia, resulting in hernias contributing to pelvic prolapse. The paravaginal defect, introduced by White and popularized by Richardson and associates over the last decade, describes lateral detachment of the pubocervical fascia from the lateral sidewall, resulting in a displacement cystocele.[2] These defects most commonly are repaired through an abdominal or laparoscopic approach, but repair also can be accomplished using a vaginal approach. A vaginal paravaginal repair is performed by reattaching the lateral edge of the detached pubocervical fascia to the white line from the ischial spine to the median aspect of the pubic symphysis using a series of interrupted sutures (Fig. 13–3). Site-specific repair of the rectocele also can be performed and is aided by rectal examination after exposure of the rectovaginal fascia. Often, discrete defects (midline, paravaginal, or tranverse) in the fascia are noted; site-specific repair can be accomplished using a series of interrupted sutures (Fig. 13–4).

Vaginal Vault Suspension Techniques

Support of the vaginal apex is thought to be the cornerstone of all successful pelvic prolapse operations. A variety of abdominal, vaginal, and laparoscopic apical support procedures are available to the gynecologic surgeon. A vaginal approach to apical prolapse often is preferred by many gynecologic surgeons because it can be routinely performed at the time of vaginal hysterectomy and colporrhaphy. Traditional and contemporary techniques require knowledge of the various support structures and surrounding relevant anatomy.

Sacrospinous Ligament Fixation

Although more than 43 different operations have been described for the surgical correction of post-hysterectomy

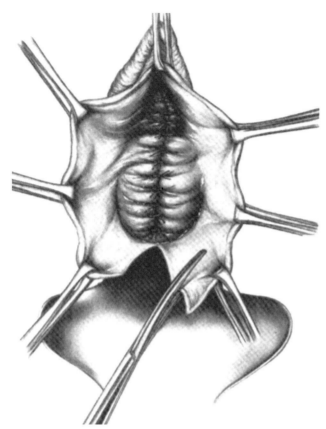

Figure 13–1 ▪ Technique of anterior repair with plication of the pubocervical fascia for cystocele repair.

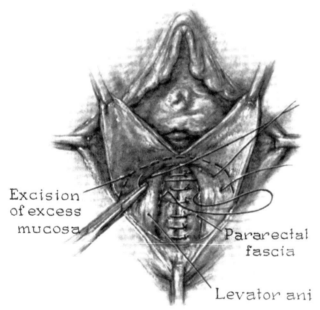

Figure 13–2 ▪ Technique of posterior repair with plication of the rectovaginal fascia for rectocele repair.

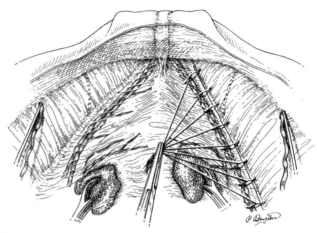

Figure 13–3 ▪ Retropubic view of paravaginal repair with reapproximation of the pubocervical fascia to the arcus tendineus fasciae pelvis (ATFP).

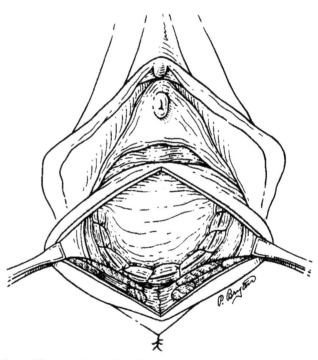

Figure 13–4 ▪ Site-specific defect repair of rectocele with closure of transverse fascial defect.

vaginal vault descensus,[3] no vaginal procedure has the extensive use and historical data comparable with those for the sacrospinous ligament fixation. In this technique, the sacrospinous space is entered through an anterior, midline, or posterior approach and the relevant pelvic anatomy is identified (Fig. 13–5). One or two sutures are taken through the upper edge of the sacrospinous-coccygeal ligament complex and then are attached to the vaginal apex using a full-thickness suture or pulley stitch (Fig. 13–6). Placement of the sacrospinous suture can be performed using a free needle holder, Miya hook, Dechamps ligature carrier, Schutt needle punch device, Endo-stitch (Ethicon, Somerville, New Jersey), or Capio needle driver (Boston Scientific, Natick, Massachusetts). Although the traditional sacrospinous ligament fixation describes unilateral suspension, many gynecologic surgeons favor bilateral sacrospinous suspension to improve cure rates and avoid unilateral deviation of the vaginal apex.

Figure 13–5 ▪ Anatomy of the sacrospinous space, including the ischial spine, sacrospinous ligament, arcus tendineus fasciae pelvis (ATFP), and coccygeus muscle. (Copyright Cleveland Clinic Foundation.)

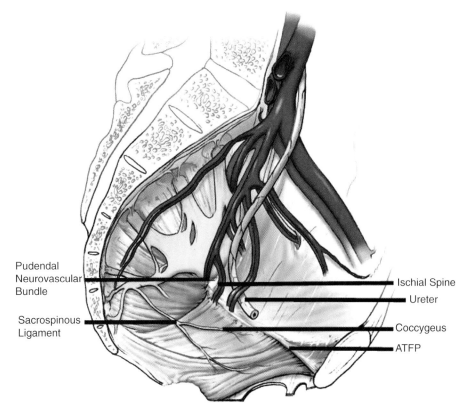

Pudendal Neurovascular Bundle

Sacrospinous Ligament

Ischial Spine

Ureter

Coccygeus

ATFP

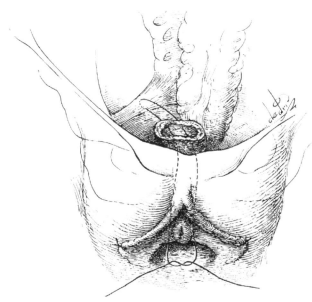

Figure 13–6 ▪ Technique of sacrospinous ligament fixation using pulley stitch to attach the vagina in the sacrospinous ligament for apical support.

Uterosacral Ligament Suspension

In an effort to provide a more anatomically correct midline suspension point, uterosacral ligament suspension, performed through a vaginal, abdominal, or laparoscopic approach, has gained recent popularity. Similar to the classically described McCall "cul-de-plasty," the uterosacral ligament suspension technique begins with adequate identification of the uterosacral ligaments through either a transperitoneal or a retroperitoneal vaginal approach. One or two sutures are then taken through the uterosacral ligament on each side and then attached to the vaginal apex. Care should be taken to identify the ureter before stitch placement, owing to its proximity and the possibility of kinking or obstruction. Tiedown of the suture results in anatomic restoration, with re-creation of the apical supports of the uterosacral ligament to the vaginal apex, as well as in closure of the anterior and posterior fascial planes (Fig. 13–7).

Iliococcygeus/Arcus Tendineus Fasciae Pelvis Fixation

To address the needs of patients with poor uterosacral ligament strength, and to avoid complications associated with sacrospinous ligament suspension such as buttock pain and pudendal neurovascular injury, iliococcygeus and arcus tendineus fasciae pelvis (ATFP) suspensions have been described. A dissection similar to that for sacrospinous ligament fixation is performed, and the relevant pelvic anatomy including the ischial spine, ATFP, and sacrospinous-coccygeal ligament complex is identified. One or two sutures are taken through either the ileococcygeus muscle or the ATFP and then attached to the vaginal apex using a full-thickness suture or pulley stitch. Unilateral or bilateral suspension can be performed.

Posterior Intravaginal Slingplasty Vault Suspension

Posterior Intravaginal Slingplasty Vault Suspension (Tyco-US Surgical, Norwalk, Connecticut) is a minimally invasive vaginal technique for vaginal vault suspension that uses needles and synthetic mesh to re-create apical support at the level of the ischial spine without midline deviation. The IVS

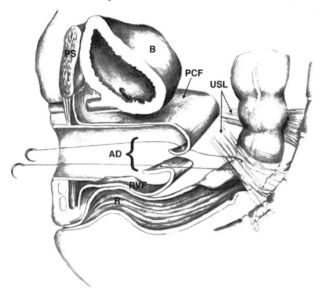

Figure 13–7 ▪ Vaginal approach to uterosacral ligament suspension with incorporation of the anterior pubocervical fascia (PCF) and posterior recto-vaginal fascia (RVF) in the uterosacral suspension suture (USL). AD, apical defect; B, bladder; R, rectum.

device consists of a trocar with a removable and reversible stylet into which a multifilament polypropylene tape can be threaded and brought up through the trocar. The procedure begins with bilateral sacrospinous space dissection and identification of the relevant anatomy, as previously described. Stab incisions in the buttocks are made bilaterally 3 cm lateral and 3 cm inferior to the anus. The trocar with tape attached is introduced through the stab wound, advanced through the ischiorectal fossa, and exited through the coccygeus muscle into the sacrospinous space under direct finger guidance. Alternatively, the needle can be exited lateral to the ischial spine near the insertion of the ATFP. The stylet with tape attached is then pulled out through the trocar. The same procedure is repeated on the other side with an empty stylus, and the free end of the tape is attached and pulled through the contralateral space. The apical portion of the tape is then attached to the vaginal apex, rectovaginal fascia, or graft material. The vaginal mucosa is closed and the traction on the free ends of the tape retracts the apex cephalad, thereby creating apical support. Excess tape is excised.

Mesh/Graft Augmentation of Prolapse Repair

Mesh or graft augmentation of prolapse repair has most recently been introduced with the hopes of improving long-term cure rates and reducing the risk of recurrence, which has been reported to be as high as 30%. In this technique, traditional colporrhaphy is performed and then a synthetic mesh or donor graft is used to reinforce the repair (Fig. 13–8). As with general surgery mesh use for hernia repairs, the augmented repair is thought to have greater strength and

Figure 13–8 ▪ Graft augmentation of rectocele repair with attachment of graft to levator muscles laterally and perineal body distally.

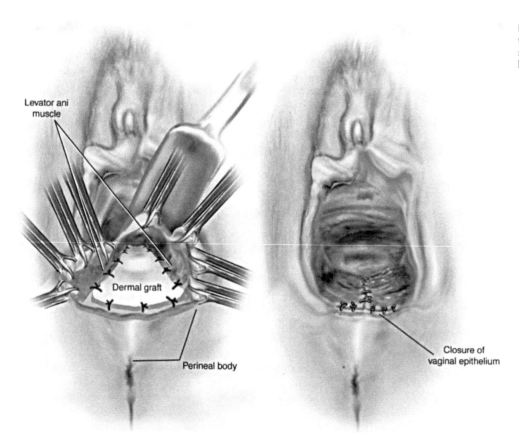

Table 13–1 ▪ Mesh and Graft Options for Prolapse

Type	Material	Trade Name	Company
Biologic	Human dermis	Repliform	Boston Scientific
Biologic	Bovine pericardium	Cytrix	Boston Scientific
Biologic	Porcine dermis	Pelvichol/Pelvisoft	CR Bard
Biologic	Porcine intestinal mucosa	SIS	Cook
Biologic	Cadaveric fascia lata	Tutoplast/Suspend	Mentor
Biologic	Porcine dermis	InteXen	AMS (American Medical Systems)
Synthetic	Polypropylene	Gynemesh	Gynecare
Synthetic	Polypropylene/porcine	Pelvitex	CR Bard
Synthetic	Polypropylene	Polyform	Boston Scientific

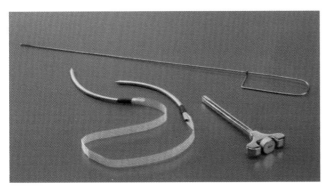

Figure 13–9 ▪ Tension-free vaginal tape (TVT) sling procedure: Instrumentation. Shown are introducer, rigid catheter guide, and TVT device (polypropylene mesh and attached trocars).

durability. A variety of graft or mesh materials are available (Table 13–1) and placement and attachment of the graft or mesh are nonstandardized. Direct mesh attachment, needle passage of the mesh, and nonattachment all have been described. Regardless of the technique, complications including mesh erosion and infection, dyspareunia or pelvic pain, and recurrence have been reported, and the gynecologic surgeon should approach this technique with caution in view of the limited data currently available.

Minimally Invasive Sling Procedures

TRANSVAGINAL RETROPUBIC SLING

Introduced in 1991, the tension-free vaginal tape (TVT) technique represents a revolutionary improvement in the suburethral sling procedure. Unique characteristics of the TVT technique include midurethral positioning of the sling, use of a polypropylene weave tape, and tension-free application without the need for large incisions or fascial attachment. Instrumentation for this procedure consists of a reusable stainless steel introducer, a reusable rigid catheter guide, and the TVT device, a single-use apparatus composed of a 1 × 40 cm strip of polypropylene mesh (Prolene, Ethicon Inc., Somerville, New Jersey) covered by a plastic sheath and held between two stainless steel needles (Fig. 13–9). The plastic sheath is designed to (1) cover the synthetic mesh during placement of the sling, thereby reducing the incidence of post-

operative infection or graft rejection, and (2) allow easy passage and placement of the tape, which is configured to stay fixed in place once the smooth protective cover is removed. This protective sheath is removed before completion of the procedure.

Two small abdominal skin incisions (0.5 to 1.0 cm) are made on each side of the midline just above the pubic symphysis. A small sagittal incision (1.5 cm) is then made in the midline of the anterior vaginal wall approximately 1 cm proximal to the external urethral meatus. The edges of this incision are grasped using tissue clamps, and minimal dissection is used to free the vaginal wall from the urethra and to develop a small paraurethral space bilaterally (Fig. 13–10). The rigid catheter guide is then inserted into the Foley catheter, facilitating identification of the urethra and the bladder neck during passage of the suspension needles. To minimize the risk of bladder or urethral perforation, the handle of the guide is deflected to the ipsilateral side just before insertion of the suspension needles.

Before placement of the sling, the introducer is attached to one of the stainless steel needles, and the speculum is removed from the vagina. The shaft of the introducer is grasped and the tip of the needle is then inserted into the previously developed paraurethral space. The needle is angulated slightly laterally, and the endopelvic fascia is perforated just behind the inferior surface of the pubic symphysis. On entry into the retropubic space, the needle is guided up to the abdominal incision while maintaining contact with the back of the pubic bone, thereby minimizing the risk of vascular or hollow viscous injury. A second layer of resistance is felt as the needle passes through the muscular and fascial layers of the abdominal wall. Passage of the needle is completed once the needle tip passes through the small abdominal incision on the corresponding side (Fig. 13–11).

Before complete extraction of the placement needle, unintentional bladder perforation should be ruled out. The rigid catheter guide is removed, and the bladder is emptied using the indwelling catheter. The catheter is then removed, and cystoscopy is performed to confirm integrity of the bladder lumen. If needle penetration of the bladder lumen is noted, the needle-introducer assembly is withdrawn, the bladder is drained, and the needle is reinserted. Once correct placement of the needle has been confirmed, the needle is detached from the introducer and passed completely through the abdominal incision. This technique is then repeated in an

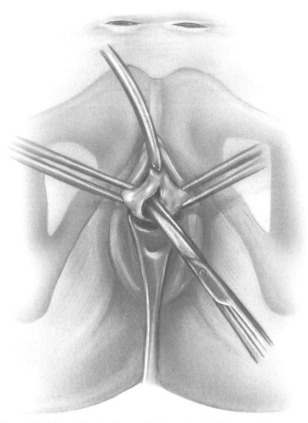

Figure 13–10 ▪ Tension-free vaginal tape (TVT) sling procedure: Vaginal dissection. Bilateral channels are created for needle insertion and mesh placement.

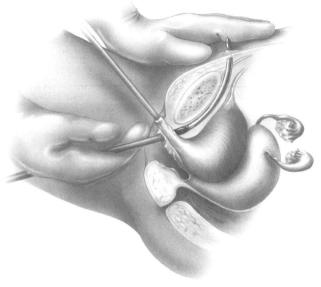

Figure 13–11 ▪ Tension-free vaginal tape (TVT) sling procedure: Passage of TVT needle and sling mesh through the retropubic space.

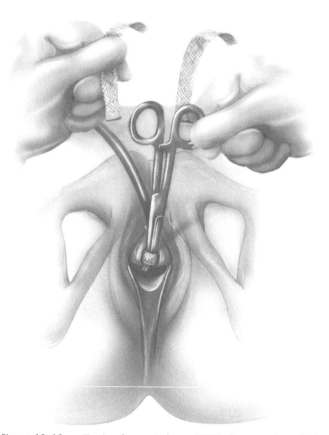

Figure 13–12 ▪ Tension-free vaginal tape (TVT) sling procedure: Final adjustment of the TVT sling after placement. This step can be performed in conjunction with a cough test to avoid overtightening the sling.

identical fashion on the contralateral side to ensure that the tape lies flat against the suburethral tissue at the level of the midurethra.

After passage of the needles has been completed, a clamp or scissors is inserted between the suburethral portion of the tape and the urethra. Gentle traction on the abdominal ends of the tape removes any excess tape material and brings the tape into contact with the instrument (Fig. 13–12). Both ends of the tape are then cut at their attachment to the needles. All instruments are removed from the surgical field, and the patient, if awake, is asked to perform a cough stress test to ensure that continence is restored without overcorrection. The tension on the tape is adjusted as appropriate. The plastic sheath of the abdominal ends of the tape is then identified and grasped with a forceps. With an instrument between the urethra and the tape, the plastic sheath is removed, leaving the Prolene tape secured under the midurethra without tension. The vaginal incision is closed. Next, the abdominal ends of the tape are cut just below the surface of the skin, without need for suture fixation. The friction between the tissues and the Prolene mesh keeps the tape in place while maintaining adequate suburethral support. Finally, the abdominal incisions are closed using either subcuticular stitches or surgical tape (Fig. 13–13).

Several TVT "me-too" products are currently available from a variety of manufacturers, using a polypropylene weave sling with slight variations in instrumentation and surgical technique (Table 13–2). Results and complications should be similar to those reported for TVT.

TRANSABDOMINAL RETROPUBIC SLING

After the introduction of the TVT procedure, an abdominal approach to the minimally invasive midurethral sling procedure was introduced by American Medical Systems (AMS). The SPARC (i.e., suprapubic arc) procedure uses Stamey-type

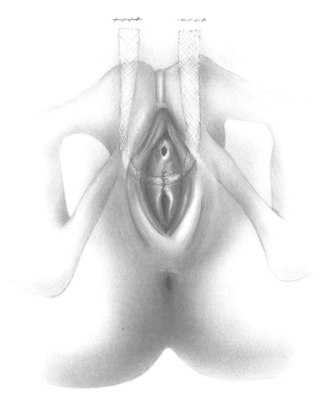

Figure 13–13 ■ Tension-free vaginal tape (TVT) sling procedure: Completed procedure with placement of suburethral hammock.

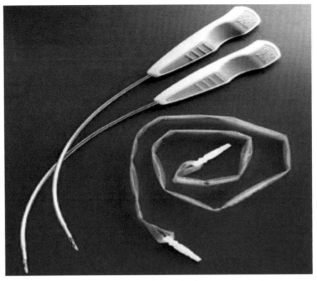

Figure 13–14 ■ Suprapubic arc (SPARC) sling procedure: Instrumentation. Shown are retropubic needles and the SPARC device (polypropylene mesh with attachment dilators).

Table 13–2 ■ Currently Available Transvaginal Retropubic Midurethral Sling Procedures

Manufacturer	Product Name
Gynecare	TVT (tension-free vaginal tape)
Boston Scientific	Advantage
CR Bard	Urotex TV
Cook	Stratasis TF Sling

Table 13–3 ■ Currently Available Suprapubic Retropubic Midurethral Sling Procedures

Manufacturer	Product Name
AMS (American Medical Systems)	SPARC
Gynecare	TVT-AG (tension-free vaginal tape–abdominal guide)
Boston Scientific	Lynx

As with TVT, several SPARC "me-too" products are currently available from a variety of manufacturers; all incorporate a polypropylene weave sling with slight variations in instrumentation and surgical technique (Table 13–3). Results and complications should be similar to those reported for SPARC.

TRANSOBTURATOR SLING

In an effort to simplify the procedure and reduce complications associated with retropubic passage of the minimally invasive midurethral sling needles, a transobturator approach has been advocated. This "outside-in" procedure initially was described in Europe and recently has been introduced in the United States. For the transobturator sling procedure, a 2-cm midline vaginal incision is made approximately 1 cm proximal to the external urethral meatus. The paraurethral tissue is bluntly dissected laterally underneath the pubic ramus until the medial edge of the obturator foramen is palpable. A small incision is made bilaterally in the skin of the groin area at the medial edge of the obturator foramen identified by palpation. This incision usually is just medial to the growing crease at the level of the clitoris. A helical or Emmet needle is then introduced through the groin incision, passed through the obtura-

needles (Fig. 13–14) to place a TVT-like mesh tape in the midurethra in an effort to be more "urology-friendly" while emulating traditional transvaginal needle suspension and traditional suburethral sling procedures. It rapidly gained popularity as an effective and familiar alternative to the TVT procedure.

The procedure begins with a similar dissection to the TVT, with a slightly larger vaginal incision used to allow finger insertion to the endopelvic fascia. The SPARC needles are inserted through each abdominal incision, guided through the retropubic space against the pubic bone, and exited through the vaginal incision under direct finger guidance. An identical procedure is performed on the contralateral side. Cystoscopy is performed to exclude bladder injury. The tape is attached to each needle, and the needles are retracted, thereby placing both arms of the sling. The sling is adjusted and the sheath removed as in the TVT procedure.

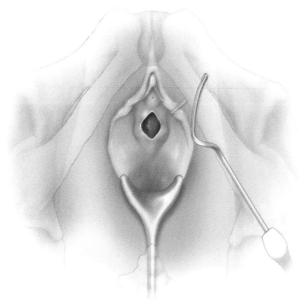

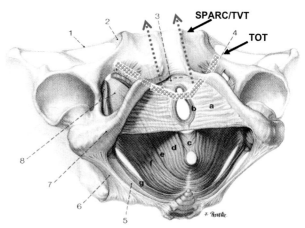

Figure 13–16 ■ Transobturator (TOT) sling procedure: Lateral placement of TOT, rather than midline attachment typical of transvaginal and retropubic approach, may result in less voiding dysfunction SPARC/TVT, suprapubic arc/tension-free vaginal tape.

Figure 13–15 ■ Transobturator sling procedure: Passage of needle through transobturator space. Bladder injury is prevented with exit of the needle through the vaginal incision under direct finger guidance.

tor foramen, and exited through the vaginal incision under direct finger guidance (Fig. 13–15). This procedure is repeated on the contralateral side. Cystoscopy is performed to rule out unintentional bladder injury. The mesh is attached in the needles, and the needles are withdrawn, placing both arms of the sling. Sling adjustment and sheath removal are similar to these steps in the TVT procedure. Avoiding passage of the needles through the retropubic space, the transobturator approach theoretically should reduce the risk of bowel, bladder, and major blood vessel injury. In addition, the transobturator technique results in gentle lateral placement, rather than midline retropubic placement, potentially reducing postoperative voiding dysfunction secondary to bladder outlet obstruction (Fig. 13–16).

Current product offerings for the outside-in approach include Obtape from Mentor (Santa Barbara, California), Monarc from AMS (Minneapolis, Minnesota), Obtryx from Boston Scientific (Natick, Massachusetts), and Urotex-transobturator from CR Bard (Covington, Georgia). Gynecare (Somerville, New Jersey) has introduced a variation of its TVT device, the TVT-Obturator, which proposes an inside-out approach to further minimize risk of vascular injury (Table 13–4).

INCIDENCE OF INJURIES

The incidence of injuries following minimally invasive procedures for correction of prolapse and incontinence is variable and highly dependent on surgical technique, clinician experience, and patient characteristics. In various studies, the incidence of major complications ranged from 0.5% to 12%. Shull and associates reported an 11% risk of perioperative morbidity including hemorrhage requiring transfusion, pelvic nerve injury, deep vein thrombosis, visceral injury, and infection,

Table 13–4 ■ Currently Available Transobturator Midurethral Sling Procedures	
Manufacturer	**Product Name**
AMS (American Medical Systems)	Monarc
Mentor	ObTape/Aris TOT Sling
Gynecare	TVT-O (tension-free vaginal tape–obturator)
CR Bard	Urotex TO
Boston Scientific	Obtryx

associated with transvaginal repair of cystocele,[4] as well as a 1% risk of transfusion requirement, 1% risk of ureteral injury or kinking, and a 0.3% perioperative death rate associated with transvaginal uterosacral ligament suspension.[5] In their review of 110 patients undergoing iliococcygeus vaginal vault suspension, Meeks and co-workers reported a 37% postoperative complication rate including postoperative transfusions, one bowel injury, and one bladder injury.[6] Buttock pain associated with placement of suture in the area of the pudendal nerve in the sacrospinous space has been reported to occur in up to 6% of patients, with resolution of the pain with conservative management in a majority.[7] The increased risk of significant bladder and ureteral injury following vaginal surgery, reported to be 2%, has prompted some gynecologic surgeons to recommend routine cystoscopy following major vaginal procedures.[8]

Mesh and graft use in prolapse surgery is still in an early stage of development, and long-term data regarding complications are scarce. In a limited series of 91 patients undergoing composite Vicryl-polypropylene mesh augmentation for rectocele repair, Lim and colleagues reported no significant intraoperative complications, except for minor hematoma, with an incidence of 2.2%. Minor vaginal protrusion was noted in 7.8% of patients (7 of 90) at 6 to 12 weeks and in 12.9% (4 of 31) at 6 months and beyond. All patients were managed by trimming the mesh, without need for removal.[9] In a small series of 52 patients undergoing polypropylene mesh augmentation for repair of cystocele or rectocele (or both), Adhoute reported a success rate of 95% or 100%, respectively, on follow-up of 27 months. Vaginal erosion occurred in only 2 patients.[10] Eglin and colleagues have similarly reported a low incidence of mesh erosion or exposure, 5% at 18 months' postoperative follow-up evaluation, using a transobturator technique to place the mesh in a subvesical position for cystocele repair.[11] Use of donor graft materials may be associated with reduced complications but also decreased cure rates. In their review of advanced cystocele repair in 33 women using Alloderm (Boston Scientific), a donor skin graft, Clemmons and associates reported a 41% objective failure rate and a 3% subjective failure rate at median 18-month follow-up evaluation. Twenty-one women (64%) were sexually active, and none complained of postoperative dyspareunia. Complications included 1 case of febrile morbidity, 1 cystotomy, and 1 anterior wall breakdown secondary to hematoma formation caused by heparin therapy. No other erosions or rejections were seen.[12]

Despite the recent introduction of the minimally invasive midurethral sling procedure, the incidence of injury with this technique has been well studied as a result of its rapid adoption and abundant literature. Significant data are available regarding the TVT procedure, with more limited data for the transabdominal retropubic sling and transobturator sling. In a review of their first 350 cases of the TVT procedure, Karram and associates reported a 4.9% incidence of bladder perforation and a 0.9% incidence of intraoperative hemorrhage. Postoperative complications included voiding dysfunction in 17 women (4.9%), requirement for anticholinergic therapy in 42 women (12%), recurrent bladder infections in 38 women (10.9%), mesh erosion or exposure in 3 patients (0.9%), and nerve injury in 3 patients (0.9%). Six women (1.7%) had persistent voiding dysfunction necessitating takedown of the sling.[13] Similar complication rates were noted in a multi-institutional review of findings in 241 patients undergoing the TVT procedure in Canada, with a bladder perforation rate of 5.8% and an intraoperative hemorrhage rate of 2.5%. Postoperative complications included urinary retention in 19.7% of patients, pelvic hematoma in 1.9%, and suprapubic wound infection in 0.4%. Rates for late complications—de novo urgency, persistent suprapubic discomfort, and mesh erosion—were 15%, 7.5%, and 0.4%, respectively.[14] In the largest study to date, a nationwide analysis of 1455 patients undergoing TVT in Finland reported that the incidence of bladder perforation was 38 per 1000, that of intraoperative blood loss greater than 200 mL was 19 per 1000, of major vessel injury 0.7 per 1000, of nerve injury 0.7 per 1000, of vaginal hematoma 0.7 per 1000, and of urethral lesion 0.7 per 1000. The incidence of minor voiding difficulty was 76 per 1000, that of urinary tract infection 41 per 1000, of complete postoperative urinary retention 23 per 1000, of retropubic hematoma 19 per 1000, of wound infection 8 per 1000, and of vaginal defect healing 7 per 1000. No case of tape rejection or life-threatening complication occurred, and the incidence of complications necessitating laparotomy was 3.4 per 1000.[15] Significant complications include bowel injury and obstruction,[16,17] bladder injury with vulvar edema,[18] and nerve injury.[19]

Data regarding complications associated with the transabdominal retropubic sling are less abundant. In a review of

their first 140 SPARC cases, Kobashi and colleagues reported 4 intraoperative transfusions, 1 retropubic hematoma requiring evacuation, and 1 case of small bowel injury. These investigators recommended caution with any technique involving blind passage of retropubic needles.[20] Tseng has reported a clinically significant greater risk of bladder injury after SPARC than after TVT (12.9% versus 0.0%; $P = .112$), although the difference was not statistically significant.[21] In a multicenter trial of 104 women undergoing SPARC in three centers, the overall complication rate was 44.2% (46 of 104 procedures). The perioperative complication rate was 10.5%, including 11 bladder injuries. A significant difference in the bladder injury rate was observed between women with and those without previous incontinence surgery (respectively, 4 of 11 [36.3%] versus 7 of 93 [7.5%]; $P < .001$). No hemorrhaging occurred. The early postoperative complication rate was 22.1%. The main complication was voiding disorders (in 11 patients), which necessitated intermittent self-catheterization for less than 15 days (1.3 ± 1.1 days, range 1 to 10 days). The late postoperative complication rate was 11.5%, including de novo urge symptoms in 12 women.[22]

Data regarding the recently introduced transobturator tape (TOT) sling procedure are limited, but initial results regarding surgical outcomes and complications are encouraging. In the earliest case reports of the procedure, Delorme reported no intraoperative complications in 32 women undergoing the procedure. One patient had prolonged urinary retention, which subsequently resolved, and de novo urge incontinence developed in two patients. In a randomized trial in 61 patients undergoing either TVT or TOT, bladder injury and postoperative voiding dysfunction were both more common after TVT than after TOT, 9.7% versus 0% and 25.8% versus 13.3%, respectively.[23] Despite direct guidance of the transobturator tape through the vaginal incision, bladder injury has been reported and intraoperative cystoscopy is recommended.[24]

PREVENTION, RECOGNITION, AND MANAGEMENT OF INJURIES

Intraoperative/Postoperative Bleeding and Hematoma

Prevention

Intraoperative hemorrhage is a common complication of pelvic surgery and can be minimized with proper dissection technique and development of proper surgical planes. During prolapse surgery, initial submucosal injection of an anesthetic-plus-epinephrine solution may reduce blood loss and facilitate entry into the proper plane. Sharp dissection allows entry into the proper plane, at which time blunt dissection can be used to extend the plane of dissection. Care should be taken in using a gauze-over-the-finger technique until a proper plane is identified, because this mode of dissection can result in greater bleeding and tissue damage.

During a minimally invasive sling procedure, bleeding can be prevented by injection of an anesthetic-plus-epinephrine solution into the retropubic and transobturator spaces, resulting in hydrodissection and decreased risk of intraoperative bleeding or hematoma. Proper dissection and correct insertion and guidance of the needles should reduce risk of excessive hemorrhage.

Recognition

Recognition of intraoperative hemorrhage often is obvious, but the source of bleeding sometimes can be difficult to determine and locate. During prolapse repair, most hemorrhage occurs with entry into the incorrect surgical plane. Risk factors include advanced prolapse with thickening of the tissue, previous vaginal surgery with resulting scarring, uterine fibroids with increased vascular supply, and menstruation. Caution is indicated with use of these procedures in patients on anticoagulant therapy or with coagulation disorders, who may require preoperative counseling and management. Location of the bleeding vessels most commonly is the paravaginal plexus, which is injured during lateral dissection and easily accessible to hemostatic suture placement. Advanced techniques using small incisions and entry into the sacrospinous space make identification of the bleeding vessels more difficult.

With minimally invasive sling procedures, bleeding most often occurs from the paravaginal plexus during retropubic needle placement and from the obturator vessels during transobturator sling procedures. Again, because of the small incisions and dissection associated with these minimally invasive procedures, localization of the bleeding source often is difficult, and conservative management is preferred. The operator must be knowledgeable of the relevant pelvic anatomy to ensure that injury to major blood vessels with passage of the retropubic needles or transobturator needles has not occurred (Fig. 13–17).

Patients with hematoma may present with abnormal vital signs suggesting anemia and hypovolemia but most commonly complain of pain in the area of the hematoma and bleeding. Retropubic and transobturator hematomas are associated with pain in the area, a palpable mass, and surrounding ecchymosis. A sacrospinous hematoma is associated with vaginal bleeding, palpable mass on rectal examination, and pelvic pain or dyschezia.

Management

Management of intraoperative hemorrhage and postoperative hematoma follows general principles of surgical hemostasis. The patient must be given colloid and blood products if bleeding is extensive or vital signs are abnormal. The source of bleeding should be located and cauterized or sutured as needed. Hemostasis should be ensured. Unfortunately, owing to the minimally invasive nature of recent prolapse and incontinence procedures, the incisions often are too small to provide adequate visualization and location of the leading source. Extension of the incision seldom improves visualization because of the inaccessible location (retropubic or sacrospinous space) of the potential bleeder. In such instances, tamponade and use of hemostatic agents (Surgicel) are preferred. Use of a 30-mL Foley catheter inserted into the bleeding area and then expanded can lead to effective tamponade. The catheter can be removed intraoperatively or sutured in place and removed in the postoperative period. In many cases, vaginal packing after the procedure is therapeutic. For cases of suspected retropubic venous bleeding, several hours of bladder distention with backfilling and clamping of an indwelling Foley catheter can be helpful. In patients with persistent postoperative bleeding indicated by vaginal bleeding or unstable vital signs or decreasing hematocrit, surgical reexploration or interventional radiology with embolization therapy is required.

Hematomas often can be managed conservatively with observation and symptomatic treatment including bedrest, pain medications, anti-inflammatory drugs, and local heat. In patients being managed conservatively, careful follow-up should be instituted for early recognition of abscess or mesh or graft erosion, if applicable. Large or expanding hematomas may require more aggressive treatment including radiologically guided drainage or surgical evacuation depending on clinical presentation.

Urinary Tract or Rectal Injury

Prevention

Prevention of viscous injury to the lower urinary tract or rectum requires good surgical technique and knowledge of the relevant anatomy. In patients with high risk for potential bowel injury, preoperative mechanical bowel preparation should be considered. Surgical dissection should be maintained in the proper plane, especially for patients at high risk for injury, including those with abnormal anatomy secondary to advanced prolapse, history of previous pelvic surgery, and attenuation of tissues secondary to vaginal atrophy. Special care should be taken in patients with enterocele, because the thinned vaginal mucosa comes into direct contact with the peritoneum and underlying bowel. Again, submucosal injection of an anesthetic-plus-epinephrine solution can reduce the chance of injury with initial incision. Correct technique of dissection and needle placement will prevent bowel or bladder injury. Care should be taken during dissection for prolapse repair and subsequent needle placement. Rectal injury has been reported with significant regularity during dissection into the sacrospinous space, especially in patients with adhe-

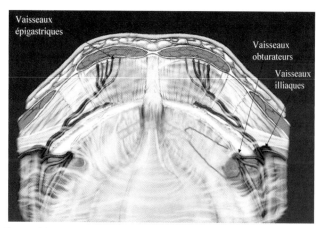

Figure 13–17 ■ Retropubic anatomy of major blood vessels and nerves potentially at risk of injury from tension-free vaginal tape (TVT) procedures.

sions secondary to previous surgery. Sharp dissection is recommended in such cases. Patients with previous retropubic surgery and alterations in the bladder anatomy are at higher risk for bladder perforation during retropubic minimally invasive sling procedures (Fig. 13–18). The risk of bowel injury can be reduced by placing the patient in Trendelenburg position.

Recognition

The most significant aspect of management of urinary tract and bowel injuries is recognition. Meticulous and methodical dissection should alert the experienced surgeon for any unintentional injury to these hollow-viscus organs. Expulsion of urine and or stool is an obvious sign, as is unexplained blood in the bladder or rectum.

To rule out bladder, ureteral, or urethral injury, cystoscopy with a 70-degree lens after intravous injection of 5 mL of indigo carmine is recommended. Examination of the entire bladder lumen, including the dome, lateral sidewalls, and trigone, is required. The ureters should demonstrate bilateral spill of dye, confirming ureteral patency. Foreign bodies including those related to stitch placement and needle injury should be excluded. The 70-degree lens can be used to evaluate the urethra during withdrawal of the cystourethroscope. Any signs of mesh or needle injury should be noted.

Rectal injury most often occurs during rectocele repair, sacrospinous dissection, or passage of the posterior IVS suspension needles. Before vaginal closure, rectal examination with digital palpation to the level of the ischial spines is recommended. Bowel injury should be suspected if a palpable

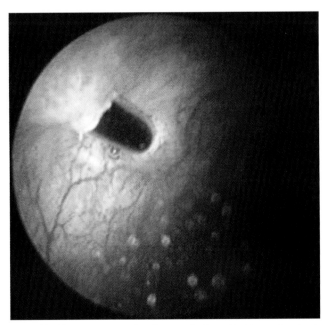

Figure 13–18 ■ Intraoperative photograph shows bladder perforation by needle during tension-free vaginal tape (TVT) procedure. The needle was removed, the bladder was decompressed, and needle passage was repeated with the needle in a more lateral position.

suture or mesh, visualized full-thickness defect, or significant alteration of the rectal anatomy is detected. In cases meriting a high index of clinical suspicion but with negative findings on examination, intraoperative anoscopy may be helpful. If the anoscope is unavailable, use of small Breisky-Navratil retractors can be helpful.

If bladder or rectal injury is suspected but not noted on cystoscopy or rectal examination or anoscopy, retrograde filling of the bladder or rectum, respectively, with approximately 200 mL of indigo carmine solution can be performed intraoperatively or postoperatively; a negative result will almost always exclude unintentional injury. Radiologic testing including a retrograde cystourethrogram and barium enema also can be helpful.

Management

Management of urinary tract and bowel injury will depend on the type and extent of the injury. Conservative measures often are the mainstay of treatment. In cases of bladder injury, any foreign body, including suture and needle or mesh, should be identified and removed as soon as possible. Repair of the cystotomy is performed using delayed absorbable suture in a double-layer closure with a watertight seal. An indwelling catheter should be left in place for constant drainage for 2 to 7 days, depending on the size and location of the bladder injury. For bladder injury associated with passage of minimally invasive sling needles, removal of the needle with completion of the procedure, followed by 24 to 48 hours of bladder drainage, should be sufficient. Ureteral injury most often involves obstruction or kinking of the ureter secondary to sutures for prolapse repair. Ureteral injury after minimally invasive sling procedures is extremely rare. Ureteral obstruction is confirmed by lack of dye extrusion from the ureteral orifice after intravenous administration of indigo carmine. An attempt to stent the nonspilling ureter will often help to identify the involved suture by indicating the level of obstruction. Suture removal is then indicated followed by confirmation of spill. Persistent or postoperative ureteral obstruction should be managed by percutaneous nephrostomy followed by surgical exploration. Urethral injury is rare after minimally invasive procedures for prolapse and incontinence. If urethral injury is noted, any surrounding foreign body must be removed, and a double-layer closure should be performed. A "vest-over-pants" repair with overlapping fascia flaps, followed by 7 to 10 days of catheterization using an indwelling catheter attached to constant drainage, is recommended to prevent subsequent fistula formation. Care should be taken with repairs close to the continence zone, because of an increased risk of postoperative urinary incontinence secondary to urethral sphincter damage.

Bowel injury is uncommon after vaginal surgery. Once identified, any foreign body should be removed from the site of injury, the area copiously irrigated with antibiotic solution, and the incision closed in a double-layer fashion perpendicular to the long axis of the bowel. Postoperative wound management including use of stool softeners and low-residue diet will facilitate wound healing, and careful follow-up should include rectal examination to exclude persistent injury or fistula.

Postoperative Voiding Dysfunction

Prevention

Postoperative voiding dysfunction, defined as urinary retention, incomplete bladder emptying, or abnormal urine stream, most commonly occurs after prolapse or incontinence surgery associated with significant pelvic floor neuropathy or bladder outlet obstruction. Patients with risk factors including older age, preoperative voiding dysfunction, previous pelvic surgery, or diabetes or history of spinal cord injury, and those undergoing incontinence procedures, should be counseled appropriately. Some clinicians advocate preoperative teaching of intermittent self-catheterization so that patients are able to appropriately manage postoperative voiding dysfunction. Prevention of postoperative voiding dysfunction includes minimizing surgical dissection and associated pelvic floor neuropathy, as well as avoiding overcorrection of the bladder neck during anterior colporrhaphy and suburethral slings.

The goal of most incontinence procedures is to prevent bladder neck descent during dynamic increases in abdominal pressure, with no elevation during static rest. "Tension-free" application minimizes risk of postoperative voiding dysfunction. Unfortunately, little standardization of proper sling adjustment has been achieved, but various surgeons have recommended use of a dilator in between the urethra and sling during sheath removal, intraoperative cough stress test, and use of a Babcock clamp to pinch off an appropriate length of tape. Most often, correct adjustment of the sling is based on clinical experience and surgical acumen.

Recognition

We recommend a postoperative voiding trial in all patients undergoing pelvic surgery for prolapse or incontinence. Various voiding protocols exist, but we use the following technique before discharge. The bladder is backfilled with 300 mL of normal saline using the indwelling Foley catheter, which is then removed. The patient is asked to spontaneously void into a "voiding hat" within 30 minutes. The amount of voided urine is measured; at least 200 mL is considered normal. Otherwise, the catheter is replaced and attached to constant drainage, and the patient is requested to return for repeat voiding trial at outpatient follow-up evaluation in 24 to 48 hours. Ideally, a uroflow and measurement of postvoid residual also should be performed on postoperative evaluation, to ensure that the quantity and quality of the patient's void are within normal parameters. This approach is especially recommended if the patient has complaints of abnormal voiding. Warning signs of voiding dysfunction include suprapubic discomfort or distention, overflow incontinence, and urinary hesitancy. On examination of affected patients, the bladder is noted to be palpable and overdistended.

Management

Management of postoperative voiding dysfunction is most commonly conservative and consists of expectant management with intermittent self-catheterization or indwelling Foley catheterization with intermittent voiding trials. Most patients will spontaneously improve, with resumption of normal pelvic floor nerve function. In patients with voiding dysfunction persisting beyond 2 to 3 weeks, further evaluation is recommended. Pain management can minimize voiding dysfunction secondary to nerve stimulation from sensory afferents. Urinalysis or urine culture should be performed to rule out infection. Examination should be performed to exclude hematoma or levator muscle spasm, which can occur after pelvic surgery. Uroflow studies with measurement of postvoid residual or multichannel urodynamic testing may help determine whether the voiding dysfunction is secondary to detrusor dysfunction or to bladder outlet obstruction. In patients with detrusor dysfunction, continued catheterization, bladder rest, and physical therapy should be initiated; symptoms usually resolve with time. In patients with persistent detrusor dysfunction, Interstim neuromodulation (Medtronic, Inc.) with placement of an indwelling electrode in the S3 foramen should be considered. In patients with bladder neck obstruction, loosening or revision of the sling should be considered.

This technique is easily performed in the outpatient surgical setting with use of local anesthesia. The previous incision is infiltrated with local anesthetic and then the skin is re-incised. Dissection exposes the area of previous surgery, and the sling often is visible. Placement of an 18 Fr Foley catheter and palpation of the sling against the catheter in the suburethral position sometimes facilitate identification of the tape. Careful dissection in the lateral portion of the tape will free the tape from the underlying suburethral tissue, and the tape can then be stretched and pulled down, thereby relieving the obstruction. In some cases, stretching of the tape is not possible, and excision is necessary. Care should be taken to avoid excessive dissection and potential urethral injury. The recurrent incontinence rate following sling takedown is approximately 20%. After completion of the repair, repeat voiding trial and uroflow studies should be performed to confirm return of normal voiding.

Postoperative Urinary Incontinence and Overactive Bladder Syndrome

Prevention

Prevention of postoperative urinary incontinence and overactive bladder syndrome depends on appropriate preoperative diagnosis. Patients with advanced pelvic prolapse can have an incidence of stress urinary incontinence as high as 83%, with an increased risk of intrinsic sphincter deficiency.[25] Often, the potential stress incontinence is masked by kinking of the urethra secondary to advanced anterior prolapse. Subsequent prolapse surgery without a concurrent incontinence procedure will result in postoperative urinary incontinence. Care must be taken during surgical dissection for prolapse and incontinence to avoid injury to the bladder or urethra and subsequent fistula formation. Correct adjustment of the suburethral sling will prevent persistent stress incontinence due to undercorrection and overflow incontinence or voiding dysfunction due to overcorrection. In patients with preoperative overactive bladder syndrome or detrusor instability, minimal pelvic dissection and loose placement of the sling are recommended, to avoid further neuropathy and bladder outlet obstruction, respectively.

Recognition

Considerations in the differential diagnosis for persistent incontinence after minimally invasive sling procedure include overactive bladder syndrome with detrusor instability, overflow incontinence secondary to bladder outlet obstruction, surgical failure with persistent stress incontinence, and urogenital fistula. Extensive evaluation should be deferred until after the immediate postoperative period, because many of the patient's symptoms will spontaneously resolve. Persistent incontinence warrants further evaluation, including urodynamic testing to exclude detrusor instability, uroflow studies and measurement of postvoid residual to exclude urinary retention, cough stress test to exclude persistent stress incontinence, and bladder filling test with dye or cystoscopy to exclude fistula or foreign body. Outpatient evaluation including a voiding diary can provide additional clinical information. Patients with frequent small voids most probably have overactive bladder or urge incontinence or overflow incontinence. Patients with constant leakage may suffer from fistula, and patients without improvement of preoperative symptoms most probably have refractory stress incontinence.

Management

Management of postoperative urinary incontinence or overactive bladder symptoms will depend on the diagnosis. Patients often will have transient overactive bladder syndrome or urge incontinence after pelvic surgery. These symptoms usually resolve spontaneously without significant intervention. For patients with persistent or bothersome symptoms, further evaluation and treatment may be warranted. Urinary tract infection should be treated and cystoscopy performed to exclude foreign body erosion. Patients with overactive bladder syndrome may benefit from a short course of bladder retraining, fluid restriction, and anticholinergic therapy.

Overflow incontinence due to bladder neck obstruction should be managed as reviewed previously. Uroflow and measurement of postvoid residual are diagnostic. Most commonly, this condition responds well to continued bladder drainage or intermittent self-catheterization. Cholinergic agents have little therapeutic value, with bladder neck obstruction and sling release indicated for persistent symptomatology.

Surgical failure following minimally invasive sling procedure is uncommon and probably is related to poor adjustment of the sling at the time of surgery. Patients with concurrent intrinsic sphincter deficiency or fixed urethra may be at increased risk for surgical failure. Treatment options will depend on the extent of persistent incontinence and the patient's symptomatology. Patients with mild refractory stress incontinence may benefit from pelvic floor exercises and physical therapy including electrical stimulation. Vaginal cones also have been recommended as a simple biofeedback technique. Patients who prefer a minor surgical procedure may benefit from injection of periurethral bulking agents, which can be performed in the office setting with use of local anesthesia. Patients with significant refractory incontinence may be candidates for either plication of the previous sling or repeat sling placement.[26]

Plication of the sling is an easy procedure that can be effectively performed in an outpatient setting. The original incision is infiltrated with anesthetic and incised. Dissection and identification of the sling are performed as previously described. With the patient awake and the bladder full, persistent stress incontinence is confirmed on cough stress test. The sling is then plicated using a permanent suture, and cough stress test is repeated. If the test result is positive, the original plication suture is removed and a larger segment of the sling is plicated. This procedure is continued until cough stress test result is just negative. Plication of the sling can be performed in the suburethral position, but lateral plication is recommended to avoid risk of urethral erosion. A voiding trial is recommended before discharge.

Fistula formation after minimally invasive prolapse and incontinence surgery is uncommon; fistula most commonly manifests 4 to 6 weeks following surgery with primary complaints of continuous and severe incontinence unrelated to activity or urgency. Diagnosis often is made on pelvic examination or cystoscopy but sometimes requires bladder instillation of dye with subsequent cough or tampon test. Management of urogenital fistula has previously been reviewed, and it is imperative to remove any foreign material in the area of the fistula before surgical correction. Timing of fistula repair is controversial, but most surgeons recommend repair 3 to 6 months after initial formation, to permit surrounding inflammation to subside, promoting improved healing. Use of an indwelling Foley catheter for 10-14 days is recommended.

Mesh Exposure/Erosion

Prevention

Prevention of mesh exposure or erosion depends on meticulous intraoperative surgical technique. Risk factors for this complication include vaginal atrophy, hemorrhage or hematoma, infection, and tension on the suture line. Preoperative and postoperative vaginal estrogen supplementation is recommended. Dissection of the vaginal mucosa should be deeper to prevent subsequent mesh erosion. Hemorrhage and risk for hematoma should be minimized to avoid infection and irritation of the mesh. We strongly recommend that redundant vaginal mucosa not be excised when a mesh or graft is placed underneath, because tension on a devascularized suture line will increase the risk of exposure or erosion. Care also must be taken to prevent unintentional "buttonholing" of the vagina, which may increase risk of mesh exposure. Postoperatively, a loosely placed vaginal packing with estrogen vaginal cream is recommended to place pressure on dead space and prevent hematoma formation, facilitate bonding of the vaginal mucosa to the underlying mesh, and provide local estrogen immediately postoperatively.

Recognition

Mesh exposure or erosion most commonly occurs in the short- to long-term postoperative period. Common presenting symptoms include vaginal discharge or bleeding, pelvic pain, dyspareunia, and protrusion or expulsion of mesh. Vaginal examination often will reveal mesh exposure or erosion on inspection. Digital vaginal examination is especially helpful to delineate the full extent of exposure or erosion and to identify any surrounding eroded filaments. Cystoscopy for anterior and examination for posterior vaginal wall mesh exposure or erosion are recommended. Of note, no generally accepted "safety time zone" for mesh exposure or erosion has been recognized, and this complication has been reported to occur as long as 10 years after mesh placement.[27] The experienced clinician will have a high index of suspicion for mesh exposure or erosion in any patient with the aforementioned symptomatology and a history of mesh placement.

Management

Management of mesh exposure or erosion begins with conservative treatment including pelvic rest and vaginal estrogen supplementation. Some clinicians also have recommended concurrent use of vaginal antibiotic cream (Cleocin or Flagyl). Close follow-up evaluation with regular examinations will reveal spontaneous healing in up to 30% of patients. In patients with persistent mesh exposure or erosion, vaginoplasty with or without excision of the eroded portion of the mesh is required. Complete removal of the mesh is not necessary and may prove difficult because of subsequent tissue and growth. The procedure can be performed using regional anesthesia on an outpatient basis. A spinal or pudendal block is preferred, to avoid injection of a vasoconstrictive agent into the surrounding inflammatory tissue. The surrounding inflammatory tissue is excised and a vaginal flap is mobilized. If possible, fascia is plicated over the eroded mesh, and then the vaginal mucosa is closed using a series of interrupted delayed absorbable sutures. Depending on the size of the mesh exposure or erosion (greater than 1 cm), the eroded portion of the mesh may have to be excised. Removal of the mesh has not been associated with recurrent prolapse or incontinence in most patients.

CONCLUSIONS

Complications associated with minimally invasive surgical procedures for prolapse and incontinence are uncommon and can readily be prevented and managed, with good outcomes. As with all surgical procedures, the key is prevention; good surgical technique and knowledge of relevant anatomy constitute the cornerstone of management. Intraoperative recognition is the next step to successful management of postoperative complications, and the experienced surgeon should be vigilant for intraoperative signs of complications. Postoperative complications occurring in the immediate and short-term postoperative period should be diagnosed and managed aggressively, to limit further risk and prevent long-term damage. With prompt recognition and management, most complications can be treated efficiently and effectively with little compromise in surgical success rates.

References

1. Kelly HA, Dumm WM. Urinary incontinence in women without manifest injury to the bladder. Surg Gynecol Obstet 1914;18:444.

2. Richardson CA, Edmonds PB, Williams NL: Treatment of stress urinary incontinence due to paravaginal fascial defect. Obstet Gynecol 1981;57:352.

3. Ridley JH. A composite vaginal vault suspension using fascia lata. Am J Obstet Gynecol 1976;126:590.

4. Shull BL, Bachofen C, Coates KW, Kuehl TJ. A transvaginal approach to repair of apical and other associated sites of pelvic organ prolapse with uterosacral ligaments. Am J Obstet Gynecol 2000;183:1365.

5. Shull BL, Bachofen C, Coates KW, Kuehl TJ. A transvaginal approach to repair of apical and other associated sites of pelvic organ prolapse with uterosacral ligaments. Am J Obstet Gynecol 2000;183:1365.

6. Meeks GR, Washburne JF, McGehee RP, Wiser WL. Repair of vaginal vault prolapse by suspension of the vagina to iliococcygeus (prespinous) fascia. Am J Obstet Gynecol 1994;171:1444.

7. Lovatsis D, Drutz HP. Safety and efficacy of sacrospinous vault suspension. Int Urogynecol J Pelvic Floor Dysfunc 2002;13:308.

8. Pettit PD, Petrou SP. The value of cystoscopy in major vaginal surgery. Obstet Gynecol 1994;84:318.

9. Lim YN, Rane A, Muller R. An ambispective observational study in the safety and efficacy of posterior colporrhaphy with composite Vicryl-Prolene mesh. Int Urogynecol J Pelvic Floor Dysfunc 2004;Sep 25.

10. Adhoute F, Soyeur L, Pariente JL, et al. Use of transvaginal polypropylene mesh (Gynemesh) for the treatment of pelvic floor disorders in women. Prospective study in 52 patients. Prog Urol 2004;14:192.

11. Eglin G, Ska JM, Serres X. Transobturator subvesical mesh. Tolerance and short-term results of a 103 case continuous series. Gynecol Obstet Fertil 2003;31:14.

12. Clemons JL, Myers DL, Aguilar VC, Arya LA. Vaginal paravaginal repair with an AlloDerm graft. Am J Obstet Gynecol 2003;189:1612.

13. Karram MM, Segal JL, Vassallo BJ, Kleeman SD. Complications and untoward effects of the tension-free vaginal tape procedure. Obstet Gynecol 2003;101(5 Pt 1):929.

14. Abouassaly R, Steinberg JR, Lemieux M, et al. Complications of tension-free vaginal tape surgery: A multi-institutional review. BJU Int 2004;94:110.

15. Kuuva N, Nilsson CG. A nationwide analysis of complications associated with the tension-free vaginal tape (TVT) procedure. Acta Obstet Gynecol Scand 2002;81:72.

16. Leboeuf L, Mendez LE, Gousse AE. Small bowel obstruction associated with tension-free vaginal tape. Urology 2004;63:1182.

17. Peyrat L, Boutin JM, Bruyere F, et al. Intestinal perforation as a complication of tension-free vaginal tape procedure for urinary incontinence. Eur Urol 2001;39:603.

18. Tseng LH, Lo TS, Wang AC, et al. Bladder perforation presenting as vulvar edema after the tension-free vaginal tape procedure. A case report. J Reprod Med 2003;48:824.

19. Geis K, Dietl J. Ilioinguinal nerve entrapment after tension-free vaginal tape (TVT) procedure. Int Urogynecol J Pelvic Floor Dysfunc 2002;13:136.

20. Kobashi KC, Govier FE. Perioperative complications: The first 140 polypropylene pubovaginal slings. J Urol 2003;170:1918.

21. Tseng LH, Wang AC, Lin YH, et al. Randomized comparison of the suprapubic arc sling procedure vs tension-free vaginal taping for stress incontinent women. Int Urogynecol J Pelvic Floor Dysfunc 2004;Oct 27.

22. Deval B, Levardon M, Samain E, et al. A French multicenter clinical trial of SPARC for stress urinary incontinence. Eur Urol 2003;44:254.

23. De Tayrac R, Deffieux X, Droupy S, et al. A prospective randomized trial comparing tension-free vaginal tape and transobturator suburethral tape for surgical treatment of stress urinary incontinence. Am J Obstet Gynecol 2004;190:602.

24. Minaglia S, Ozel B, Klutke C, et al. Bladder injury during transobturator sling. Urology 2004;64:376.

25. Veronikis DK, Nichols DH, Wakamatsu MM. The incidence of low-pressure urethra as a function of prolapse-reducing technique in patients with massive pelvic organ prolapse (maximum descent at all vaginal sites). Am J Obstet Gynecol 1997;177:1305.

26. Riachi L, Kohli N, Miklos J. Repeat tension-free transvaginal tape (TVT) sling for the treatment of recurrent stress urinary incontinence. Int Urogynecol J Pelvic Floor Dysfunc 2002;13:133.

27. Kohli N, Walsh PM, Roat TW, Karram MM. Mesh erosion after abdominal sacrocolpopexy. Obstet Gynecol 1998;92:999.

Complications of Pediatric and Adolescent Laparoscopy

14

Ryan J. Zlupko and Joseph S. Sanfilippo

Operative laparoscopy in children has continued to gain wider acceptance in the surgical community. Work by international and domestic pioneers in the field of pediatric surgery demonstrated the feasibility of these procedures.[1] Pathologic conditions involving the adnexa commonly may be found at the time of laparoscopy in patients presenting with abdominal pain. Adnexal torsion and ovarian cysts may manifest with abdominal pain with or without a pelvic mass.[2,3] Solid neoplasms in the abdomen are being approached laparoscopically as well, for both diagnostic and therapeutic interventions.[4,5] As the volume of these procedures has increased, so has the database of reported complications. This chapter reviews key technical considerations for the gynecologic surgeon who performs minimally invasive procedures and also examines the current evidence regarding operative complications for procedures in the pediatric population.

SPECIAL CONSIDERATIONS IN THE PEDIATRIC AND ADOLESCENT POPULATION

Patient Selection

Despite the growing range of clinical problems being addressed endoscopically, basic surgical principles still apply. Choosing appropriate candidates for a minimally invasive approach is an essential first step for the clinician. Patients should be hemodynamically stable. Underlying medical conditions that may contribute to morbidity associated with the procedure, such as sepsis, coagulopathy, or other derangements of metabolism, should be medically corrected or stabilized before any surgical intervention is undertaken. Emergency procedures deemed necessary in the unstable patient may still remain an indication for traditional open surgery. Oncologic procedures that traditionally were always performed through a laparotomy incision are a subject of ongoing study.[5,6]

Diagnosis of surgical disease remains a cornerstone of good medical practice. History and physical examination are fundamental to correct diagnosis and proper patient selection. Imaging techniques such as computed tomography (CT) scan, magnetic resonance imaging (MRI), and ultrasonography

often are valuable additions that may confirm or refute clinical suspicions before operative intervention. Such a scenario is illustrated in cases of pelvic pain with or without the presence of a mass. For the female patient, adnexal masses may result in ovarian torsion. The differential diagnosis for lower quadrant right-sided pain usually includes appendicitis. Clinical presentations in older children and adolescents will be similar to those in adults with regard to symptoms of both ovarian torsion and appendicitis. Abdominal pain with or without nausea or vomiting is common to both. Depending on the age of the patient, more focus may be placed on the physical examination to determine the etiology of symptoms, especially in the very young child. Demeanor and body language can be telling with signs of irritability or abdominal guarding.

Surgical teaching has traditionally followed a motto of "See one, do one, teach one." Increasing evidence in the laparoscopic literature shows that the associated learning curve for these procedures can be both steep and extended. Various reviews for procedures such as splenectomy and Nissen fundoplication demonstrate that complications are minimized and efficiency maximized at close to 20 to 40 procedures.[7,8] Formal laparoscopic training during hospital residency has been shown to increase accuracy and speed of procedures.[9,10] Specialized training and mentoring should be undertaken as needed. As always, surgeons must be acutely aware of the level of their own surgical skill and experience to ensure the best outcomes for their patients.

Consent for a laparoscopic approach is vital to the ethical treatment of all patients. In discussing surgical approaches with the family, advantages of a laparoscopic versus a laparotomic approach to be mentioned include decreased postoperative pain, shorter hospitalization, faster return to normal activity, and a better cosmetic result. Efficacy in most series seems equivocal. Discussion of conversion to laparotomy is standard.

Anesthesia

Laparoscopy in the pediatric patient presents some special concerns for the anesthesiologist.[11-13] Carbon dioxide (CO_2) insufflation and the rise in intra-abdominal pressure can exert deleterious effects on normal physiology and must be addressed in these patients.

The increased intra-abdominal pressure from insufflation will decrease preload after 10 mm Hg and increase afterload in the heart causing decreased cardiac output. Pressures greater than 10 mm Hg may actually increase venous return by emptying splanchnic beds. Increased intra-abdominal pressure also increases intracranial pressure, thereby decreasing cerebral perfusion.

CO_2 is better absorbed from the thin abdominal cavity in these patients, leading to hypercapnia. Likewise, the increased intra-abdominal pressure in concert with the head-down position leads to increased peak airway pressures, decreased diaphragmatic excursion, decreased thoracic compliance, and decreased forced respiratory capacity, resulting in decreased oxygenation.

The high body surface area–to-mass ratio and minimal subcutaneous fat in the pediatric patient allow for rapid loss of heat in the operating room, especially with circulation of cold CO_2 in the peritoneal cavity. Monitoring of core body temperature is essential, and use of external warmers should be almost routine. Warmed, humidified CO_2 systems also may be of some benefit.

The value of preoperative medication in the pediatric patient is still debated in the literature. If needed, preoperative medication with midazolam is preferred over opiates or barbiturates because of the risk of hypoventilation with the latter two. Anticholinergic premedication also may blunt the vagal response seen with entry into the peritoneal cavity. Induction of anesthesia may be achieved with intravenous or inhalational agents. Routine American Society of Anesthesiologists (ASA) monitoring should be maintained.

Induction of anesthesia may be performed in any of several ways. Induction with isoflurane has been shown to have less effect on pulmonary vasculature than occurs with either halothane or enflurane. Newer agents such as desflurane and sevoflurane seem to be equivalent to isoflurane. Intravenous induction with a barbiturate or propofol may lead to hypotension secondary to negative inotropic and vasodilatory properties. Etomidate will provide effective anesthesia without the negative cardiovascular effects. The maintenance phase of anesthesia should generally avoid halothane because of concerns over increased cardiac sensitivity with hypercarbia. Decreased hepatic blood flow also may predispose the patient to increased halothane hepatotoxicity. Nitrous oxide also is avoided because of increased postoperative nausea and vomiting associated with its use. Typically, anesthesia is maintained with an inhalational agent (isoflurane, desflurane, or sevoflurane), supplemented by intravenous opioids. Neuromuscular blockade can be provided by any of the nondepolarizing agents. Preemptive intravenous antiemetics, such as metoclopramide, are used routinely.

Endotracheal intubation with controlled ventilation is preferred. Prevention of hypercarbia may require up to a 20% to 60% increase in minute ventilation. Use of positive end-expiratory pressure (PEEP) may help decrease the incidence of atelectasis and shunting, thereby improving oxygenation.

Maintaining adequate ventilation and perfusion requires an appreciation for these changes with specific interventions as outlined previously. The anesthesiologist may safely maintain patients in this age group for laparoscopic procedures.

Several series have shown the safety of anesthesia using these principles.[12-14]

Equipment

Early pioneers in the field of pediatric laparoscopy were limited to procedures in older children and adolescents because of the availability of only adult-sized laparoscopes and instruments. These instruments were ill suited to the small working spaces and delicate tissues found in young children. Advances in rod-lens technology and brighter light sources have allowed the development of laparoscopes with diameters of less than 2 mm. Advanced digital systems have added to the ability to gain adequate visualization without increasing the size of the instrument. Operative graspers and scissors also have been miniaturized for operation on the smallest of patients. Of note, smaller equipment usually is more delicate and may break easily during surgery or, more commonly, during postoperative care and cleaning. Having backup instruments readily available is likely to avoid major surgical delays when problems with equipment occur. Most cases can be accomplished with 5- to 10-mm scopes and 3- to 5-mm instruments in all pediatric patients except infants.[14,15]

Laparoscopic resolution is intimately linked to lighting. The best optical equipment will fail to provide adequate visualization if connected to an inferior light source. A general rule of thumb is to obtain the brightest source available and to carefully monitor the fiberoptic cords. General wear and tear eventually snaps the individual fiberoptic strands bundled in the cord. Cord replacement generally is recommended if more than 25% of the fibers are broken.

The adult abdomen may require 2.5 to 4.0 L of insufflation gas for adequate distention. Children may only require 0.9 L. Absolute volumes are generally meaningless in view of the wide variation in patient size. End point pressure is the key element to monitor because pressure, not volume, will dictate the physiologic changes in the patient. Insufflator pressure should be set to 6 to 8 mm Hg for smaller infants, 10 to 12 mm Hg in older children, and absolutely less than 15 mm Hg in almost all patients. Use of newer systems that provide warmed, humidified CO_2 should be considered, because they may decrease the incidence of lens fogging inside the abdominal cavity. Fogging of the lens during a procedure will severely limit visualization, which may lead to inadvertent injury. Anti-fog solutions generally do not work well. A "low-tech" alternative is a thermos of warmed water to dip the scope into, to both warm and clean the scope lens. This measure will decrease condensation once the scope is placed back in the abdominal cavity.

The primary and secondary trocar-cannula systems should match the size of the patient. The anterior abdominal wall of the child is thinner, with little to no subcutaneous fat in most cases. An excessive cannula length will serve only as an impediment to the scope and to the operative instruments in the restricted space of the pediatric cavity. Wide spacing of the port sites is essential to gain adequate angles between instruments for effective surgery.

Operative cannulas often need to be fixed to the abdominal wall to prevent both advancing into and withdrawing from the port site. Various methods have been described, ranging from suturing with a spacer to more basic methods of taping the cannula in place.[14-16]

Anatomy

As mentioned previously, the abdominal wall of the child is thinner and more elastic than that of the adult. Nevertheless, the same relative anatomic considerations exist.

Because of the child's smaller body size, positioning the patient with the arms outstretched will leave less room for the surgeon. Raising the arms higher or increased pressure from a crowded surgeon's body may lead to upper extremity nerve damage. Generally, such injury can be avoided by tucking the arms in a neutral position at the patient's side. Liberal use of foam padding also will aid in protecting the arms.

The smaller vagina and uterus also pose challenges when uterine manipulation is needed during a procedure. Uterine positioning may be accomplished with an assistant's finger in the vagina or, alternatively, with a small cervical dilator affixed to a tenaculum—most commercial manipulators are too large.

The inferior epigastric vessels and the ureter usually are very well visualized through the peritoneum. Depending on the age of the patient, the bladder dome may rest higher up on the anterior abdominal wall, and umbilical remnants may be present that can interfere with the visual field or be injured during the procedure. Such variation is especially likely in neonates, and some authors recommend primary trocar placement at Munro's point, lateral to the rectus sheath, in a line between the umbilicus and the anterior superior iliac spine.[17]

In the confined space of a pediatric abdomen, relative distances between structures such as bowel, vessels, and ureter may be decreased. These relationships must be respected to avoid inadvertent injury during dissection or with use of energy sources in the abdomen. Bipolar electrocautery instruments may certainly be used safely when consideration is made for the degree of thermal spread. Some authors suggest that laser energy or ultrasonic sources have less thermal spread, with fewer consequent complications. Another alternative is suture ligation with pre-tied endoloops or free suture.

A mean decrease in blood loss is an often-cited advantage of laparoscopic surgery. Strict hemostasis becomes even more important in the pediatric patient because total blood volume is lower. Blood volume in the pediatric patient has been estimated (Table 14–1).

Indications for transfusion are similar to those of adults, but the indications are somewhat more stringent (Table 14–2).

Most healthy children will compensate for hemoglobin concentrations as low as 8 g/dL and will regenerate their red cell mass quickly with simple iron therapy, thereby avoiding the complications associated with transfusion.

COMPLICATIONS OF LAPAROSCOPY

Published reviews of complications of minimally invasive surgery in this age group have focused mainly on the general surgical patient. Much of this information can be extrapolated to the practice of gynecologic surgery, because the basic techniques of entry, tissue dissection, and closure are universal to minimally invasive methods.

In 1996 Peters published the results of a survey of pediatric urologists.[18] The information collected from more than 5400 procedures revealed a complication rate of 5.38%. When complications such as subcutaneous emphysema and preperitoneal insufflation were excluded, the rate fell to 1.18%. Of all complications, only 0.39% necessitated any surgical repair. Injuries to the bowel (0.17%), bladder (0.17%), and vasculature (0.43%) all were reported, along with a 0.15% hernia rate at the trocar sites. Use of a closed entry, with a Veress-type needle, was associated with a complication rate of 2.6%, versus 1.2% for an open technique. Entry technique and experience of the operator were concluded to be the major determinants of a safe outcome. Specific procedures, that is,

Table 14–2 ▪ Guidelines for Pediatric Red Blood Cell Transfusions

Children and Adolescents

Acute loss > 25% circulating blood volume
Hemoglobin < 8.0 g/dL* in perioperative period
Hemoglobin < 13.0 g/dL and *severe* cardiopulmonary disease
Hemoglobin < 8.0 g/dL and *symptomatic* chronic anemia
Hemoglobin < 8.0 g/dL and *marrow failure*

Infants within First 4 Months of Life

Hemoglobin < 13.0 g/dL and *severe* pulmonary disease
Hemoglobin < 10.0 g/dL and *moderate* pulmonary disease
Hemoglobin < 13.0 g/dL and *severe* cardiac disease
Hemoglobin < 10.0 g/dL and major surgery
Hemoglobin < 8.0 g/dL and *symptomatic* chronic anemia

Words in *italics* must be defined for local transfusion guidelines.
*Hematocrit estimated by Hb g/dL × 3.
From Nelson's pediatrics, 17th ed., p 1647.

Table 14–1 ▪ Approximate Blood Volume

Age	Total Blood Volume (mL/kg)	Age	Total Blood Volume (mL/kg)
Preterm infants	90-105	4-6 yr	80-86
Term newborns	78-86	7-18 yr	83-90
1-12 mo	73-78	Adults	68-88
1-3 yr	74-82		

From Nathan D, Oski FA. Hematology of infancy and childhood. Philadelphia: WB Saunders, 1998.

diagnostic versus operative, did not seem to alter these results.

Chen and associates, also in 1996, published a retrospective review of data on endoscopic procedures in 636 pediatric patients (574 laparoscopies and 62 thoracoscopies) during a 5-year period. The mean age of the patients was 6.7 years (standard deviation [SD] ±4.9 years).[19] The overall complication rate was 2%. This number does not include 10 cases requiring conversion to laparotomy for technical reasons. An omental hernia developed at the umbilical trocar site in 2 children. Wound cellulitis developed around a gastrostomy tube brought out through an operative port site in 2 other children. Of the 5 children requiring laparotomy for management of intraoperative complications, 4 had significant hemorrhage and 1 experienced an esophagotomy during a Nissen fundoplication. The authors noted that a majority of complications occurred during the surgeon's first 5 to 10 procedures performed.

Esposito and colleagues described 10 years' experience at an Italian center, reporting 430 cases in children with a mean age of 5 years. Of eight complications (1.8%), only one was severe, a major vascular injury with a Veress needle.[20] A follow-up publication in 2000, specifically looking at laparoscopic Nissen fundoplications in 289 children, showed a slightly higher rate of intraoperative complications associated with the more complex dissection (5.1%); however, only 1.3 % of the cases required conversion to open surgery.[21] Similar results were reported in a multicenter retrospective review covering 1689 procedures in 2002 and another series looking at urologic procedures in 2003.[22,23] No fatalities were reported in any of these reviews.

A majority of all laparoscopic complications still occur during the process of obtaining access to the peritoneal cavity.[24] These complications include vascular injury, injury to the gastrointestinal or urinary tract, and subcutaneous emphysema. Postoperative wound complications including wound infection, hernia, and port site metastasis also have been reported. Various reviews of injuries associated with creation of a pneumoperitoneum have been summarized for the adult population. Overall, the incidence of major vascular injury ranges from 0.04% to 0.5%, and injury to the gastrointestinal tract occurs in 0.06% to 0.83% of procedures. Although various injury rates are quoted in the literature, the overall trend is for open techniques, such as that described by Hasson, which reduce the injury rate by about half, with the major vascular injury rate plummeting.[24]

The anatomy of the pediatric abdominal cavity, with a thinner anterior abdominal wall and close approximation of major retroperitoneal vessels, raises the possibility of increasing the incidence of injury with a closed technique. Additionally, the peritoneum is much more elastic in these patients, which may mislead the surgeon to believe that entry has been achieved despite deep penetration of the Veress needle. Many authors recommend open entry to avoid the complications of a blind insertion.[14,15,18,25] An orogastric tube to decompress the stomach should be standard. Emptying the bladder either with a Foley catheter or by a Credé maneuver also will assist in visualization and decrease inadvertent injury with placement of operative trocars.

The incidence of hernia is estimated to be approximately 0.02% or more and much higher with use of 10-mm or larger trocars.[24] Multiple case reports describe herniation with smaller trocar sizes.[24,26-28] In some of these cases, manipulation of the port site during surgery may have widened the fascial opening. Most of the smaller-site hernias involved only omental fat or intestinal epiploica, as reported in the aforementioned studies. In some patients, management with only local anesthesia at the bedside may be adequate. In view of the smaller caliber of the bowel in the pediatric patient, however, the chance of a Richter's hernia may be increased. Therefore, it probably is prudent to close all site wounds 5 mm or more in diameter in this age group.

Secondary trocars should always be placed under direct vision to avoid injury to underlying structures. Suprapubic trocar sites can perforate the dome of the bladder if placed too low or angled too caudally.[29,30] These injuries may be of the through-and-through type, which may not be recognized intraoperatively. Inferior epigastric vessels may be injured if their course is not confirmed during placement or if the angle of insertion is too shallow. This angle may allow the sharp trocar to lacerate the vessel even if the skin incision is placed well lateral. Generally, the angle of insertion should be perpendicular to the curve of the inflated abdomen. The insertion also may require additional stabilization, because it may deflect the abdominal wall to a greater degree than in an adult patient. The abdomen may be grasped externally, graspers placed through existing ports may provide resistance internally, or the trocar may be aimed directly at the primary cannula, effectively providing a safety sheath. Management of these complications is the same as in the adult and is covered more extensively in other chapters (see Chapters 4 and 5).

No good published data are available on postoperative wound infection in pediatric endoscopic cases. In several reports, the rate of intra-abdominal abscess in laparoscopically managed ruptured appendicitis was higher than that in open cases. This finding is balanced somewhat by the decreased rate of superficial wound complications in patients undergoing laparoscopic appendectomy. The main advantage of this technique is an improved cosmetic result, with a more rapid return to normal activities. Some authors dispute the more rapid recovery, noting no difference in analgesic use or time to return to normal diet. Certainly the ideal candidate would be a patient with acute appendicitis uncomplicated by rupture or with abdominal pain for which the cause is less clear, because laparoscopic survey of the abdomen in such cases is far improved from the open mini-laparotomy. Otherwise, wound infection overall is rare and would be managed the same as in the adult.

SUMMARY

Laparoscopy has proved to be an invaluable tool for the treatment of both adult and pediatric patients. Overall, the safety of laparoscopy in children is equivalent to or better than that in the adult patient. Ongoing study is needed to better define the patients that will benefit the most from this approach. Skills applied in open surgery do not always translate to the maneuvers performed with laparoscopic surgery, although the anatomy may be the same. The longer instrumentation and more limited degrees of freedom can be frustrating. Laparoscopic skills are now developed during residency but may not fully mature until later because of the extended learning curve.

This is an important consideration for credentialing physicians in advanced laparoscopic techniques.

References

1. Gans SL. Historical development of pediatric endoscopic surgery. In: Holcomb GW III, ed. Pediatric endoscopic surgery. Norwalk, CT: Appleton & Lange, 1994;1.
2. Jawad AJ, Al-Meshari A. Laparoscopy for ovarian pathology in infancy and childhood. Pediatr Surg Int 1998;14:62.
3. Lee KH, Yeung CK, Tam YH, Liu KK. The use of laparoscopy in the management of adnexal pathologies in children. Aust N Z J Surg 2000;70:192.
4. Sandoval C, Strom K, Stringel G. Laparoscopy in the management of pediatric intraabdominal tumors. JSLS 2004;8:115.
5. Sailhamer E, Jackson CC, Vogel AM, et al. Minimally invasive surgery for pediatric solid neoplasms. Am Surgeon 2003;69:566.
6. Holcomb GW III, Tomita SS. Minimally invasive surgery in children with cancer. Cancer 1995;76:121.
7. Cusick RA, Waldhausen JHT. The learning curve associated with pediatric laparoscopic splenectomy. Am J Surg 2001;181:393.
8. Meehan JJ, Georgeson KE. The learning curve associated with laparoscopic antireflux surgery in infants and children. J Pediatr Surg 1997;32:426.
9. Whitted RW, Pietro PA, Martin G, et al. A retrospective study evaluating the impact of formal laparoscopic training on patient outcomes in a residency program. J Am Assoc Gynecol Laparosc 2003;10:484.
10. Rosser JC, Rosser LE, Savalgi RS. Objective evaluation of a laparoscopic surgical skill program for residents and senior surgeons. Arch Surg 1998;133:657.
11. Pennant JH. Anesthesia for minimally invasive surgery: Laparoscopy, thoracoscopy, hysteroscopy. Anesthesiol Clin North Am 2001;19.
12. Tobias J. Anaesthesia for minimally invasive surgery in children. Best Pract Res Clin Anaesthesiol 2002;16:115.
13. Wedgewood J, Doyle E. Anaesthesia and laparoscopic surgery in children. Paediatr Anaesth 2001;11:391.
14. Lobe TE. Laparoscopic surgery in children. Curr Prob Surg 1998;35:861.
15. Sanfilippo JS, Lobe TE. Operative laparoscopy in the pediatric patient. In: Vitale GC, Sanfilippo JS, Perissat J, eds. Laparoscopic surgery: An atlas for general surgeons. Philadelphia: JB Lippincott, 1995;75.
16. Bax NMA, van der Zee DC. Trocar fixation during endoscopic surgery in infants and children. Surg Endosc 1998;12:181.
17. Waldschmidt J, Schier F. Laparoscopic procedures in neonates and infants. In: Holcomb GW III, ed. Pediatric endoscopic surgery. Norwalk, CT: Appleton & Lange, 1994;67.
18. Peters CA. Complications in pediatric urological laparoscopy: Results of a survey. J Urol 1996;155:1070.
19. Chen MK, Schropp KP, Lobe TE. Complications of minimal-access surgery in children. J Pediatr Surg 1996;31:1161.
20. Esposito C, Ascione G, Garipoli V, et al. Complications of pediatric laparoscopic surgery. Surg Endosc 1997;11:655.
21. Esposito C, Montupet P, Amici G, Desruelle P. Complications of laparoscopic antireflux surgery in childhood. Surg Endosc 2000;14:622.
22. Esposito C, Mattioli G, Monguzzi GL, et al. Complications and conversions of pediatric videosurgery: The Italian multicentric experience on 1689 procedures. Surg Endosc 2002;16:795.
23. Esposito C, Lima M, Mattioli G, et al. Complications of pediatric urological laparoscopy: Mistakes and risks. J Urol 2003;169:1490.
24. Munro MG. Laparoscopic access: Complications, technologies, and techniques. Curr Opin Obstet Gynecol 2002;14:365.
25. Holcomb GW III. Diagnostic laparoscopy: Equipment, technique, and special concerns in children. In: Holcomb GW III, ed. Pediatric endoscopic surgery. Norwalk, CT: Appleton & Lange, 1994;9.
26. Montz FJ, Holshneider CH, Munro MG. Incisional hernia following laparoscopy: A survey of the American Association of Gynecologic Laparoscopists. Obstet Gynecol 1994;84:881.
27. Plaus WJ. Laparoscopic trocar site hernias. J Laparoendosc Surg 1993;3:567.
28. Mark SD. Omental herniation through a small laparoscopic port. Br J Urol 1995;76:137.
29. Lamaro VP, Broome JD, Vancaillie TG. Unrecognized bladder perforation during operative laparoscopy. J Am Assoc Gynecol Laparosc 2000;7:417.
30. Ostrzenski A, Ostrzenska KM. Bladder injury during laparoscopic surgery. Obstet Gynecol Surv 1998;53:175.

Unusual Complications during Gynecologic Laparoscopic Surgery

15

James K. Robinson III and Keith Isaacson

COMPLICATIONS OF LAPAROSCOPY IN PREGNANT PATIENTS

Pregnancy presents a unique set of challenges to the surgeon. Not only must the surgeon be concerned with both maternal and fetal well-being, but maternal physiology is appreciably altered during pregnancy, affecting cardiopulmonary parameters, clotting factors, hemoglobin levels, and blood volume. As gestation progresses, surgical visualization becomes more difficult regardless of surgical approach. It is estimated that surgery is necessary during the course of pregnancy in as many as 1 of every 150 pregnancies.[1] Traditionally, pregnancy was considered an absolute contraindication to laparoscopy; however, over the last decade, laparoscopy for the management of gynecologic and nongynecologic conditions has emerged as a safe and often preferable alternative to laparotomy. The most common surgical procedures during pregnancy are cholecystectomy (45% to 48.1% of procedures), adnexal surgery (28% to 34%), and appendectomy (15% to 16.2%),[2,3] all of which have been shown to be safely amenable to the laparoscopic approach in experienced hands.[2-18]

Gynecologic surgery during pregnancy is warranted for a number of reasons, including ectopic pregnancy, persistent adnexal cysts, ovarian torsion, malignancy, and in rare cases, degenerating or obstructing myomas. It is estimated that in up to 1 of every 81 pregnancies, an adnexal cyst will be found,[7] a diagnosis that has increased in recent years with the widespread performance of perinatal ultrasonography. Perhaps as many as 1 in 600 pregnancies will demonstrate an adnexal cyst persisting into the second trimester of pregnancy and requiring surgery.[12] A majority of sonographically identified ovarian cysts are in fact corpus luteal cysts and will resolve spontaneously if followed into the second trimester.[19] Unfortunately, in many instances, the clinical presentation requires immediate intervention before spontaneous cyst resolution occurs. Ovarian torsion occurs more frequently in the first trimester of pregnancy than at any other time, at a rate of approximately 1 per 5000 pregnancies.[6,14]

Two overriding issues argue strongly for adnexal surgery during pregnancy. First, the overall malignancy rate of ovarian cysts in pregnancy ranges from 1% to 8%[6]; therefore, any persistent cyst deserves pathologic evaluation. The other concern driving surgical management is the long-term risk associated with observation (i.e., expectant management). Stepp and colleagues[7] recently reviewed the relevant data, which suggest the cumulative risk of significant morbidity from torsion, rupture, infection, and hemorrhage to be in the range of 10% to 42%. In view of the significantly higher rate of preterm labor and birth in patients who undergo emergent surgery than in those whose cysts are treated electively, the risk of nonsurgical management becomes substantial.

Benefits of Laparoscopy

For the treatment of disorders occurring in pregnancy, laparoscopy may be preferable to laparotomy for many reasons. Initially, laparoscopy has been shown to confer the same benefits in pregnant patients as in nonpregnant patients. These include significant decreases in hospital stay and convalescence,[4,10,11] decreased postoperative complications,[10,11] and decreased narcotic usage, with its adverse effects on the fetus.[11] Although a single early report suggested that laparoscopy may increase the risk of fetal death compared with laparotomy,[20] the bulk of the international literature does not support this finding. In a large Swedish retrospective review of 2181 laparoscopies and 1522 laparotomies performed during pregnancy over a 20-year period, no differences in birth weight, gestational duration, frequency of intrauterine growth restriction, congenital malformations, stillbirths, or neonatal deaths were found.[5] Two retrospective reviews from Israel confirm these findings.[9,10]

Theoretically, laparoscopy affords better visualization than laparotomy and may result in less uterine manipulation and subsequent preterm contractions.[14] It also acts as an excellent diagnostic tool when the diagnosis is in question. This point may be especially important with regards to appendicitis. From 35% to 50% of explorations for presumed appendicitis yield negative findings in the third trimester. Despite this poor yield, most morbidity associated with appendicitis in pregnancy can be attributed directly to a delay in diagnosis.[11] The decreased morbidity associated with diagnostic laparoscopy makes it the ideal surgical modality to resolve the dilemma inherent in these conflicting data.[12] Muench and coworkers also found that delaying surgery for biliary disease led to increased morbidity, again arguing for timely laparoscopic treatment.[21]

One final possible benefit of laparoscopy over laparotomy is a presumed relative protection against thromboembolic events. Venous stasis and physiologic changes in clotting factors associated with pregnancy place pregnant patients at higher risk for these potentially catastrophic complications than persons in the general public. Surgery only compounds this risk. Most surgeons believe that early ambulation associated with minimally invasive surgery helps reduce this risk.

Prevention of Complications

The long-standing prohibition against laparoscopy in pregnancy was based in large part on theoretical risks associated with insufflation and pneumoperitoneum. Pregnancy, like obesity, alters pulmonary mechanics. Specifically, metabolic demand increases and functional residual lung capacity (FRC) diminishes as pregnancy progresses. The stresses of general anesthesia, supine positioning, head-down (Trendelenburg) positioning, and increased intra-abdominal pressure from carbon dioxide (CO_2) pneumoperitoneum all exacerbate this problem. As FRC falls below closing pressure in the dependent airways, atelectasis results in ventilation-perfusion mismatch, with ensuing maternal respiratory acidosis and hypoxemia. If these disturbances are not corrected, fetal acidosis and ultimately hypoxemia may follow. Pregnant patients respond to induction of anesthesia and surgery in similar fashion to that observed in nonpregnant patients with respect to cardiac parameters. Cardiac index decreases with induction of anesthesia, and both mean arterial pressure (MAP) and systemic vascular resistance (SVR) decrease.[22] These changes contribute to decreases in uterine artery blood flow in this setting.

Fetal acidosis during insufflation pressures of 10 to 15 mm Hg has been documented in pregnant ewes[23]; however, fetal hypoxemia did not ensue, presumably because of the rightward shift in the oxygen dissociation curve associated with acidosis. Other possible causes of fetal acidosis associated with increased intra-abdominal pressure include decreases in maternal venous return and cardiac output, decreased uterine artery blood flow, and transperitoneal or placental absorption of CO_2. These hypothetical concerns have been either corroborated or refuted by a number of well-designed animal studies[23-25] making reliable conclusions difficult. Despite the conflicting evidence, none of these studies documented any adverse pregnancy outcomes associated with their findings, suggesting that at least in pregnant sheep, the fetal acid-base alterations possibly associated with laparoscopy are well compensated and do not appear to adversely jeopardize the well-being of the fetus.

Armed with this information, the prudent surgeon will take a number of precautions to prevent the sequelae of fetal hypoxia. Initially, rotating the operative table to the left will take pressure off the inferior vena cava, increasing venous return and cardiac output or cardiac index.[6,11,12,14] Maintenance of intraperitoneal pressure at or below 12 mm Hg will allow for adequate surgical visualization while decreasing ventilatory, intra-abdominal, and intrauterine pressures and maximizing uterine artery blood flow.[4,6,14] Mathevet and co-workers also recommend the routine use of intraoperative ephedrine to maintain MAP at or above 80% of baseline, to

help maintain uteroplacental perfusion.[6] Some authors also recommend intraoperative transvaginal fetal ultrasound evaluation.[11,12,14] If intraoperative fetal evaluation becomes nonreassuring, abdominal insufflation pressures can be reduced and maternal pressures stabilized before surgery is resumed.

Another major risk factor associated with laparoscopy in pregnancy is Veress needle or trocar injury to the gravid uterus. A number of case reports have documented Veress needle injury to the gravid uterus, without subsequent complications[2,9,12]; however a single case report of pneumoamnion with subsequent fetal loss after second-trimester laparoscopy has been reported.[26] As pregnancy progresses, safe placement of the initial trocar becomes increasingly difficult.

To avoid uterine injury, a number of different recommendations have been made. The open (Hasson) approach is advocated by many authors to minimize the risk of Veress needle injury.[2,4,6,11,12,26] After 18 weeks of gestation, use of an alternative laparoscope site between the umbilicus and xyphoid process should be considered.[2,4,11,14,26] Use of the left upper quadrant[2,6,7,12,26] and ultrasound guidance for placement of the initial Veress needle[12,14] also are reasonable precautions.

A hypothetical risk of operative laparoscopy during pregnancy is fetal carbon monoxide (CO) poisoning from the transperitoneal absorption of intra-abdominal smoke after thermal desiccation. The use of electrosurgery and laser during laparoscopy in a highly anoxic environment results in incomplete combustion and the generation of significant amounts of CO, which is readily absorbed across the peritoneal membrane.[27] Presumably, sublethal maternal CO poisoning with the high affinity of CO for maternal hemoglobin, could adversely affect oxygen delivery to the fetus. Two separate studies on nonpregnant patients have demonstrated absorption of CO using either CO oximetry or serum carboxyhemoglobin (COHb) monitoring in patients undergoing laparoscopy with significant smoke generation.[28,29] A study by Nezhat and colleagues demonstrated that by preoxygenating patients and by maintaining end-tidal CO_2 levels in the range of 30 mm Hg, serum levels of COHb were unchanged from pre- to postoperative levels despite the generation of significant intra-abdominal CO.[27] We concur that maintaining optimal patient oxygenation and end-tidal CO_2 levels, along with aggressive evacuation of smoke from the surgical field, is important and especially relevant in operating on pregnant patients. The use of ultrasonic energy generates mostly water vapor, and this modality may be a better choice than laser or electrosurgery in pregnant patients, to minimize the risks of CO poisoning to the fetus.

Laparoscopic surgery during pregnancy is ideally performed in the second trimester, when most organogenesis has been achieved and the background miscarriage rate has fallen. Although visualization is more difficult than in first-trimester surgery, the miscarriage rate is 5.6%, compared with a first-trimester rate of 12%. Deferring surgery to the third trimester should be avoided if possible, in view of significant visualization issues and a potentially higher rate of preterm labor necessitating tocolysis. Most authorities do not routinely administer tocolytic agents after laparoscopic surgery, although indomethacin,[4] ketoprofen,[6] and ritodrine[14] have been used successfully when persistent uterine contractions follow laparoscopic surgery.

Recognition and Management of Complications

Once the decision to pursue laparoscopy in the pregnant patient has been made and all of the relevant precautions have been taken, complications will still occur. Recognition and management are the next most crucial steps. Although many laparoscopic surgical procedures can be performed in an outpatient setting, it is prudent to observe all pregnant patients at least overnight. Fetal monitoring for fetal well-being and uterine activity, both intraoperatively and postoperatively, is warranted. In cases of postsurgical contractions, the evidence suggests that aggressive tocolysis is warranted.

Intraoperative use of pneumatic compression boots and early postoperative ambulation are important measures to help mitigate the risk of thromboembolism. Any evidence of postoperative maternal hypoxia, pleuritis, tachycardia, or hypertension should be aggressively evaluated. Spiral computed tomography (CT) scanning delivers a lower radiation dose than that from a ventilation-perfusion ($\dot{V}$/Q) scan, and with appropriate shielding, CT-associated radiation exposure is well within the fetal safety limits. For this reason CT is the diagnostic modality of choice for evaluation of pulmonary embolism. Lower-extremity Doppler ultrasound evaluation also can be a useful tool in the workup of thromboembolic disease, with no risk to the fetus. The importance of prompt recognition and rapid anticoagulation in this scenario for both mother and fetus cannot be overstated.

In cases of uterine trauma during surgery, CT evaluation can readily diagnose pneumoamnion. In the single case report of this complication, the patient's lower abdominal pain worsened postoperatively, and her amniotic membranes ruptured shortly thereafter.[26]

Given that no intracervical uterine manipulation should ever be used in pregnancy, the risk of postoperative chorioamnionitis in the absence of ruptured membranes is remote. Any evidence of intrauterine infection, however, must be evaluated fully. Amniocentesis is warranted if no other obvious infectious source surfaces, with emergent delivery if the diagnosis is confirmed.

UTERINE RUPTURE AFTER LAPAROSCOPIC MYOMECTOMY

Uterine rupture or dehiscence in pregnancy following surgery on the uterine corpus is well described. Semm and Metler performed the first laparoscopic myomectomy in 1979.[30] Since that time, at least 13 cases of spontaneous rupture in the late second or early to middle third trimester after laparoscopic myomectomy or myolysis have been described in the English-language literature.[31-43] These cases, all occurring before the onset of labor, make many authorities wary of the laparoscopic approach, especially in patients who wish to conceive in the future. Given that the primary indication for myomectomy in approximately 30% of patients is otherwise unexplained infertility,[44,45] the question of approach is important. Benefits of the laparoscopic approach over laparotomy include decreases in complications, blood loss, length of hospital stay, length of recovery, overall cost, and rate of adhesion formation.[46] In cases in which infertility is the primary indication,

subsequent pregnancy rates are 71%, with a live birth rate of 73% based on an analysis of nine large pregnancy series after laparoscopic myomectomy (Table 15–1). Counter to conventional wisdom and classical cesarean section data, of the 284 live births reviewed, 113 (38%) were delivered vaginally without any evidence of rupture. Miscarriage rates after laparoscopic myomectomy are identical to the rate following laparotomy, at approximately 19%.[45,47]

Unfortunately, although both the overall benefits of laparoscopy and the pregnancy outcomes are impressive after laparoscopic myomectomy, the true incidence of uterine rupture remains unclear. All but three of the cases previously reported were from individual case reports, and only one of the three remaining cases reported in a large series occurred at the site of a previous laparoscopic myomectomy. This single case represented 1% of all pregnancies occurring after the procedure in Dubuisson and associates' series.[48] Because no other uterine ruptures are found in our series review, we calculate the uterine rupture rate to be 0.33%. Uterine rupture after laparotomic myomectomy is also rare; however, one review placed the subsequent dehiscence rate as high as 2.5%.[49]

Because of the paucity of case reports, it is difficult to know with any certainty which etiologic factors contribute most to subsequent rupture. Three theories appear to hold the most favor. The use of electrosurgery, particularly monopolar electrocautery with its subsequent thermal tissue damage, may predispose tissue to necrosis and poor wound healing. This in turn may predispose patients to uterine rupture in the later stages of pregnancy.[32,38,45,48,50-52] This theory is supported by the preponderance of monopolar electrosurgical dissection techniques used in the cases in which subsequent rupture occurred (Table 15–2). Another contributing factor is likely to be the difficulty of appropriately reapproximating tissue planes in laparoscopic surgery.[32,36,38,45,48,50-53] Laparoscopic suturing is an advanced technique not mastered by many gynecologic surgeons. An inability to replicate open myomectomy closure techniques also appears to play a role. Finally, poor closure of dead space predisposes patients to intrauterine hematoma formation that also is likely to delay and hamper wound healing.[48,51,54] A review of the existing case reports suggests that electrosurgery, inadequate tissue reapproximation, and possibly posterior fibroid location all may play a role in subsequent uterine rupture (see Table 15–2).

Prevention

In view of the uterine stresses of pregnancy, infertile patients and women desiring future fertility who undergo laparoscopic myomectomy must be selected carefully and their surgical treatment meticulously performed. In cases in which more than four myomas are present or the dominant myoma is greater than 7 to 10 cm in diameter, laparotomy should be considered as the most efficacious route. Posterior fibroids also must be approached with caution, because these defects are more difficult to reapproximate than anterior or fundal myomas. Reapproximation is especially difficult when the posterior fibroid is in the lower uterine segment. In all posterior ruptures previously reported, closure has been either serosal or nonexistent (see Table 15–2). If criteria are favorable, however, the laparoscopic approach to myomectomy in the patient desiring future fertility is desirable.

Table 15–1 ■ Series Review: Pregnancy after Laparoscopic Myomectomy

Study	Total Cases	Infertility	Pregnant Patients	Total Pregnancies	Live Births	C Section	Vaginal Delivery	Rupture	Mean Largest (cm)	Mean #	Pedunculated	Subserosal	Intramural	Submucous (cavity entered)
Hasson et al, 1992[44]	56	17	15	15	11	2	9	0	NR	NR	NR	NR	NR	NR
Darai, 1997[135]	143	44	17	19	11	3	8	0	NR	NR	NR	NR	NR	NR
Nezhat et al, 1999[45,121]	115	34	31	42	30	22	6 (2)	0	6.27	3.04	NR	47%	42%	NR
Ribeiro et al, 1999[136]	161	28	18	18	14	8	6	0	6	NR	NR	NR	NR	1
Dubuisson et al, 2000[48]	263	NR	98	145	100	42	58	1	4.8	1.8	25	41	32	6
Seinera et al, 2000[51]	202	NR	54	65	56	45	9	0	3.9	NR	NR	26	28	1
Stringer et al, 2001[47]	7	5	7	7	5	4	1	0	8	4	0	0	0	7
Rosetti, 2001[137]	29	29	17	19	14	10	4	0	5.4	NR	NR	NR	NR	NR
Landi et al, 2003[50]	359	92	72	76	57	26	31	0	NR	NR	33	108	82	6
TOTALS	1335	126	329	406	298	162	109	1	NA	NA	NA	NA	NA	NA

Combined pregnancy rate (excluding Dubuisson and Seinera)   71%
Combined live birth rate   73%
Uterine rupture rate (live births)   0.033%

Table 15–2 ▪ Uterine Rupture after Laparoscopic Myomectomy

Case Report	Gestational Age (wk)	Energy Source	Closure	Myoma Type	Myoma Location
Harris, 1992[38]	34	"Electrosurgery"	Serosal	Subserous ?Endometrial entry	Posterior
Mecke et al, 1995[42]	28	NR	NR	NR	NR
Friedmann et al, 1996[39]	28 3/7	NR	"Sutured"	Intramural	Fundal
Pelosi and Pelosi, 1997[36]	33	Mono/bipolar	None	Subserous Superficial	Posterior
Arcangeli and Pasquarette, 1997[37]	26	Bipolar myolysis	None/NA	Intramural	Fundal
Dubuisson et al, 2000[48]	32	NR	Single layer figure-of-eight at 2nd look	NR	NR
Foucher et al, 2000[33]	32	Mono/bipolar	none	3 subserous, 1 intramural	Posterior
Nkemayim et al, 2000[35]	28	NR	NR	Subserous, intramural	Fundal
Hockstein, 2000[40]	29	Monopolar	Multilayer interrupted via minilap	Intramural	Fundal
Oltem et al, 2001[43]	17	Monopolar	None	Subserous	Corneal
Hasbargen et al, 2002[32]	29	Monopolar	None	Pedunculated	Posterior
Asakura et al, 2004[41]	NR	NR	NR	Intramural	Anterior fundal
Lieng et al, 2004[31]	35 5/7	Bipolar	None	Pedunculated	Posterior

NR, not reported.

The importance of technique in the prevention of subsequent uterine rupture cannot be overstated. Minimizing thermal tissue damage during myoma enucleation is the first important step.[31,32,36,47,50,51] The routine use of monopolar energy, especially at low power settings and with intermittent "coagulation" waveforms, leads to prolonged contact with tissue and wide thermal injury margins. The use of scissors, ultrasonic energy, laser, or monopolar high-watt continuous "cutting" waveforms minimizes thermal damage on entry into the myometrium and are preferable. Maintenance of hemostasis is another important rule of successful laparoscopic myomectomy. To this end, most surgeons advocate subserous injections of dilute vasopressin before making a uterine incision, and many recommend preoperative treatment with a gonadotropin-releasing hormone (GnRH) agonist for 1 to 3 months. Obviously, the use of cold scissors or high-power monopolar cutting makes maintenance of hemostasis challenging, so some surgeons advocate the use of either ultrasonic energy or laser for the initial entry into the uterus. Once the myoma has been identified and the pseudocapsule developed, the enucleation is accomplished for the most part using a combination of traction and countertraction and blunt dissection. One of the benefits of high-magnification laparoscopy is exceptional visualization of vascular pedicles. When these are encountered, they should be skeletonized and desiccated with the lowest-power bipolar forceps available. If all vascular pedicles are treated in this manner, bleeding should be minimal after removal of the myoma. If significant bleeding persists, broad-base cautery fulguration should be avoided. Hemostasis is better obtained with well-placed sutures.

Perhaps the most daunting technical challenge is adequate closure of the myometrial defect. All tissue planes must be reapproximated and dead space closed. The serosa layer should always be closed, even in the case of pedunculated and superficial subserous myomas.[32,36] This generally requires a two-to-four–layer closure. When the endometrial cavity is entered, endometrium should be closed separate from the overlying myometrium. Absorbable suture material should always be used, but preference as to type varies. The use of either interrupted or running sutures is acceptable so long as the resulting closure is strong and intact. The difficulty of laparoscopic suturing appears to be the limiting factor for most surgeons, some of whom have begun to use laparoscopic suture devices. In one series, seven patients with full-thickness myomas entering the endometrial cavity underwent laparoscopic myomectomy with multilayer closure using the Endo Stitch device (Auto Suture Company, Division of US Surgical Corp., Norwalk, Connecticut).[47] All became pregnant, with five opting to continue their pregnancies. No ruptures were reported. With use of one of the suturing devices, it is important to make certain tissue purchase is adequate, because numerous smaller bites tend to strangulate tissue, potentially leading to necrosis and subsequent rupture.

Patients in whom the endometrial or myometrial defects have not healed well are presumably at the highest risk of subsequent rupture. To identify this cohort, some authors advocate a second-look laparoscopy with intracervical injection of methylene blue.[44,47,48,55] One case report of rupture occurred after a postoperative fistula was identified at second look and repaired with a single figure-of-eight suture.[48] This highlights the importance of adequate repair at the initial surgery. Other investigators use postoperative ultrasound examination[52] or magnetic resonance imaging (MRI)[32,48] to assess the integrity of the uterine repair and myometrial thickness before advocating pregnancy.

The question of how long patients should wait after myomectomy before attempting pregnancy is not established.

Fascial closures attain their full preoperative strength 6 to 12 weeks postoperatively. Waiting a period of at least 3 months after myomectomy before attempting pregnancy seems prudent.

Recognition

No cases of uterine rupture after laparoscopic myomectomy have been reported during labor. Prelabor ruptures are reported from 17 to 35 5/7 weeks of gestation (see Table 15–2) with preponderance in the late second to early third trimesters. Any pregnant patient with a previous history of myomectomy regardless of type or approach who presents with acute onset of abdominal pain after 20 weeks' gestation should be evaluated for the possibility of uterine rupture. Symptoms of rupture vary and can be nonspecific, so a high level of clinical suspicion is warranted. Patients generally present with abdominal pain, often acute in onset, and fetal heart rate changes may accompany the pain or may be an ominous development later in the course. In the case of dehiscence, the fetal heart rate pattern may remain reassuring. Of greatest concern for both mother and fetus is evidence of hemoperitoneum or hypovolemic shock. Table 15–2 summarizes the presenting symptoms in all cases reported to date. In cases in which the diagnosis is in question, the most reliable modality for evaluation of the entire myometrium is MRI.[32,48]

Management

Uterine rupture constitutes an emergency necessitating immediate cesarean delivery. The site of uterine rupture should be repaired in multiple layers in the same fashion as for open myomectomy. Patients with multilayer closures after laparoscopic myomectomy will inevitably face the question of whether or not to undergo labor. Although most obstetricians will extrapolate from classical cesarean section data and recommend a scheduled cesarean section before the onset of labor, no direct evidence indicates that this approach is safer than a trial of labor. In the cumulative experience of the trials summarized in Table 15–1, the successful vaginal delivery rate was 38%, and no uterine ruptures during labor have ever been reported after laparoscopic myomectomy.

URINARY RETENTION

Postoperative urinary retention is a common problem in men and women after both laparotomy and laparoscopy. The complication is most prevalent after anorectal surgery, with reported incidence rates as high as 52%.[56] Gynecologic surgery also predisposes patients to retention at a rate of approximately 9% of cases.[57] In view of its relative frequency, the limited understanding of this phenomenon is of some interest. Complications resulting from urinary retention include bladder dilatation with subsequent temporary or permanent atony, urinary tract infection, sepsis, prolonged catheterization, increased pain and analgesic requirements, and prolonged hospital stay. Numerous studies and reports in the surgical literature have attempted to identify predisposing factors and to develop preoperative and postoperative

algorithms in an attempt to mitigate the substantial costs to patients and the health care delivery system. Unfortunately, findings have been contradictory, with little interstudy consistency.

The factor that obscures meaningful analysis of the literature to the greatest extent is the absence of any consistent definition. Definitions of urinary retention range from an inability to spontaneously void within 3 hours of surgery to the necessity of prolonged indwelling catheter placement. One of the most regularly implicated factors in the development of postoperative urinary retention is the administration of high volumes of perioperative fluids[58-65]; however, numerous studies have determined that high fluid volumes do not make a difference.[66-69] Similarly, advanced age has been implicated in some studies[58,60,62,65,69-71] and refuted in others.[61,67,68,72-74] General anesthesia contributes to postoperative urinary retention[60,72,73,75]; regional anesthesia also is a risk factor.[61,75,76] Most studies identify high postoperative narcotic usage as a contributing factor,[67-72,74] with specific emphasis on patient-controlled analgesia, although this is not universally agreed on.[58,63] In some studies, males experience retention more frequently than females,[77-79] whereas in others, no significant difference has been found.[61,69,72-74] Laparotomy is consistently implicated more frequently than laparoscopy,[56,74] and the intraoperative use of both sympathomimetic and anticholinergic drugs appears to consistently increase the risk of postoperative urinary retention.[58,64]

A growing body of evidence suggests that in the absence of an obvious infectious or obstructive cause, some cases may stem from an intrinsic failure of the striated external urethral sphincter to relax appropriately.[77-81] Fowler's syndrome, the most extreme manifestation of this phenomenon, occurs in young women with electromyography (EMG)-confirmed abnormalities of the urethral sphincter in whom prolonged or unremitting urinary retention develops that is otherwise unexplained. In 65% of these patients, an inciting event is identified, with gynecologic surgery representing almost half of these events.[77] This is an interesting finding in view of the unexplained concurrent diagnosis of polycystic ovarian syndrome in 66% of patients with Fowler's syndrome.[56] A postoperative EMG study of patients undergoing surgery for stress urinary incontinence demonstrated persistent EMG activity in the striated external urethral sphincter in all patients in whom retention developed; such activity was not evident in patients in whom retention did not develop.[81] In other studies, a history of obstructive symptoms was reported retrospectively by up to 80% of patients in whom postoperative retention developed.[58,82] These studies lend support to the theory that subsets of patients with physiologic hyperactive external urethral sphincters are at highest risk for postoperative urinary retention. In the most extreme cases, the retention may not resolve spontaneously (Fowler's syndrome).

The bladder and urethra are innervated by both sympathetic and parasympathetic fibers. Sympathetic stimulation of alpha-1 receptors in the distal bladder and proximal urethra increases outflow resistance, whereas parasympathetic stimulation of the detrusor fibers increases bladder contractility. Anesthesia, pain, and anxiety all contribute to increased sympathetic stimulation and urinary retention. Obviously sympathomimetic and anticholinergic drugs also predispose patients to retention.

Prevention

Patients undergoing laparoscopic surgery are at lower risk for the development of postoperative urinary retention than those undergoing laparotomy; however, the complication occurs more than 1% of the time even in patient populations at the lowest risk. A meta-analysis of patients undergoing laparoscopic cholecystectomy without intraoperative catheterization found an overall rate of 1.4%.[83] Gynecologic laparoscopy regularly uses bladder catheterization to avoid trocar injury to the bladder, presumably placing the incidence above that found for laparoscopic cholecystectomy but below the estimated overall rate of 9.2% after all gynecologic surgery. In view of the frequency of this complication and its sequelae, a preventive strategy is prudent.

Preoperative voiding histories are useful in identifying patients at highest risk for the development of postoperative retention. A history of previous or subclinical obstructive symptoms was present in 80% of surgical patients in whom urinary retention developed in a study of 5220 consecutive surgical patients (overall rate 3.8%).[58] Specifically, previous obstruction, frequent voiding, feelings of incomplete voiding, straining to void, and frequent urinary tract infections all appear to predispose patients to obstruction postoperatively. With any of these historical risk factors, postvoid residual capacities should be obtained before surgery, and every effort should be made to minimize intraoperative risk factors. Although consensus on risk factors is elusive, minimizing unnecessary catheterization, excessive intraoperative fluid administration, anticholinergic and sympathomimetic medications, and postoperative narcotics are good practice. Consideration should be given to preoperative treatment with cyclooxygenase-2 (COX-2) inhibitors and benzodiazepines, as well as the liberal use of intraoperative local anesthetics to reduce postoperative pain and anxiety. These measures should reduce both sympathetic stimulation and postoperative narcotic needs. All patients should be encouraged to ambulate as soon as safely possible postoperatively, and indwelling catheters should be removed at the soonest reasonable time. Any patient who undergoes surgery at the level of the trigone, bladder neck, or urethra, or who reports a positive history of obstructive symptoms, must be considered to be at high risk for urinary retention and should not be sent home postoperatively without first demonstrating a successful, spontaneous, and complete void.

Prophylactic pharmacologic therapy is also well described. Alpha blockade in high-risk patients, achieved historically with the nonselective phenoxybenzamine and more recently with selective alpha-1 blockers such as prazosin, shows mixed results; however, a meta-analysis of randomly controlled trials researching the prophylactic use of phenoxybenzamine demonstrated a 29.1% reduction in incidence.[84] Results with postoperative prophylactic use in patients undergoing vaginal and abdominal gynecologic surgery have been encouraging.[85,86] One successful dosing regimen was 10 mg orally given 6 to 8 hours postoperatively and again in 18 hours.[85] A randomized study using 2 mg of oral prazosin preoperatively and every 12 hours postoperatively during hospitalization demonstrated a decrease in urinary retention from 75% to 7% in catheterized patients undergoing joint replacement surgery compared with patients who received no drug.[87]

Of note, the manufacturer's recommended starting dose of prazosin is 1 mg two or three times daily for the treatment of hypertension, in order to avoid postural hypotension and syncope. Preoperative prophylaxis with either phenoxybenzamine or one of the selective alpha-1 blockers such as prazosin in high-risk patients undergoing minimally invasive surgery may be of benefit but has not been clearly demonstrated as of yet. Any use in this capacity is currently off label and may predispose patients to hypertension.

Recognition

Urinary retention classically manifests with excruciating abdominal pain, marked hypertension, tachycardia, and a palpable bladder. Postoperatively, sensation is potentially decreased, along with the normal physiologic manifestations. This is especially true after regional anesthesia. Patients should be followed closely postoperatively and encouraged to void. If the patient is unable to void within 3 hours of surgery, evaluation of bladder volume must ensue. Ultrasonic bladder scanners provide a reasonable estimation of volume and are available in most hospitals. At a volume of 300 mL, a majority of patients will demonstrate an urge to void. If this response is absent, catheterization is important to avoid unrecognized bladder distention.

Management

A majority of people with postoperative urinary retention respond well to conservative helping measures including ambulation, privacy, and the application of a warm bottle to the suprapubic region.[74,88] If these measures fail to relieve the retention, bladder drainage is important before overdistention develops. Most patients requiring catheterization will resume normal voiding after a single temporary catheterization. Twelve to 24 hours of bladder rest with an indwelling catheter in place generally is sufficient to reverse the retention if a single catheterization fails to correct the problem. In the rare case of a patient who returns to the hospital emergently with a massively dilated bladder, a week of bladder rest with either intermittent self-catheterization or an indwelling catheter is advised to avoid long-term post-traumatic atony.

Pharmacologic therapy for urinary retention has a long history. Bethanechol, a parasympathomimetic with selective bladder and gut action, has been in use for longer than 50 years. Although it certainly is capable of eliciting bladder smooth muscle tone, it does not appear to reproduce physiologic bladder contractions[89] and generally is found to be ineffective for treatment of postoperative retention when other factors are controlled.[56,90] Its significant side effect profile includes flushing, nausea, vomiting, diarrhea, gastrointestinal upset, bronchospasm, headache, salivation, sweating, and difficulties with visual accommodation, making its modern-day use unattractive. Alpha blockade is well studied for prophylaxis in high-risk patients but is not well described for treatment of postoperative urinary retention. Earlier concerns regarding possible gastrointestinal carcinogenic properties of phenoxybenzamine have been largely abandoned, and no such concerns exist for the selective alpha-1 antagonists. In view of the minimal and anticipated side effect profile of postural hypotension, syncope, tachycardia, nasal congestion, and drowsiness, alpha blockers may be a reasonable therapeutic alternative in patients with difficult and refractory postoperative urinary retention. The use of prostaglandins also is described under the hypothesis that they contribute to maintenance of bladder tone and contractile activity. Prostaglandin E_2 (PGE_2) also has been shown to cause a net decrease in urethral smooth muscle tone.[89] Numerous studies using different concentration of intravesicular preparations of both PGE_2 and $PGF_{2\alpha}$ show mixed results, making any therapeutic recommendations difficult.

Any patient who fails to respond to conservative measures, bladder rest, or pharmacologic management requires urodynamic evaluation and possibly EMG evaluation of the external striated urethral sphincter. In the rare case of Fowler's syndrome, sacral neuromodulation may represent the only efficacious therapy.[77-79]

OVARIAN REMNANT SYNDROME

Ovarian remnant syndrome (ORS), first described by Kaufman in 1962,[91] is defined as persistent functional ovarian tissue after bilateral oophorectomy. It occurs after incomplete ovarian dissection and removal after a difficult procedure in which adhesions from previous surgery, endometriosis, previous pelvic infection, neoplasm, or irradiation make ovarian mobilization difficult. It also is described after vaginal hysterectomy and oophorectomy, when pelvic support mechanisms make isolation of the infundibulopelvic ligament difficult, with subsequent clamp placement across the ovarian stroma. The ovarian remnant syndrome is not the same as the residual ovary syndrome, in which ovarian tissue is intentionally preserved, ultimately leading to symptomatology. Supernumerary ovaries are rarely encountered. These extra ovaries are derived from the germinal ridge or caudal yolk sac endoderm during embryogenesis.[92] With rising gonadotropin levels after bilateral oophorectomy in premenopausal patients, supernumerary ovaries are stimulated and can mimic ovarian remnants. They typically are located in omentum, mesentery, or the retroperitoneum and theoretically are less frequently associated with extensive adhesive disease.

Ovarian remnant syndrome can occur in the adnexal region after incomplete excision of the ovary or in ectopic locations after ovarian morcellation or fragmentation. Numerous reports of devascularized ovarian stromal implantation and regrowth exist.[93-96] Animal models have demonstrated ovarian revascularization and return of ovarian function after devascularized ovarian tissue was placed in contact with both intact and denuded peritoneum.[97,98] It is likely that rising levels of stimulatory gonadotropins after oophorectomy contribute to the development of this functional ovarian residual tissue.[99]

The true incidence of ovarian remnant syndrome is not known. In a cohort study involving 119 women with previous hysterectomy bilateral salpingo-oophorectomy (BSO) and chronic pelvic pain, the diagnosis was confirmed in 18% of the women.[93] Recurrence after previous resection reportedly occurs in approximately 8% to 30% of cases.[100] Most cases of histologically confirmed ovarian remnant syndrome occur in patients who have undergone multiple previous laparotomies or laparoscopies. No single surgical approach or method of

isolating ovarian tissue and occluding the ovarian vessels appears preferable to another.[99] Cases are reported after laparotomy, vaginal surgery, and laparoscopy when loops, staplers, sutures, or cautery devices have been used.

Prevention

Given the high morbidity of numerous surgeries and chronic pain associated with ovarian remnant syndrome, as well as its relative frequency after difficult bilateral oophorectomy, the conscientious gynecologist will take precautions to prevent its occurrence at the time of initial oophorectomy. Recommendations include dividing ovarian pedicles well beyond the interface with ovarian stroma and removing ovaries in one piece if possible. The use of an Endo bag with laparoscopy is highly recommended, to reduce the risk of fragmentation and port site remnants. Ovarian tissue should not be removed through unsheathed trocar sites. If morcellation or fragmentation is unavoidable, the surgeon must pay meticulous attention to the removal of all ovarian stroma from the peritoneal cavity. With this in mind, some practitioners recommend copious suction irrigation with the patient in reverse Trendelenburg position to facilitate migration of minute fragments of tissue into the posterior cul-de-sac, where they can be easily identified and removed.

The most difficult scenario, unfortunately, is the classic presentation in which extensive adhesive disease predates the original oophorectomy. In such cases, severe endometriosis, pelvic inflammatory disease, inflammatory bowel disease, previous surgery, or neoplasm may have made ovarian mobilization difficult. Adhesions to bowel, bladder, ureter, or pelvic vessels give the prudent surgeon pause and may lead to incomplete ovarian resection. In these cases, the same principles that apply to the successful surgical resection of ovarian remnants should be applied preemptively.

Any patient at risk for extensive preexisting adhesive disease should be counseled appropriately and undergo effective bowel preparation before surgery. Numerous authors advocate a retroperitoneal approach to adherent ovaries and remnants.[99,101-104] This approach allows for identification and mobilization of the ureter and major vessels before extensive ovarian surgery. In the case of a difficult ureterolysis, initiating the process at the pelvic brim appears safest,[101] and placement of a ureteral stent may aid in the dissection.[93,100,104-106] Ligation and resection of the hypogastric vessels can be useful to assist in ureterolysis or to extirpate all functional ovarian tissue.[101,104] With a retroperitoneal approach, the ovarian vessels also can be identified and secured well away from the ovarian tissue. Once the vital sidewall structures have been mobilized, the ovary can be removed en bloc with any adherent peritoneum[102,104] (Fig. 15–1). In the case of dense adhesions to the bowel or bladder, the surgeon must be prepared to make and repair any enterotomies or cystotomies that may result from complete ovarian resection. In the case of enterotomy repair, the site should be inspected for leakage under water, and sigmoidoscopy can be employed to further evaluate the integrity of the repair.[99] Cystotomy repairs in proximity to the trigone should be inspected cystoscopically.

An optimal initial oophorectomy is the best approach to avoiding the development of ovarian remnant syndrome. By

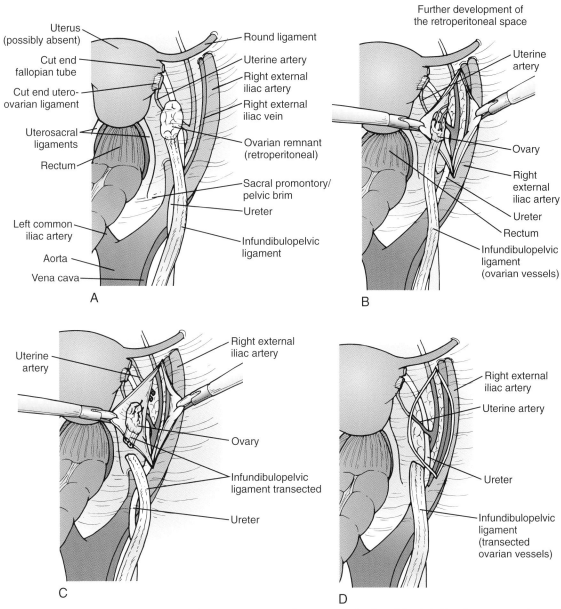

Figure 15–1 ▪ **Laparoscopic repair for management of ovarian remnant syndrome. A,** Relationship of the vital sidewall structures to the ovarian remnant with initial surgical approach. **B,** Retroperitoneal dissection starting at the pelvic brim allows ureteral mobilization. **C,** Isolation and transection of the infundibulopelvic ligament. **D,** Removal of the ovarian remnant en bloc with associated peritoneum.

routinely employing these meticulous steps, even the most difficult oophorectomies can be completed successfully, decreasing the risk of this highly morbid, long-term, postoperative complication.

Recognition

Ovarian remnant syndrome should be included in the differential diagnosis for any patient with chronic or cyclic pelvic pain following bilateral oophorectomy. Other typical evidence includes multiple previous pelvic surgery procedures, history of severe endometriosis or pelvic infection, evidence of a pelvic mass, and premenopausal levels of follicle-stimulating hormone (FSH), luteinizing hormone (LH), and estradiol in the absence of hormone replacement therapy.[99,100,102,104] Pain can be described as constant and dull or cyclic and sharp. It can be well localized, bilateral, or diffuse. Most patients describe intermittent, sharp, localized, stabbing pain, which may be aggravated by intercourse or defecation, in addition to their primary complaint.[104]

In atypical cases the presenting symptoms can be associated with a secondary diagnosis. Ureteral obstruction is well described[100,104,105] and typically manifests as flank pain, with radiographic evidence of hydronephrosis or ureteral narrowing. Constipation or symptoms of complete bowel obstruction[93] can be the presenting complaint, as can urinary retention.[107] Constitutional symptoms consistent with ascites and ovarian malignancy after bilateral oophorectomy also can be the first sign that an ovarian remnant exists.[108,109] Retrospectively, most patients diagnosed with these atypical secondary presentations report a history of less severe typical symptomatology predating the actual diagnosis.

Although premenopausal levels of gonadotropin after bilateral oophorectomy are virtually diagnostic of the condition, not all histologically confirmed remnants are active enough to maintain low gonadotropin levels. Further complicating this test is the fact that most young women take hormone replacement therapy after their surgical menopause, making FSH, LH, and PGE_2 levels unreliable.

Most patients with an ovarian remnant will have a palpable mass or thickening in the adnexa on examination; however, in Pettit and Lee's series of 31 histologically confirmed cases, 9 patients had masses discovered sonographically, which could not be palpated.[104] This highlights the importance of ultrasound examination in the evaluation of pelvic pain in patients who fit the profile for ovarian remnant syndrome. A number of case reports describe preoperative stimulation of suspected ovarian remnants that are neither radiographically or palpably apparent, to help both diagnostically and surgically. Specifically, clomiphene citrate, gonadotropin, and GnRH agonists all have been used to stimulate follicular growth in unlocalized ovarian remnants.[110-112] In all reported cases, follicular stimulation before surgery confirmed the diagnosis of ovarian remnant syndrome and aided the surgeon in identification and excision of the remnant.

Management

The management of ovarian remnant syndrome is primarily surgical, utilizing the principles described under "Prevention." The question of approach, however, generates significant debate. Many authorities believe that the intrinsic difficulty of the surgery, in view of the level of adhesive disease and potential for blood loss and adjacent organ injury, precludes laparoscopy as a reasonable approach. As equipment and expertise in minimally invasive surgery continue to improve, however, a growing number of advanced endoscopists feel that a laparoscopic approach offers some significant advantages over traditional laparotomy.[93,99,102,103,105,113] Magnification in laparoscopy assists in identification of major structures, and the pressures of pneumoperitoneum may help develop better dissection planes. Finally, fine coagulating and vessel sealing instruments aid in the maintenance of hemostasis and further improve visualization. The choice of surgical approach must ultimately rest with the surgeon, based on comfort and the specifics of each individual case.

In view of the complexity of surgery for ovarian remnant syndrome, medical management is an attractive alternative. Early reports used castrating levels of pelvic radiation, which were successful in a number of cases.[93,98,107] This approach has been largely abandoned because of the associated risks of future malignancy and long-term radiation colitis and obstruction. In the most refractory of cases, collaboration with a radiation oncologist continues to be a last-choice option. Hormonal therapy with combined contraceptives, progestins, and danazol has had limited success[93]; however, suppression of persistent ovarian remnants with long-term GnRH agonist therapy is reported with some success.[93,100] GnRH agonist therapy also may help confirm the diagnosis

before surgery, because the early agonist surge should have a stimulatory effect on the mass and long-term suppression should result in shrinkage of the mass. This approach is particularly appealing in patients who are otherwise approaching a menopausal age and whose pain is primarily cyclic in nature. A role for GnRH antagonist therapy may exist but has not as of yet been evaluated.

Currently the standard of practice for the management of ovarian remnant syndrome is extirpative surgery. As noted previously, all patients should be counseled about possible blood loss and damage to bowel, bladder, ureter, and blood vessels. In the case of laparoscopy, patients need to understand the distinct possibility of conversion to laparotomy. All patients, regardless of approach, should receive preoperative mechanical bowel preparation. Complete resection of ovarian remnants demands wide surgical margins after mobilization of adherent organs. This typically favors a retroperitoneal approach initiated at the level of the pelvic brim. In the case of laparoscopy, the use of an Endo bag to remove the remnant, thereby avoiding spillage and subsequent seeding, is important. All fragments must be meticulously removed from the abdomen to reduce the significant risk of recurrence.

CHEMICAL PERITONITIS AFTER RUPTURED DERMOID

Mature ovarian teratomas or dermoid cysts constitute approximately 15% of all ovarian neoplasm and are the most common benign ovarian tumors. They are the single most common ovarian tumor in women younger than 20 years of age.[114] Spontaneous rupture occurs infrequently, generally after torsion, with an estimated incidence of 0.7% to 4.6%.[115] Spillage of dermoid contents may result in widespread granulomatous chemical peritonitis, manifested by peritoneal and visceral implants, omental cake, and ascites. This presentation mimics ovarian malignancy. In most cases the diagnosis is made after pathologic review following total abdominal hysterectomy, BSO, and extensive tumor debulking for presumed cancer. Dermoid cysts generally are asymptomatic and are diagnosed incidentally on physical or radiographic examination or during surgery for an unrelated reason.

In view of their slow rate of growth with increasing risks of torsion, and a 0.3% to 1% rate of malignancy,[116] management generally is surgical. Laparoscopic ovarian cystectomy in premenopausal patients and laparoscopic oophorectomy in postmenopausal patients is well described[114,117-128] and has become the standard of care in many institutions with experienced surgeons. The two strongest arguments against a laparoscopic approach both stem from the risk of cyst spillage. In cases of malignancy, rupture potentially upgrades the cancer stage, changing subsequent management. In the case of benign mature cystic teratomas, intraoperative rupture and spillage could lead to the subsequent development of granulomatous chemical peritonitis. Only four cases of chemical peritonitis after laparoscopic dermoid cystectomy have been described in the English literature.[123,129-131] A review of all reported cases of laparoscopic dermoid management as of 1999 by Nezhat and associates calculated a 0.3% incidence of chemical peritonitis after laparoscopy as a result of dermoid content spillage.[121] Despite the paucity of case reports, numerous recommendations exist to minimize the risk of this uncommon complication.

Prevention

Avoiding intraoperative spillage of cyst contents is the most reliable approach to prevention of postoperative chemical peritonitis. Unfortunately, reported spillage rates after laparoscopy run the spectrum from 0% to 100% depending on the surgeon, selected technique, and the premium placed on avoidance of spill. Surgical techniques aimed at consistently avoiding cyst rupture require longer operative times even in the hands of expert gynecologic laparoscopists. Remorgida and co-workers reported the successful intact removal of 44 consecutive dermoid cysts over the course of 4 years using a technique that emphasized (1) development of a cleavage plane; (2) dissection by a combination of water, scissors, and gravity without traction on the cyst wall; and (3) removal of the intact cyst through an impermeable endoscopic bag.[132] Their average operating time was longer than 2 hours, and by their own admission, the technique requires a high level of expertise. If an unruptured ovarian cystectomy can be performed, removal of the cyst in an impermeable bag or through posterior colpotomy helps to minimize subsequent rupture and peritoneal contamination.

Perhaps the most important factor to consider is the complete removal of all spilled contents from the peritoneal cavity. Copious saline suction lavage is widely utilized to decrease the subsequent risk of peritonitis.[114,124,128,133] In a randomized, blinded, controlled rat model study, Fielder and colleagues demonstrated a massive inflammatory response with the development of widespread adhesions after the introduction of human dermoid contents into the rat abdomen. A similar response was not noted after the introduction of human follicular fluid, suggesting that the response was not entirely antigenic in nature.[133] Copious saline lavage was found to clinically ameliorate the response despite the histologic persistence of inflammatory mediators.[133] The difficulty encountered with suctioning dermoid contents from the cyst cavity or peritoneum stems from its thick sebaceous nature, which is not easily suspended after copious lavage. Erian and Goh advocate the use of warmed dilute povidone-iodine solution for the suction irrigation of any sebaceous material.[134] The iodine solution decreases the interfluid surface tension between the saline and cyst fluid, and warming the fluid prevents solidification of the sebaceous material.[134] To prevent gross cyst rupture with the need for subsequent prolonged "cleanup," many authors advocate intraoperative cyst drainage or controlled spillage into the posterior cul-de-sac.[114,117,120,122,124,126,128,134] Regardless of the technique, copious irrigation and lavage must be performed after dermoid spillage until no further evidence of sebaceous material or hair exists.

In view of the possibility of malignancy, many authorities recommend frozen section at the time of surgery. The decision to pursue extensive debulking surgery should wait until definitive permanent pathologic review has been completed. This renders frozen section results moot. If malignancy is confirmed on final pathologic review, prompt debulking and staging should ensue after consultation with an oncologist and the patient.

Recognition and Management

In a majority of the reports in the literature, dermoid-associated chemical peritonitis follows spontaneous cyst rupture not associated with surgery. Because most cases result from slow cyst leakage, the symptoms of abdominal discomfort generally are mild and vague, initially without associated changes in abdominal girth. As the peritonitis progresses, a variety of symptoms can ensue, depending on the involved locale. These manifestations are often associated with ascites.[115] The acute abdomen presentation, although described, is less likely to follow surgery in which an attempt to remove spilled material has already taken place. Although uncommon, chemical peritonitis should be a consideration in the differential diagnosis if symptoms mimicking ovarian carcinoma manifest shortly after surgery for a dermoid cyst. This benign complication requires unilateral salpingo-oophorectomy but does not require extensive removal of all granulomatous lesions, except for diagnostic purposes. More extensive surgery is warranted only to relieve associated symptoms.[115]

Summary

Dermoid cysts represent the most common benign ovarian tumors and can be successfully managed laparoscopically. The risk of chemical peritonitis after cyst rupture at the time of surgery is very low and can be minimized by containment of cyst contents and copious suction lavage. In the rare case of postrupture peritonitis, the clinical presentation can mimic epithelial ovarian carcinoma, but management should be focused on alleviating symptoms. Conservative surgical management generally is sufficient. No evidence is available to support the routine use of laparotomy for the management of a presumed dermoid cyst.

References

1. Mazze RI, Kallen B. Reproductive outcome after anesthesia and operation during pregnancy: A registry study of 5405 cases. Am J Obstet Gynecol 1989;161:1178.
2. Lachman E, Schienfeld A, Voss E, et al. Pregnancy and laparoscopic surgery. J Am Assoc Gynecol Laparosc 1999;6:347.
3. Reedy MB, Galan HL, Richards WE, et al. Laparoscopy during pregnancy. A survey of laparoendoscopic surgeons. J Reprod Med 1997;42:33.
4. Carter JF, Soper DE. Operative laparoscopy in pregnancy. JSLS 2004;8:57.
5. Reedy MB, Kallen B, Kuehl TJ. Laparoscopy during pregnancy: A study of five fetal outcome parameters with use of the Swedish Health Registry. Am J Obstet Gynecol 1997;177:673.
6. Mathevet P, Nessah K, Dargent D, Mellier G. Laparoscopic management of adnexal masses in pregnancy: A case series. Eur J Obstet Gynecol Reprod Biol 2003;108:217.
7. Stepp KJ, Tulikangas PK, Goldberg JM, et al. Laparoscopy for adnexal masses in the second trimester of pregnancy. J Am Assoc Gynecol Laparosc 2003;10:55.
8. Stepp K, Falcone T. Laparoscopy in the second trimester of pregnancy. Obstet Gynecol Clin North Am 2004;31:485.
9. Soriano D, Yefet Y, Seidman DS, et al. Laparoscopy versus laparotomy in the management of adnexal masses during pregnancy. Fertil Steril 1999;71:955.

10. Oelsner G, Stockheim D, Soriano D, et al. Pregnancy outcome after laparoscopy or laparotomy in pregnancy. J Am Assoc Gynecol Laparosc 2003;10:200.

11. Curet MJ, Allen D, Josloff RK, et al. Laparoscopy during pregnancy. Arch Surg 1996;131:546.

12. Fatum M, Rojansky N. Laparoscopic surgery during pregnancy. Obstet Gynecol Surv 2001;56:50.

13. Geisler JP, Rose SL, Mernitz CS, et al. Non-gynecologic laparoscopy in second and third trimester pregnancy: Obstetric implications. JSLS 1998;2:235.

14. Wang CJ, Yen CF, Lee CL, Soong YK. Minilaparoscopic cystectomy and appendectomy in late second trimester. JSLS 2002;6:373.

15. Lyass S, Pikarsky A, Eisenberg VH, et al. Is laparoscopic appendectomy safe in pregnant women? Surg Endosc 2001;15:377.

16. Rizzo AG. Laparoscopic surgery in pregnancy: Long-term follow-up. J Laparoendosc Adv Surg Tech A 2003;13:11.

17. Rollins MD, Chan KJ, Price RR. Laparoscopy for appendicitis and cholelithiasis during pregnancy: A new standard of care. Surg Endosc 2004;18:237.

18. Barnes SL, Shane MD, Schoemann MB, et al. Laparoscopic appendectomy after 30 weeks pregnancy: Report of two cases and description of technique. Am Surg 2004;70:733.

19. Bernhard LM, Klebba PK, Gray DL, Mutch DG. Predictors of persistence of adnexal masses in pregnancy. Obstet Gynecol 1999;93:585.

20. Amos JD, Schorr SJ, Norman PF, et al. Laparoscopic surgery during pregnancy. Am J Surg 1996;171:435.

21. Muench J, Albrink M, Serafini F, et al. Delay in treatment of biliary disease during pregnancy increases morbidity and can be avoided with safe laparoscopic cholecystectomy. Am Surg 2001;67:539.

22. Steinbrook RA, Bhavani-Shankar K. Hemodynamics during laparoscopic surgery in pregnancy. Anesth Analg 2001;93:1570.

23. Curet MJ, Vogt DA, Schob O, et al. Effects of CO_2 pneumoperitoneum in pregnant ewes. J Surg Res 1996;63:339.

24. Hunter JG, Swanstrom L, Thornburg K. Carbon dioxide pneumoperitoneum induces fetal acidosis in a pregnant ewe model. Surg Endosc 1995;9:272.

25. Barnard JM, Chaffin D, Droste S, et al. Fetal response to carbon dioxide pneumoperitoneum in the pregnant ewe. Obstet Gynecol 1995;85:669.

26. Friedman JD, Ramsey PS, Ramin KD, Berry C. Pneumoamnion and pregnancy loss after second-trimester laparoscopic surgery. Obstet Gynecol 2002;99:512.

27. Nezhat C, Seidman DS, Vreman HJ, et al. The risk of carbon monoxide poisoning after prolonged laparoscopic surgery. Obstet Gynecol 1996;88:771.

28. Ott DE. Carboxyhemoglobinemia due to peritoneal smoke absorption from laser tissue combustion at laparoscopy. J Clin Laser Med Surg 1998;16:309.

29. Esper E, Russell TE, Coy B, et al. Transperitoneal absorption of thermocautery-induced carbon monoxide formation during laparoscopic cholecystectomy. Surg Laparosc Endosc 1994;4:333.

30. Semm K. New methods of pelviscopy (gynecologic laparoscopy) for myomectomy, ovariectomy, tubectomy and adnectomy. Endoscopy 1979;11:85.

31. Lieng M, Istre O, Langebrekke A. Uterine rupture after laparoscopic myomectomy. J Am Assoc Gynecol Laparosc 2004;11:92.

32. Hasbargen U, Summerer-Moustaki M, Hillemanns P, et al. Uterine dehiscence in a nullipara, diagnosed by MRI, following use of unipolar electrocautery during laparoscopic myomectomy: Case report. Hum Reprod 2002;17:2180.

33. Foucher F, Leveque J, Le Bouar G, Grall J. Uterine rupture during pregnancy following myomectomy via coelioscopy. Eur J Obstet Gynecol Reprod Biol 2000;92:279.

34. Dubuisson JB, Chavet X, Chapron C, et al. Uterine rupture during pregnancy after laparoscopic myomectomy. Hum Reprod 1995;10:1475.

35. Nkemayim DC, Hammadeh ME, Hippach M, et al. Uterine rupture in pregnancy subsequent to previous laparoscopic electromyolysis. Case report and review of the literature. Arch Gynecol Obstet 2000;264:154.

36. Pelosi MA 3rd, Pelosi MA. Spontaneous uterine rupture at thirty-three weeks subsequent to previous superficial laparoscopic myomectomy. Am J Obstet Gynecol 1997;177:1547.

37. Arcangeli S, Pasquarette MM. Gravid uterine rupture after myolysis. Obstet Gynecol 1997;89:857.

38. Harris WJ. Uterine dehiscence following laparoscopic myomectomy. Obstet Gynecol 1992;80:545.

39. Friedmann W, Maier RF, Luttkus A, et al. Uterine rupture after laparoscopic myomectomy. Acta Obstet Gynecol Scand 1996;75:683.

40. Hockstein S. Spontaneous uterine rupture in the early third trimester after laparoscopically assisted myomectomy. A case report. J Reprod Med 2000;45:139.

41. Asakura H, Oda T, Tsunoda Y, et al. A case report: Change in fetal heart rate pattern on spontaneous uterine rupture at 35 weeks gestation after laparoscopically assisted myomectomy. J Nippon Med Sch 2004;71:69.

42. Mecke H, Wallas F, Brocker A, Gertz HP. [Pelviscopic myoma enucleation: Technique, limits, complications.] Geburtshilfe Frauenheilkd 1995;55:374.

43. Oktem O, Gokaslan H, Durmusoglu F. Spontaneous uterine rupture in pregnancy 8 years after laparoscopic myomectomy. J Am Assoc Gynecol Laparosc 2001;8:618.

44. Hasson HM, Rotman C, Rana N, et al. Laparoscopic myomectomy. Obstet Gynecol 1992;80:884.

45. Nezhat CH, Nezhat F, Roemisch M, et al. Pregnancy following laparoscopic myomectomy: Preliminary results. Hum Reprod 1999;14:1219.

46. Stringer NH, Walker JC, Meyer PM. Comparison of 49 laparoscopic myomectomies with 49 open myomectomies. J Am Assoc Gynecol Laparosc 1997;4:457.

47. Stringer NH, Strassner HT, Lawson L, et al. Pregnancy outcomes after laparoscopic myomectomy with ultrasonic energy and laparoscopic suturing of the endometrial cavity. J Am Assoc Gynecol Laparosc 2001;8:129.

48. Dubuisson JB, Fauconnier A, Deffarges JV, et al. Pregnancy outcome and deliveries following laparoscopic myomectomy. Hum Reprod 2000;15:869.

49. Georgakopoulos PA, Bersis G. Sigmoido-uterine rupture in pregnancy after multiple myomectomy. Int Surg 1981;66:367.

50. Landi S, Fiaccavento A, Zaccoletti R, et al. Pregnancy outcomes and deliveries after laparoscopic myomectomy. J Am Assoc Gynecol Laparosc 2003;10:177.

51. Seinera P, Farina C, Todros T. Laparoscopic myomectomy and subsequent pregnancy: Results in 54 patients. Hum Reprod 2000;15:1993.

52. Seinera P, Arisio R, Decko A, et al. Laparoscopic myomectomy: Indications, surgical technique and complications. Hum Reprod 1997;12:1927.

53. Ribeiro SC, Reich H, Rosenberg J, et al. Laparoscopic myomectomy and pregnancy outcome in infertile patients. Fertil Steril 1999;71:571.

54. Landi S, Zaccoletti R, Ferrari L, Minelli L. Laparoscopic myomectomy: Technique, complications, and ultrasound scan evaluations. J Am Assoc Gynecol Laparosc 2001;8:231.

55. Dubuisson JB, Fauconnier A, Chapron C, et al. Second look after laparoscopic myomectomy. Hum Reprod 1998;13:2102.

56. Burger DH, Kappetein AP, Boutkan H, Breslau PJ. Prevention of urinary retention after general surgery: A controlled trial of carbachol/diazepam versus alfuzosine. J Am Coll Surg 1997;185:234.

57. Bodker B, Lose G. Postoperative urinary retention in gynecologic patients. Int Urogynecol J Pelvic Floor Dysfunct 2003;14:94.

58. Tammela T, Kontturi M, Lukkarinen O. Postoperative urinary retention. I. Incidence and predisposing factors. Scand J Urol Nephrol 1986;20:197.

59. Kulacoglu H, Dener C, Kama NA. Urinary retention after elective cholecystectomy. Am J Surg 2001;182:226.

60. Petros JG, Rimm EB, Robillard RJ, Argy O. Factors influencing postoperative urinary retention in patients undergoing elective inguinal herniorrhaphy. Am J Surg 1991;161:431.

61. Petros JG, Bradley TM. Factors influencing postoperative urinary retention in patients undergoing surgery for benign anorectal disease. Am J Surg 1990;159:374.

62. Tammela T, Kontturi M, Lukkarinen O. Postoperative urinary retention. II. Micturition problems after the first catheterization. Scand J Urol Nephrol 1986;20:257.

63. Rosseland LA, Stubhaug A, Breivik H, et al. [Postoperative urinary retention.] Tidsskr Nor Laegeforen 2002;122:902.

64. Tammela T. Postoperative urinary retention—why the patient cannot void. Scand J Urol Nephrol Suppl 1995;175:75.

65. Zaheer S, Reilly WT, Pemberton JH, Ilstrup D. Urinary retention after operations for benign anorectal diseases. Dis Colon Rectum 1998;41:696.

66. Pavlin DJ, Pavlin EG, Fitzgibbon DR, et al. Management of bladder function after outpatient surgery. Anesthesiology 1999;91:42.

67. Walts LF, Kaufman RD, Moreland JR, Weiskopf M. Total hip arthro-plasty. An investigation of factors related to postoperative urinary reten-tion. Clin Orthop 1985;Apr:280.

68. Petros JG, Alameddine F, Testa E, et al. Patient-controlled analgesia and postoperative urinary retention after hysterectomy for benign disease. J Am Coll Surg 1994;179:663.

69. Petros JG, Mallen JK, Howe K, et al. Patient-controlled analgesia and postoperative urinary retention after open appendectomy. Surg Gynecol Obstet 1993;177:172.

70. O'Riordan JA, Hopkins PM, Ravenscroft A, Stevens JD. Patient-controlled analgesia and urinary retention following lower limb joint replacement: Prospective audit and logistic regression analysis. Eur J Anaesthesiol 2000;17:431.

71. Petros JG, Rimm EB, Robillard RJ. Factors influencing urinary tract retention after elective open cholecystectomy. Surg Gynecol Obstet 1992;174:497.

72. Stallard S, Prescott S. Postoperative urinary retention in general surgi-cal patients. Br J Surg 1988;75:1141.

73. Stricker K, Steiner W. [Postoperative urinary retention.] Anaesthetist 1991;40:287.

74. Kulacoglu H, Dener C, Kama NA. Urinary retention after elective chole-cystectomy. Am J Surg 2001;182:226.

75. Finley RK Jr, Miller SF, Jones LM. Elimination of urinary retention fol-lowing inguinal herniorrhaphy. Am J Surg 1991;57:486.

76. Mahan KT, Wang J. Spinal morphine anesthesia and urinary retention. J Am Podiatr Med Assoc 1993;83:607.

77. Swinn MJ, Wiseman OJ, Lowe E, Fowler CJ. The cause and natural history of isolated urinary retention in young women. J Urol 2002;167:151.

78. Swinn MJ, Fowler CJ. Isolated urinary retention in young women, or Fowler's syndrome. Clin Auton Res 2001;11:309.

79. DasGupta R, Fowler CJ. Urodynamic study of women in urinary reten-tion treated with sacral neuromodulation. J Urol 2004;171:1161.

80. Barone JG, Cummings KB. Etiology of acute urinary retention follow-ing benign anorectal surgery. Am Surg 1994;60:210.

81. FitzGerald MP, Brubaker L. The etiology of urinary retention after surgery for genuine stress incontinence. Neurourol Urodyn 2001; 20:13.

82. Ringdal M, Borg B, Hellstrom AL. A survey on incidence and factors that may influence first postoperative urination. Urol Nurs 2003;23:341.

83. Shea JA, Healey MJ, Berlin JA, et al. Mortality and complications asso-ciated with laparoscopic cholecystectomy. A meta-analysis. Ann Surg 1996;224:609.

84. Velanovich V. Pharmacologic prevention and treatment of postoperative urinary retention. Infect Urol 1992;3:87.

85. Livne PM, Kaplan B, Ovadia Y, Servadio C. Prevention of post-hysterectomy urinary retention by alpha-adrenergic blocker. Acta Obstet Gynecol Scand 1983;62:337.

86. Lose G, Lindholm P. Prophylactic phenoxybenzamine in the prevention of postoperative retention of urine after vaginal repair: A prospective randomized double-blind trial. Int J Gynaecol Obstet 1985;23:315.

87. Peterson MS, Collins DN, Selakovich WG, et al. Postoperative urinary retention associated with total hip and knee arthroplasties. Clin Orthop Rel Res 1991;269:102.

88. Gonullu NN, Gonullu M, Utkan NZ, et al. Postoperative retention of urine in general surgical patients. Eur J Surg 1993;159:145.

89. Wein AJ. Neuromuscular dysfunction of the lower urinary tract and its management. In: Walsh PC, Retik AB, Vaughan ED Jr, Wein AJ, eds. Campbell's urology, 8th ed. Philadelphia: WB Saunders, 2002.

90. Tammela T. Prevention of prolonged voiding problems after unexpected postoperative urinary retention: Comparison of phenoxybenzamine and carbachol. J Urol 1986;136:1254.

91. Kaufman JJ. Unusual causes of extrinsic ureteral obstruction. I. J Urol 1962;87:319.

92. Cruikshank SH, Van Drie DM. Supernumerary ovaries: Update and review. Obstet Gynecol 1982;60:126.

93. Abu-Rafeh B, Vilos GA, Misra M. Frequency and laparoscopic manage-ment of ovarian remnant syndrome. J Am Assoc Gynecol Laparosc 2003;10:33.

94. Payan HM, Gilbert EF. Mesenteric cyst-ovarian implant syndrome. Arch Pathol Lab Med 1987;111:282.

95. Marconi G, Quintana R, Rueda-Leverone NG, Vighi S. Accidental ovarian autograft after a laparoscopic surgery: Case report. Fertil Steril 1997;68:364.

96. Wood C, Hill D, Maher P, Lolatgis N. Laparoscopic adnexectomy—indications, technique and results. Aust N Z J Obstet Gynaecol 1992;32:362.

97. Minke T, DePond W, Winkelmann T, Blythe J. Ovarian remnant syndrome: Study in laboratory rats. Am J Obstet Gynecol 1994;171:1440.

98. Shemwell RE, Weed JC. Ovarian remnant syndrome. Obstet Gynecol 1970;36:299.

99. Nezhat CH, Seidman DS, Nezhat FR, et al. Ovarian remnant syndrome after laparoscopic oophorectomy. Fertil Steril 2000;74:1024.

100. Koch MO, Coussens D, Burnett L. The ovarian remnant syndrome and ureteral obstruction: Medical management. J Urol 1994;152:1580.

101. Unger JB, Paul RA. Ovarian remnant excision necessitating resection of the anterior hypogastric system. Am J Obstet Gynecol 2001;184:235.

102. Kamprath S, Possover M, Schneider A. Description of a laparoscopic technique for treating patients with ovarian remnant syndrome. Fertil Steril 1997;68:663.

103. Lafferty HW, Angioli R, Rudolph J, Penalver MA. Ovarian remnant syn-drome: Experience at Jackson Memorial Hospital, University of Miami, 1985 through 1993. Am J Obstet Gynecol 1996;174:641.

104. Pettit PD, Lee RA. Ovarian remnant syndrome: Diagnostic dilemma and surgical challenge. Obstet Gynecol 1988;71:580.

105. Klutke J, Kavoussi LR, Albala DM, Clayman RV. Laparoscopic treatment of ureteral obstruction secondary to ovarian remnant syndrome. J Urol 1993;149:827.

106. Berek JS, Darney PD, Lopkin C, Goldstein DP. Avoiding ureteral damage in pelvic surgery for ovarian remnant syndrome. Am J Obstet Gynecol 1979;133:221.

107. Bryce GM, Malone P. The ovarian remnant syndrome presenting with acute urinary retention. Postgrad Med J 1989;65:797.

108. Bruhwiler H, Luscher KP. [Ovarian cancer in ovarian remnant syndrome.] Geburtshilfe Frauenheilkd 1991;51:70.

109. Glaser D, Burrig KF, Mast H. [Ovarian cancer in ovarian remnant syndrome?] Geburtshilfe Frauenheilkd 1992;52:436.

110. Kaminski PF, Sorosky JI, Mandell MJ, et al. Clomiphene citrate stimu-lation as an adjunct in locating ovarian tissue in ovarian remnant syndrome. Obstet Gynecol 1990;76:924.

111. Scott RT, Beatse SN, Illions EH, Snyder RR. Use of the GnRH agonist stimulation test in the diagnosis of ovarian remnant syndrome. A report of three cases. J Reprod Med 1995;40:143.

112. Kosasa TS, Griffiths CT, Shane JM, et al. Diagnosis of a supernumerary ovary with human chorionic gonadotropin. Obstet Gynecol 1976;47:236.

113. Nezhat F, Nezhat C. Operative laparoscopy for the treatment of ovarian remnant syndrome. Fertil Steril 1992;57:1003.

114. Berg C, Berndorff U, Diedrich K, Malik E. Laparoscopic management of ovarian dermoid cysts. A series of 83 cases. Arch Gynecol Obstet 2002;266:126.

115. Waxman M, Boyce JG. Intraperitoneal rupture of benign cystic ovarian teratoma. Obstet Gynecol 1976;48:9S.

116. Comerci JT Jr, Licciardi F, Bergh PA, et al. Mature cystic teratoma: A clinicopathologic evaluation of 517 cases and review of the literature. Obstet Gynecol 1994;84:22.

117. Lin P, Falcone T, Tulandi T. Excision of ovarian dermoid cyst by laparoscopy and by laparotomy. Am J Obstet Gynecol 1995;173:769.

118. Canis M, Mage G, Pouly JL, et al. Laparoscopic diagnosis of adnexal cystic masses: A 12-year experience with long-term follow-up. Obstet Gynecol 1994;83:707.

119. Mecke H, Savvas V. Laparoscopic surgery of dermoid cysts—intraoper-ative spillage and complications. Eur J Obstet Gynecol Reprod Biol 2001;96:80.

120. Nezhat C, Winer WK, Nezhat F. Laparoscopic removal of dermoid cysts. Obstet Gynecol 1989;73:278.

121. Nezhat CR, Kalyoncu S, Nezhat CH, et al. Laparoscopic management of ovarian dermoid cysts: Ten years' experience. JSLS 1999;3:179.

122. Reich H, McGlynn F, Sekel L, Taylor P. Laparoscopic management of ovarian dermoid cysts. J Reprod Med 1992;37:640.

123. Mendilcioglu I, Zorlu CG, Trak B, et al. Laparoscopic management of adnexal masses. Safety and effectiveness. J Reprod Med 2002;47:36.

124. Hessami SH, Kohanim B, Grazi RV. Laparoscopic excision of benign dermoid cysts with controlled intraoperative spillage. J Am Assoc Gynecol Laparosc 1995;2:479.

125. Luxman D, Cohen JR, David MP. Laparoscopic conservative removal of ovarian dermoid cysts. J Am Assoc Gynecol Laparosc 1996;3:409.

126. Zanetta G, Ferrari L, Mignini-Renzini M, et al. Laparoscopic excision of ovarian dermoid cysts with controlled intraoperative spillage. Safety and effectiveness. J Reprod Med 1999;44:815.

127. Chapron C, Dubuisson JB, Samouh N, et al. Treatment of ovarian dermoid cysts. Place and modalities of operative laparoscopy. Surg Endosc 1994;8:1092.

128. Campo S, Garcea N. Laparoscopic conservative excision of ovarian dermoid cysts with and without an endobag. J Am Assoc Gynecol Laparosc 1998; 5:165.

129. Cristoforoni P, Palmeri A, Walker D, et al. Ovarian cystic teratoma: To scope or not to scope? J Gynecol Tech 1995;1:153.

130. Clement D, Barranger E, Benchimol Y, Uzan S. Chemical peritonitis: A rare complication of an iatrogenic ovarian dermoid cyst rupture. Surg Endosc 2003;17:658

131. Leonard F, Lecuru F, Rizk E, et al. Perioperative morbidity of gynecological laparoscopy. A prospective monocenter observational study. Acta Obstet Gynecol Scand 2000;79:129.

132. Remorgida V, Magnasco A, Pizzorno V, Anserini P. Four year experience in laparoscopic dissection of intact ovarian dermoid cysts. J Am Coll Surg 1998;187:519.

133. Fielder EP, Guzick DS, Guido R, et al. Adhesion formation from release of dermoid contents in the peritoneal cavity and effect of copious lavage: A prospective, randomized, blinded, controlled study in a rabbit model. Fertil Steril 1996;65:852.

134. Erian MM, Goh JT. A new laparoscopic aspiration technique for ovarian dermoid cysts. J Am Assoc Gynecol Laparosc 1994;2:71.

135. Darai E, Dechaud H, Benifla JL, et al. Fertility after laparoscopic myomectomy: preliminary results. Hum Reprod 1997;12:1931.

136. Ribeiro SC, Reich H, Rosenberg J, et al. Laparoscopic myomectomy and pregnancy outcome in infertile patients. Fertil Steril 1999;71:571.

137. Rossetti A, Sizzi O, Soranna L, et al. Fertility outcome: Long-term results after laparoscopic myomectomy. Gynecol Endocrinol 2001;15:129.

Complications of Hysteroscopic Surgery

Morris Wortman

16

As with any other area of surgery, the incidence and severity of complications attributable to hysteroscopic surgery are inversely related to operator skill. Additionally, the accumulation of experience and the scholarly recognition of one's limits are paramount in avoidance of unnecessary complications. Airplane pilots often say that good judgment comes from "experience"—the experience of making bad judgments *and* surviving them. The same can be said of hysteroscopic surgery. Complication avoidance is a function of training, supervision, experience, accumulating wisdom from errors committed, and understanding the limits of technology and personal skill levels. Many complications occur in a setting in which the surgeon's desire to meet a patient's expectations (or personal ones) collides with intraoperative reality—when unanticipated fluid absorption occurs or when visualization is limited by excessive bleeding. Even the most dedicated physician has at one time felt pressured to complete a procedure that in hindsight should have been abandoned in favor of a more reasoned approach.

In the original 1977 *Star Wars* film, Obi-Wan Kenobi warned young Luke Skywalker to beware the "dark temptations of human personality." Likewise, to avoid complications of hysteroscopic surgery requires not only knowledge and experience but a disciplined approach to patient selection and sound intraoperative decision making.

Surgical complications are rarely the result of a single error. More often than not they are the end product of an "error chain." Excessive fluid absorption seldom occurs suddenly. Instead, it results from ignoring information regarding patient risk factors, minor fluid imbalances, or excessive hydrostatic pressures—not unseen just by a single person but by the surgeon, anesthesiologist, and operating room staff. Many uterine perforations occur during mechanical cervical dilatation and often result from a combination of relative cervical stenosis, excessive force, failure to properly prepare the uterine cervix, and incorrect assessment of uterine position. Injuries to bowel or bladder have occurred in the setting of unexplained fluid imbalance and poor visualization.

Complications of hysteroscopic surgery can be divided into *immediate* and *delayed*. Immediate complications are related to cervical stenosis, cervical lacerations, poor visualization, uterine perforation and rupture, fluid overload, hemorrhage, infection, gas emboli, intraoperative bradycardia, and unintended vaginal and vulvar burns. Delayed complications include pregnancy, symptomatic hematometra, persistent and recurrent vaginal bleeding, post-ablation tubal sterilization syndrome, and the delayed diagnosis of endometrial cancers.

IMMEDIATE COMPLICATIONS

Cervical Stenosis

A majority of hysteroscopic surgical procedures involve the introduction of instruments that range from 7 to 9 mm in diameter. Once the instrument is introduced into the uterine cavity, the operator must be able to move the instrument freely within the confines of the uterus. Serden and Brooks[1] advocate a fairly tight seal around the cervix, whereas other investigators[2,3] prefer to operate with an overdilated cervix. All authorities agree, however, that significant cervical stenosis is an impediment to successful hysteroscopic surgery. This is especially true in the course of resecting large myomas. During hysteroscopic myomectomy, the resectoscope may be introduced and withdrawn many times in order to remove tissue fragments and strips. Significant cervical stenosis is a relative contraindication to hysteroscopic myomectomy.

Cervical stenosis often can be anticipated by a careful history and physical examination—still, its presence cannot always be predicted. A history of cryosurgery, a loop excision procedure, or laser vaporization of a lesion should alert the gynecologist to the possibility of this surgical obstacle. In addition, cervical stenosis should be anticipated in women who are nulliparous or menopausal or who have a history of obstetric trauma.

Up to 10% of my patients have some element of relative cervical stenosis, making the introduction of a 26F resectoscope difficult and in some instances impossible. In most cases the stenosis can be overcome with a combination of slow methodical dilatation, intracervical vasopressin, and enough force. The use of excessive force, however, is undesirable and increases the risks of external and internal cervical lacerations, as well as uterine perforation. Most intraoperative surprises can be avoided, however, by employing one or more of the following methods.

Use of *Laminaria* Tents

Preoperative visits are scheduled the day before surgery. After reviewing the procedure and answering any questions the patient still has, a speculum examination is performed to assess the cervix. The cervix is grasped with a single-toothed tenaculum. Paracervical block anesthesia does not reduce the pain of cervical dilatation,[4] but a small wheal of xylocaine placed on the anterior cervix with a 24-gauge needle can eliminate the pain from the tenaculum placement. A single 2- to 4-mm diameter of *Laminaria japonica* is inserted into the endocervical canal. If the cervix is relatively stenotic, a single 200-μg misoprostol tablet is inserted into the vagina.

Misoprostol

Misoprostol can be administered either orally or by vaginal insertion. Thomas and associates[5] found that the administration of 400 μg of oral misoprostol 12 to 24 hours before surgery provides excellent cervical softening and reduces the pain of dilatation. Preutthipan and Herabutya[6] reported similar results using vaginal administration of misoprostol in similar doses.

Unfortunately, not all cases of cervical stenosis can be avoided even with the aforementioned interventions. In those rare circumstances other intraoperative tools can be utilized.

Intraoperative Vasopressin

Phillips and associates[7] reported that the use of 4 units (U) of vasopressin given intracervically at 4 o'clock and 8 o'clock produced a very significant reduction in both the peak linear force required and the time necessary to accomplish cervical dilatation. In my practice I prepare a solution of vasopressin containing 10 U in 80 mL of sterile saline. Using a 21-gauge 1½-inch needle on a 3-inch needle extender, I inject 10 mL each at the 3 o'clock and 9 o'clock positions for a total dose of 2.5 U in a total volume of 20 mL.

Endocervical Resection

It is rare that the aforementioned methods will not adequately address the problem of cervical stenosis. Nonetheless, circumstances will arise in which cervical stenosis has not been anticipated, and the physician is then faced with this intraoperative challenge. Provided that the cervix can be dilated to 8 mm, an extended-loop electrode can be placed into the endocervical canal[8] (Fig. 16–1); then, under sonographic guidance, the anterior or posterior endocervical canal is resected.

Small-Diameter Resectoscopes

Most major instrument manufacturers now produce a small, 7-mm-diameter resectoscope that can be introduced to accomplish many hysteroscopic procedures. Although these instruments are very helpful, they generally are inadequate for

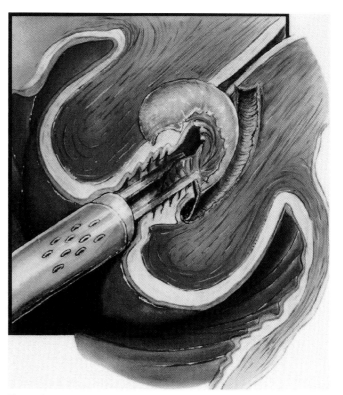

Figure 16–1 ■ Endocervical resection showing removal of posterior endocervical canal.

accomplishing the resection of large myomas or the surface area of an enlarged uterus.

It is worthwhile mentioning that an improperly dilated cervix is a contraindication to hysteroscopic surgery. It is a courageous and wise physician who, with a patient under anesthesia and in stirrups, will cancel the planned surgery in favor of placing a *Laminaria* or vaginal misoprostol tablet and allowing the cervix to adequately ripen, rather than dealing with the complications consequent to pressing onward in an attempt to complete a procedure under adverse conditions.

Cervical Lacerations

Two types of cervical lacerations are encountered during the course of hysteroscopic surgery: those that occur on the exocervix and those that occur in the endocervical canal. *Exocervical lacerations* generally occur from the excessive countertraction force applied to a single-toothed tenaculum used to stabilize the cervix during surgery. Careful preoperative evaluation and preparation of the cervix with the agents and techniques described previously can reduce the incidence of this complication. Another technique involves placing *two* separate tenacula on the anterior cervical lip to distribute countertraction forces over a broader surface area. Exocervical lacerations are rarely serious and easily repaired by placing interrupted absorbable sutures across them. Almost all lacerations can be avoided by the judicious use of *Laminaria*, misoprostol, vasopressin, small-diameter scopes, and the technique of endocervical resection.

Endocervical lacerations, though rare, are potentially serious because they may result in uncontrollable bleeding or

Figure 16–2 ▪ Deeply septated uterus. Note that the deep uterine septum creates two smaller cavities that do not allow distention fluid to recirculate.

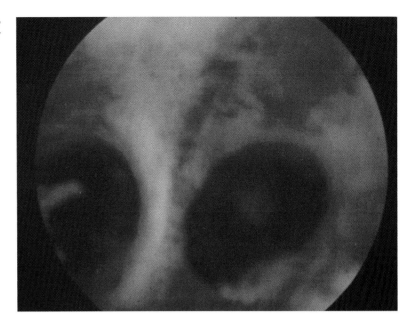

increased fluid absorption during the course of surgery. These lacerations almost always are the result of the use of excessive force during the course of cervical dilatation. Lacerations that extend laterally can produce profound bleeding that requires careful suturing of the cervical branches of the uterine artery. In extreme situations, an emergency hysterectomy may be the only method to control a larger endocervical laceration.

Poor Visualization

Although not in itself a complication, poor visualization often is the first link in an error chain. It is impossible to know how many complications of hysteroscopic surgery begin with poor visualization of the operative field. At the very least, failure to adequately visualize the uterine cavity leads to incomplete resection of myomas, polyps, and endometrium. Failure to establish adequate visualization of the uterine cavity can thwart efforts to even begin the procedure.

Two categories of visualization problems are recognized: those caused by *inadequate circulation* of distention fluid within the uterine cavity and those caused by *inadequate uterine distention*. Most commonly, poor visualization results from inadequate circulation of distention fluid allowing blood, mucus, and debris to collect within the uterine cavity. One cause is inadvertently reversing the resectoscope's inflow and outflow port attachments. Poor visualization also is common in the setting of a functionally small uterus. Even experienced hysteroscopists do not always anticipate this surgical impediment. Functionally small uteri include ones that are anatomically small (less than 7 cm) and those with large cavity-filling myomas, large polyps, or deep septa. A uterus with large septa (Fig. 16–2) or a bicornuate uterus may appear large but is functionally small, inasmuch as the narrow horns block distention fluid from entering the resectoscope's suction ports, thereby preventing the normal ingress and egress of fluid.

Faced with the problem of poor visualization resulting from inadequate circulation of distention fluid, the gynecolo-

gist must first avoid uterine perforation or activation of electrosurgical current until intrauterine landmarks have been established. Remedies for poor visualization include the following:

- Checking that inflow and outflow tubing are properly connected and functioning
- Checking the resectoscope's outer sheath to ascertain that the outflow ports are free of debris
- Increasing the pressure head of fluid entering the uterine cavity
- Overdilating the cervix to allow distention fluid to egress from the cervix

In the presence of sonographic guidance, poor visualization can easily be remedied by resection of the anterior or posterior endocervical canal (see Fig. 16–1). This maneuver creates an alternate outflow tract, thereby improving fluid circulation within the uterine cavity (Fig. 16–3).

Once fluid circulation begins, allowing debris to be cleared from the field of view, an important surgical obstacle has been overcome. Of course, endocervical resection is contraindicated in any situation in which continued fertility is desired.

Less commonly, poor visualization may be associated with an inadequately distended uterus. Inadequate distention probably is responsible for many suboptimal outcomes of endometrial ablation or endomyometrial resection (EMR) procedures. Without visualizing the tubal ostium, the physician may unwittingly leave significant areas of endometrium untreated at the uterine cornual areas. The consequences of this oversight include failure to achieve control of abnormal uterine bleeding and the delayed formation of hematometra. Common factors associated with inadequately distention of the uterus include the following:

- Large size of the uterus (length greater than 10 cm as measured by transvaginal ultrasound study)
- Presence of intramural or submucous leiomyomas
- Presence of large endometrial polyps

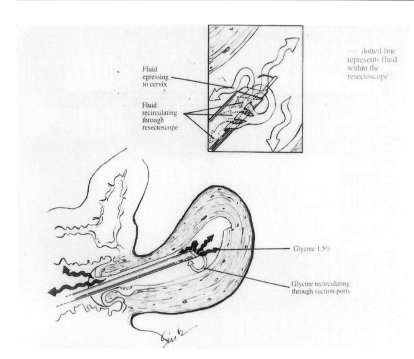

dotted line
represents fluid
within the
resectoscope

Fluid
egressing
to cervix

Fluid
recirculating
through
resectoscope

Glycine 1.5%

Glycine recirculating
through suction ports

Figure 16–3 ▪ Endocervical resection: Creating an alternate outflow tract.

• Cervical overdilatation sufficient to allow distention fluid to extravasate, thereby reducing intrauterine pressure
• Presence of a uterine septum
• Significant central obesity

Ironically, although the technique of overdilating the cervix may solve the problem of clearing the operative field of blood and debris, it may contribute to the problem of limiting visualization at the cornua, because intrauterine pressure is decreased. This problem can be remedied by placing a second tenaculum on the uterine cervix at its 3 o'clock position once adequate fluid circulation has been established (Fig. 16–4). When additional intrauterine pressure is required, the tenaculum at 3 o'clock position is turned 90 degrees and held together with the tenaculum at the 12 o'clock position. This causes the cervix to fit snugly against the resectoscope, thereby eliminating any fluid extravasation from that source.

Three other techniques for improving uterine distention include (1) raising the height of the distention media, (2) increasing distention pressure directly from a fluid management system, and (3) reducing the egress of fluid by partially closing the valve from the suction port.

The presence of a significant uterine septum (see Fig. 16–2) can pose a challenging surgical obstacle in performing an endometrial ablation or EMR procedures. Oftentimes, the septum must be incised or removed before the uterine cornua can be adequately visualized. Incision of a deep uterine septum is ideally performed with the adjuvant use of real-time sonographic guidance. In the absence of real-time sonography, some practitioners prefer the use of simultaneous laparoscopy. Unfortunately, laparoscopy poorly visualizes the myometrial thickness that remains during incision of a septum.

Uterine Perforation and Uterine Rupture

Uterine perforations occur in approximately 0.76% to 2%[9-11] of all hysteroscopic procedures. The risk factors include cervical stenosis, previous cervical surgery (cryocautery, cone biopsy, loop electrosurgical excision procedure [LEEP]), marked retroversion of the uterus, small uterine cavity size (menopausal), and excessive force, poor visualization, and lack of ultrasound guidance. In 1997, Jansen and co-workers[9] conducted a prospective study involving 82 hospitals in the Netherlands. The study included 13,600 hysteroscopies of which 11,085 were diagnostic hysteroscopies and 2,515 were operative procedures. The former group sustained 14 (0.13%) perforations, whereas the operative group sustained 19 (0.76%) perforations. Of the 33 uterine perforations, 18 (55%) occurred during introduction of a dilator or a hysteroscope; the remaining 15 were caused by technique-related issues. Of interest, 10 of the 15 cases were stopped because of the perforations; the remaining 5 were completed.

Two types of uterine perforation are recognized: those in which a "cold" surgical device (e.g., dilator, resectoscope, obturator, or cold electrode) passes through the uterine musculature and those in which a "hot" or thermoactive electrode perforates the uterus with the potential to injure other pelvic organs and viscera.

Perforation with a uterine dilator or other "cold" surgical device generally necessitates cessation of the procedure. In the presence of a small uterine perforation I have occasionally continued the procedure and retrieved the remaining distention fluid by passing a transcervical catheter through the uterine perforation and collecting the remaining fluid under ultrasound guidance. Such decisions are based on experience and operator comfort. In general, it is prudent to discontinue the case and reoperate (with the patient's consent) in 6 to 10 weeks. If possible, such procedures after a uterine perforation should be performed under sonographic guidance. In any event, uterine perforations should be managed *expectantly*. A baseline ultrasound study and complete blood count should be performed and repeated in 12 to 24 hours. Patients should be kept under close observation. Any signs of peritonitis should be aggressively investigated to rule out the possibility of a bowel injury.

Figure 16–4 ▪ "Two-tenaculum" technique to control egress of distention fluid.

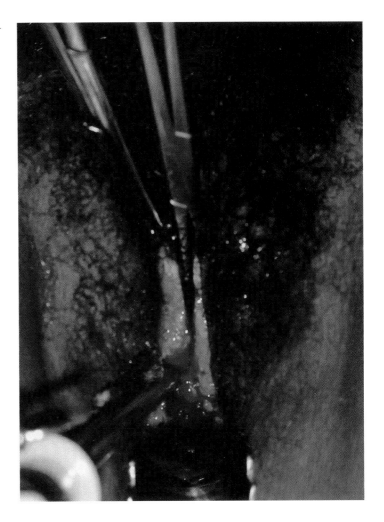

Uterine *rupture* also can occur during hysteroscopic surgery and results from the interplay of increased hydrostatic forces and excessive thinning of the myometrium—usually in the setting of hysteroscopic myomectomy or endomyometrial resection.

At least one author[12] recommends a diagnostic laparoscopy after uterine perforation, to rule out any damage to adherent or adjacent structures. This may well be an example of the treatment being worse than the disease! There has been at least one medical malpractice case in which an uncomplicated uterine perforation was followed by a diagnostic laparoscopy during which the patient sustained multiple bowel injuries from a Veress needle.

Diagnostic laparoscopies are advised only when clinical signs indicate the likelihood of adjacent bowel or bladder injury. Routine laparoscopy for uterine perforation is strongly discouraged in view of the fact that laparoscopy carries its own risks of bowel and vascular injuries. In addition, laparoscopy is not sensitive in detecting early bowel injuries, and the postoperative pain that accompanies laparoscopy may obscure early signs of peritonitis.

Uterine perforation with a thermoactive electrode is less common and does carry with it the risk of thermal damage to adjacent organs and structures including large bowel, small bowel, bladder, blood vessels, and even ureters. Not all surgeons videotape their procedures. When a videotape or recording disk is available, however, viewing the tape may be

very helpful after a uterine perforation with an active electrode. If the patient is stable, a prudent first course of action would be replaying the videotape or digital recorder *in slow motion*. In my practice, examination using this method has saved several women an unnecessary laparoscopy or laparotomy. One case involved the use of a wire-loop electrode used to resect the uterine endomyometrium. Within seconds it was clear that the fundus was perforated in the midline. On replaying the videotape it also was obvious that the apparent "perforation" actually occurred as a result of extreme uterine "thinning" and subsequent rupture. The tape recording revealed that the uterine fundus ruptured only *after* the electrode had been withdrawn toward the cervix—the result of increased intrauterine hydrostatic force coupled with excessive thinning of the fundal myometrium. The active electrode never passed through the uterine wall. Because uterine rupture carries little if any risk of adjacent thermal injury to pelvic viscera, I elected to hospitalize this patient, rather than expose her to an unnecessary laparoscopy. After 24 hours of observation involving serial blood counts and sonograms, she was discharged with careful instructions. Because bowel injuries from thermoactive electrodes may not produce clinical signs or symptoms for up to 1 to 2 weeks, patients should be advised to contact the physician with any symptoms of increasing abdominal pain, nausea, fever, or chills. Early laparotomy is strongly suggested if any signs of peritonitis are present.

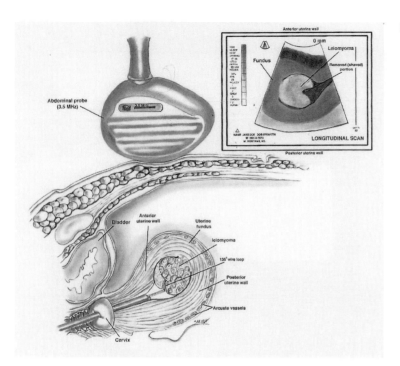

Figure 16–5 ▪ Ultrasound-guided hysteroscopic surgery.

Routine use of *Laminaria japonica* to improve cervical dilatation, with the judicious use of real-time ultrasonography to monitor the course of hysteroscopic surgery, has all but eliminated uterine perforations from my practice. Simultaneous ultrasound monitoring may be helpful whenever a hysteroscopic myomectomy[13] is anticipated in which a significant intramural component is present. In addition, sonographic monitoring during any surgical procedure in the presence of an anatomically small uterus (length less than 6 cm), cervical stenosis, uterine septa, multiple previous cesarean sections, or synechiae will help reduce the risk of uterine perforation. Sonographic guidance is a requirement for any reoperative hysteroscopic surgery in which a previous endometrial ablation or resection procedure has been performed.[14]

Still other techniques have been recommended to minimize the possibility of uterine perforation with an active electrode. Most authors suggest that the rollerball electrode be "fired" only as the electrode is withdrawn from the uterine fundus and toward the endocervical canal. Another important technique is to avoid re-treating the same area of the uterus—particularly the fundus and uterine cornual areas. It is important to appreciate that the uterus is being distended under pressure, and re-treatment with either coagulating, cutting, or blended current also results in tissue cutting and thinning that is not obvious without ultrasound guidance. With enough thinning, clinically normal levels of intrauterine distention pressure can overcome uterine wall integrity, resulting in a uterine rupture.

In my experience, no significant modality has been more important in reducing the incidence of perforation than simultaneous ultrasound guidance (Fig. 16–5). Early advocates of hysteroscopic myomectomy or excision of a uterine septum often recommended simultaneous diagnostic laparoscopy. Unfortunately, laparoscopy merely confirms that a uterine perforation *already happened*—it provides little, if any, guidance and provides no information regarding uterine

wall thickness. Several key points are worth noting for clinicians learning to use simultaneous ultrasound guidance. Working with the same technician is recommended, to help develop a team approach (Fig. 16–6) toward sonographically guided surgery.

The ultrasound monitor should be placed adjacent to the video monitor, allowing the operator to easily view both the hysteroscopic and the sonographic images. Transabdominal scanning is generally carried out with a 3.0-MHz transducer in both sagittal and transverse planes. Before the procedure, the bladder is filled with several hundred milliliters of sterile saline to create an adequate *anterior acoustic window* (Fig. 16–7). In selected cases, saline may be infused through an 18-gauge needle placed in the cul-de-sac to create a *posterior acoustic window*. As fluid is allowed to flow into the uterine cavity, an operative sonohysterogram is observed clearly delineating uterine wall thickness at all times. Communication between the surgeon and the ultrasound technician will ensure that proper guidance occurs at the operative site. As in all surgical ventures, experience is gained by beginning with relatively simple cases before progressing to more challenging ones.

Clinicians who are still learning sonographically guided surgery are reminded that patients do not present themselves in order of increasing complexity! To facilitate learning and self-confidence, it is prudent to select relatively simple cases at the start—those involving largely submucous leiomyomas or ones with a minimal intramural component. Having successful experience with relatively simple cases is essential in gaining confidence in oneself and in the operative team before progressing to more difficult and challenging cases.

Fluid Overload

In 1993 Baggish and co-workers[15] reported four cases of acute glycine and sorbitol toxicity during operative hysteroscopy.

Figure 16–6 ▪ Operative team for ultrasound-guided surgery.

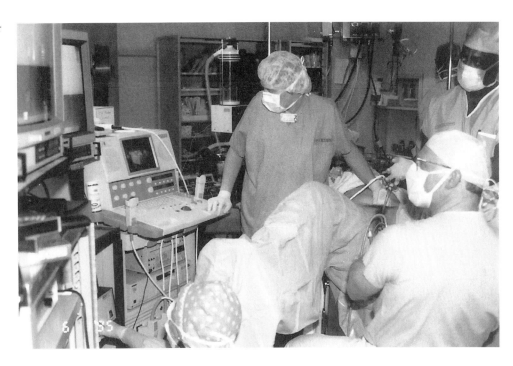

Figure 16–7 ▪ Demonstration of an anterior acoustic window.

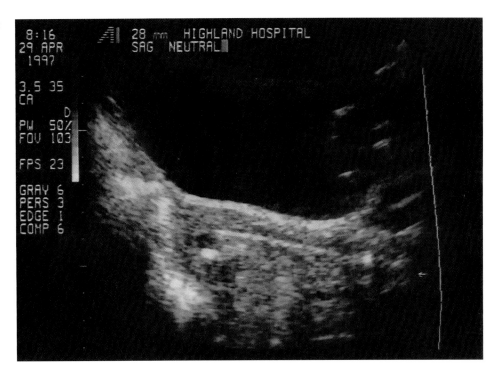

Two of the four patients died as a result of this complication. Fluid overload is the most feared and lethal complication of hysteroscopic surgery. In Propst and co-workers' series of 925 women undergoing hysteroscopic surgery, excessive fluid absorption was the most frequent complication, occurring in 7 (0.42%).[16] Fluid overload happens in the setting of lack of experience, in either the surgeon or the operating room staff, and complex cases involving the resection of myomas. Propst and co-workers reported the risk of excess fluid absorption in women undergoing myomectomy to be 4.7%—greater than a 10-fold increase compared with women without myomas.

Hysteroscopic surgery demands critical attention to uterine distention. A balance must be reached that allows the operator to obtain maximum intrauterine visualization while limiting the risk of fluid absorption. Diminished intrauterine pressure, the result of fluid extravasation from the cervix or a diminished hydrostatic pressure infused into the resectoscope, results in poor or incomplete visualization, as noted earlier. Excessive uterine pressure, often required to distend a larger uterus, may result in the intravasation of large volumes of distention fluid.

In inexperienced hands, hysteroscopic surgery has been associated with the intravasation of substantial volumes of distention medium into the intravascular compartment. I reviewed one case of operative mortality in which a woman undergoing a hysteroscopic myomectomy was allowed to absorb as much as 11 L of low-viscosity distention fluid! This complication represented a true failure on the part of the surgeon, the anesthesiologist, and operating room staff to prevent one of the most easily avoided complications of hysteroscopic surgery.

Before beginning any hysteroscopic surgery, the surgeon, the anesthesiologist, and operating room staff should agree on a maximum allowable fluid absorption limit (MAFA$_{limit}$) At any given time during the course of surgery, one should be able to calculate the patient's net fluid absorption by subtracting the amount of fluid recovered from the fluid infused. Modern fluid monitoring systems (Fig. 16–8) calculate this volume automatically and display it on the video monitor. Once this predetermined net fluid absorption limit has been reached, it should *not* be renegotiated.

A word about MAFA$_{limit}$: It has been our practice for many years to calculate this limit using the equation MAFA$_{limit}$ = 17.6 mL/kg × body weight (kg). This formula was based on a regression analysis of a large number of data points comparing fluid absorption and body mass with serum sodium change (ΔNa$^+$). The MAFA$_{limit}$ predicts that a healthy woman without cardiac, liver, or renal disease may absorb a volume of glycine 1.5% equal to 17.60 mL/kg without experiencing a fall in serum sodium concentration greater than 10 mmol/L. For instance, a healthy 37-year-old woman weighing 67.3 kg may absorb up to 1184 mL of glycine 1.5% without concern for symptomatic hyponatremia. Although MAFA$_{limit}$ has not been analyzed with other low-viscosity fluids, we continue to employ this formula even after switching to mannitol 5%. I have performed greater than 1500 cases using this formula and can attest to its value in preventing serum sodium changes greater than 10 mEq/L. This study, carried out before the advent of accurate fluid monitoring systems, bears repeating now that newer and more accurate technology is available for fluid measurement. Of note, because few data points are available for women weighing more than 125 kg, the operator should not risk allowing fluid absorption beyond 2 L under any circumstance! Once the patient absorbs her MAFA$_{limit}$, the procedure is brought to a halt. This figure is *never* renegotiated in the futile hope that a few more minutes of operative time will produce surgical rewards beyond the dire consequences to which the patient is exposed.

Inattention to net fluid absorption may lead to the most serious complications of hysteroscopic surgery—an error chain resulting in fluid and electrolyte imbalances, hypoosmolarity, hyponatremia, generalized edema, encephalopathy, pontine herniation, and death.[17,18]

Three low-viscosity anionic distention fluids are commonly used for monopolar hysteroscopic surgery: glycine 1.5% (178 mOsm/L), sorbitol 3% (165 mOsm/L), and mannitol 5% (280 mOsm/L). Glycine and sorbitol are hypoosmolar relative to human serum (280 mOsm/L). Excess fluid absorption of any of these low-viscosity fluids may cause dilutional hyponatremia, encephalopathy, fluid overload, and cardiac failure. Additionally, the hypo-osmolarity of glycine and sorbitol may cause life-threatening generalized tissue edema, pontine herniation, and respiratory center death. Glycine has additional disadvantages—it is metabolized to ammonia by the liver; it is liposoluble and passes through the blood-brain barrier, and it is metabolized into serine and glyoxylic acid, which are false neurotransmitters. Although all of these fluids must be carefully monitored, mannitol has several advantages including its iso-osmolarity with serum and its self-regulating diuretic properties. In 1998 Indman and coworkers[19] suggested the use of mannitol 5% as the preferred distention medium for all hysteroscopic surgery. This suggestion represents the best standard of care available at this time.

Recently, bipolar resectoscopes have been introduced in the United States and Canada. The advantage of such resectoscopes is that they allow the operator to use normal saline (0.9%) for uterine distention. The use of physiologic saline for uterine distention, however, does not obviate the risks of fluid overload, and several reports of severe pulmonary edema and death have emerged because of inattention to fluid management with the use of normal saline.

Operating rooms around the country are rapidly adopting automated fluid monitoring systems (see Fig. 16–8), and within a few years, this will become the only acceptable standard of care for hysteroscopic surgery. Hamou and associates[20]

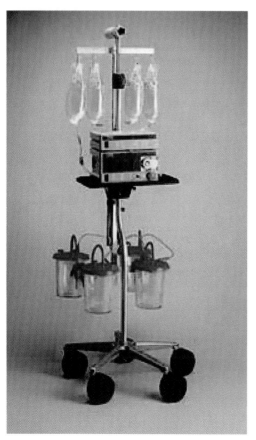

Figure 16–8 ▪ Fluid monitor system (Karl Storz Endoscopy—America, Culver City, California).

showed in an elegant study that the use of the Endomat fluid monitoring system (Karl Storz Endoscopy, Culver City, Califormia) provided a 56% reduction in fluid intravasation compared with a gravity-fed system. It is hoped that the widespread use of these systems will eliminate some of the avoidable tragedies that accompany fluid overload.

Even the best fluid monitoring systems will be confounded by unaccounted-for fluid losses—from fluid trapped in the drapes, for example, or spilled onto the floor. The major disadvantage of these mishaps will be a falsely elevated total for fluid absorption, which may cause the surgeon to stop the case prematurely. Fluid overload should rarely happen, however, so long as these systems and their safeguards are in place.

For surgeons not yet using automatic fluid management systems, the circulating nurse should obtain careful input and output records at 5-minute intervals and communicate the findings to the surgeon. Once the predetermined $MAFA_{limit}$ has been reached, the procedure should be halted and a serum sodium concentration should be checked.

Severe hyponatremia (serum sodium level ≤110 mEq/L) is uncommon and is most likely to be seen with an inexperienced operating room team, poor attention to input and output records, and prolonged procedures requiring large volumes of distention fluid. Arieff and Ayus[18] noted that although men and women are equally prone to develop hyponatremia and resultant encephalopathy, women of reproductive age are 25 times more likely to die of encephalopathy than men or postmenopausal women who experience similar serum sodium changes. Of importance, Arieff[17] did report one death after an endometrial ablation that lasted nearly 3 hours and resulted in a serum sodium level of 121 mEq/L several hours postoperatively.

The following guidelines are useful for avoiding and managing fluid overload and hyponatremia:

- Consider overdilating the cervix. Place a 2- to 4-mm length of *Laminaria* before all hysteroscopic procedures (with the exception of treatment failures). This practice was first advocated by Townsend and colleagues[2] and is very effective in promoting excellent cervical dilatation. It is difficult to obtain excessive intrauterine pressures when fluid is allowed to escape through the cervical canal.
- Unless specifically contraindicated, administer intracervical vasopressin. Vasopressin has a potent uterine constriction effect that lasts for at least 20 minutes after its administration. I place 10 U of vasopressin in 80 mL of normal saline and inject 10 mL of solution each at the 3 o'clock and 9 o'clock positions for a total of 2.5 U. Corson and associates[21] reported that patients who received vasopressin during hysteroscopic surgery had approximately one third the risk of fluid intravasation compared with patients who received placebos.
- Establish an $MAFA_{limit}$ before every procedure. When the $MAFA_{limit}$ is reached, the procedure is concluded—no exceptions.
- Procedures should not be allowed to continue beyond 1 hour. The risk of dilutional hyponatremia increases with operative time. (It is better to halt the procedure wishing you had completed it, than to complete the procedure wishing you had halted!)

PROBLEM

A 42-year-old woman undergoes a hysteroscopic EMR. Her postoperative serum sodium is 112 mEq/L. The patient weighs 100 kg. How should her serum sodium concentration be corrected using a 3% solution of sodium chloride? a 5% solution of sodium chloride?

First, calculate total body water.

Total body water in most women between 30 and 50 years of age is approximately 45%. In markedly obese women, the total body water may approach 50%.

100 kg × % body water (0.45) = 45 L of total body water

Second, determine how many mmol of sodium should be administered per hour.

To correct serum sodium from 112 to 130 mEq/L, a total of 1 to 2 mEq/L per hour, or 45 L × 1 to 2 mmol, may be given. If 1.5 mmol per hour is chosen, this translates to 67.5 mEq per hour.

Hypertonic saline is available in 3% (513 mmol/L) and 5% (856 mEq/L) concentrations. A 3% saline solution would contain 513 mEq/L. A 5% saline solution would contain 856 mEq/L.

For correction of serum sodium:

To infuse 67.5 mEq per hour using a *3% solution*, a rate of 132 mL/hour will be required. The rate of flow set at the infusion pump is determined as follows:

Desired infusion of sodium in mmol/hour × mL/mmol (desired solution) = desired flow rate of the infusion pump

67.5 mEq/hour × 1000 mL of 3% sodium solution/513 mEq = 132 mL/hr of 3% sodium solution

To infuse 67.5 mmol using a *5% solution*, a rate of 78.9 mL/hour is required. The infusion pump setting is calculated as follows:

67.5 mEq/hr × 1000 mL of 5% sodium solution/856 mEq = 78.9 mL/hr of 5% saline solution

- Consider placing an absolute limit on the amount of low-viscosity fluids that are used before a procedure is brought to halt—10 to 15 L.
- When postoperative serum sodium concentrations are between 130 and 140 mEq/L, no treatment is necessary. Restoration of normal serum sodium should occur in 12 to 24 hours if the absorption is from slow peritoneal effusion.
- When postoperative serum sodium concentrations fall between 120 and 130 mEq/L, absent signs or symptoms of encephalopathy, fluid restrictions and furosemide (10 to 20 mg intravenously) constitute the mainstay of management. Careful intake and output records should be kept, and serum sodium should be checked every 4 hours until a level greater than 130 mEq/L is attained. An intensivist should be consulted for any serum sodium concentration below 120 mEq/L.
- Patients whose serum sodium concentration falls below 120 mEq/L may require hypertonic saline unless this measure is clearly contraindicated.
- Patients who show clear evidence of encephalopathy, *regardless* of their serum sodium concentration, should receive hypertonic saline. The signs and symptoms of encephalopathy include tremulousness, dilated pupils, decreased oxygen saturation, hypothermia, grand mal seizures, lethargy, and clonus.

• Before administration of hypertonic saline, furosemide should be given to prevent circulatory overload. The risk of central pontine myelinolysis can be minimized by correcting serum sodium concentration with sodium repletion at a rate of 1 to 2 mEq/L per hour. The goal should be to correct serum sodium to 130 to 135 mEq/L, but to not exceed 25 mEq/L per 24 hours. Although most gynecologists will never encounter or treat this problem, it is worthwhile reviewing, as set out in the accompanying box.

Hemorrhage

The incidence of intraoperative or postoperative hemorrhage resulting from hysteroscopic surgery is difficult to estimate. Hill and colleagues[22] reported 7 instances of immediate or postoperative hemorrhage in 850 women undergoing operative hysteroscopy (0.8%), whereas the Scottish Hysteroscopy Audit Group[11] places the incidence of significant intraoperative and immediate postoperative bleeding at 3.6%. Hysteroscopic myomectomy, endomyometrial resections, and the division of uterine septa all are associated with greater blood loss than with endometrial ablation. No single method or technique is adequate to avoid excessive intraoperative bleeding. The skilled and experienced operator vigilantly anticipates this and other complications, using methods to minimize its occurrence. Once bleeding is encountered, the burden of judgment falls to the surgeon in deciding whether to continue or stop short of completing the planned procedure. The goal is to prevent what started out as a minimally invasive operation from becoming an unplanned hysterectomy.

Preoperative and intraoperative measures to reduce bleeding include the use of gonadotropin-releasing hormone agonists such as leuprolide acetate, *Laminaria japonica*, and intracervical vasopressin. The use of intraoperative sonographic guidance can be very helpful in avoiding significant bleeding associated with uterine septum division, endomyometrial resection, and myomectomy.

The management of intraoperative bleeding generally involves point coagulation of arterioles and small venous sinuses. During the course of performing myomectomies, bleeding often can be minimized by the use of high-power settings of cutting current (100 to 150 watts) while drawing the loop electrode slowly through the tissue to promote the desiccation of small blood vessels.

The individual physician must decide when excessive intraoperative bleeding precludes safe continuation of a procedure. Fortunately, hysteroscopic surgery, unlike most other gynecologic surgery, can be halted at almost any point. In the presence of significant intraoperative bleeding, a 16F or 18F Foley catheter is inserted with a 30-mL balloon (the tip is first removed); under sonographic guidance, saline is instilled until the catheter fills and slightly distends the uterine walls enough to compress the bleeding vessels—this generally requires anywhere from 10 to 50 mL. The catheter is left in for 2 to 4 hours. After that period of time has elapsed, half the volume of saline in the balloon is removed and the patient is observed. If after 30 minutes the bleeding has been controlled, the remaining half of the fluid is removed, along with the catheter. The patient is observed for at least another hour before being discharged.

In those rare instances in which bleeding persists after removal of the catheter, the physician should reinsert the catheter and arrange for the patient to undergo uterine artery embolization. Rarely will this procedure fail—when it does, a hysterectomy may be the only reasonable therapy.

Infection

Infection is an uncommon complication of hysteroscopic surgery. In a review of greater than 600 cases from 1988 to 1995, a total of 4 infections (0.67%) were reported. The first case occurred before use of prophylactic antibiotics and involved a woman who presented 12 hours postoperatively with an obvious myometritis and sepsis. A cervical culture was positive for group A beta-streptococci. A second patient presented 7 weeks postoperatively with a tubo-ovarian abscess and required a salpingo-oophorectomy. Two other patients presented with low-grade fever, leukocytosis, and increasing abdominal pain. Both of these women had myometritis that responded quickly to oral antibiotics.

I recommend the use of prophylactic antibiotics—Monocid 1 g given as an intravenous infusion to patients who are not allergic to penicillin. For patients with known or suspected penicillin allergies, I recommend gentamicin 80 to 120 mg or clindamycin 300 to 600 mg, both administered intravenously solution set.

Gas Emboli

Gas embolism has been reported in many kinds of gynecologic surgery, including tubal insufflation[23] procedures, cesarean section,[24] and dilatation and curettage. Since the popularization of hysteroscopic surgery, several case reports[4,25,26] have described its association with gas emboli. Potential sources of gas emboli during hysteroscopic surgery include the gaseous products of electrosurgical tissue vaporization and room air introduced into the uterus. Once thought to be infrequent, gas embolization is a common occurrence during resectoscopic surgery and can be detected using precordial Doppler evaluation. Fortunately, however, these emboli are rarely symptomatic—a happy result of the fact that the volume of gas produced by electrosurgery is small, under normal circumstances, compared with the capacity of the uterine venous blood flow to solubilize the potentially harmful gas bubbles. Brooks[27] reported 7 cases of venous gas embolism during the course of hysteroscopic surgery, resulting in 5 deaths (71.4%). In each instance, the earliest signs of problems were dramatic signs observed by the anesthesiologist. These signs included a sudden fall in end-tidal CO_2, decreased oxygen saturation, bradycardia, and a "millwheel" type of murmur auscultated over the precordium—the classic sign of air in the heart.

Whether the culprit in these operative fatalities is gas produced from electrosurgical tissue vaporization or room air is unknown. In either case, however, the mechanism involved in clinically significant gas embolism is well known.

Air or electrosurgically created gases can enter the venous circulation slowly by diffusion or, in some cases, rapidly through surgically exposed venous sinuses. The gas entering the uterine veins is carried by the venous system to the right side of the heart and into the pulmonary circulation. The pressure gradient responsible for carrying gases to the right side of the heart is proportional to the difference between intrauterine pressure and the venous pressure. The presence of bubbles or foam mechanically blocks small pulmonary arteries. In rare cases the volume of these bubbles is large enough to increase pulmonary vascular resistance, resulting in pulmonary hypertension. The hypertension may be mild, detectable only with a pulmonary artery catheter, or severe, leading to right ventricular failure and signs of acute cor pulmonale. Because pulmonary vascular obstruction diminishes the number of pulmonary capillaries available for gas exchange, carbon dioxide elimination is blocked, resulting in a decrease in end-tidal CO_2, and oxygen intake is limited, resulting in hypoxemia. Clinically, the anesthetized and ventilated patient experiences a decrease in end-expiratory CO_2. Munro and co-workers[28] describe at least six findings that may follow venous gas embolization: pulmonary hypertension, hypercarbia, hypoxia, arrhythmias, tachypnea, and systemic hypotension. Brooks[27] adds a seventh—a "millwheel murmur" that can be auscultated over the heart.

Resuscitative efforts include stopping the source of air inflow, turning the patient on her left side, attempting to aspirate as much of the gas as possible from the right side of the heart, and flushing the circulation with a large saline bolus. Although this modality is not available in most hospitals, transfer to a hyperbaric oxygen chamber can be critically important to a patient's survival. Unfortunately, the events of venous air embolism are so sudden and catastrophic that they are extremely difficult to manage and often result in either death or severe disability. Therefore, the physician's attention must be directed toward prevention.

The mainstays of prevention include measures to prevent room air from entering the venous system, to minimize excessive gas formation within the uterus, and to decrease the possibility of inadvertent cervical lacerations:

- Avoid putting the patient in Trendelenburg position.
- Suction accumulated gas bubbles whenever possible.
- Avoid leaving an exposed and dilated cervix open to room air longer than necessary.
- Dilate the cervical canal with care. The use of *Laminaria* tents and cervical ripening agents such as misoprostol and vasopressin is strongly encouraged.

Intraoperative Bradycardia and Vasopressin

It is difficult to estimate the incidence of bradycardia after paracervical vasopressin infiltration. Most bradycardias are transient and resolve spontaneously or with the administration of atropine. The risk of bradycardia is difficult to assess, because physicians tend to administer varying concentrations of vasopressin. Martin and Shenk[29] reported one case of acute myocardial infarction after paracervical administration of 5 mL of vasopressin in a solution containing 4.29 U/mL. Most hysteroscopists recommend the administration of solutions that contain no more than a maximum of 6 U. My practice is to alert the anesthesiologist just before vasopressin administration. Any bradycardia may be a warning sign of impending cardiac deterioration and warrants prompt intervention. The administration of vasopressin to any patient with a known history of cardiovascular disease should be carefully considered.

Unintended Vaginal and Vulvar Burns

In 1997 Vilos and colleagues[30] reported 3 cases of vaginal burns resulting from "stray" currents during the course of hysteroscopic surgery; 3 years later this investigative group[31] reported 10 additional cases. A careful analysis of these cases, however, reveals the following: More than half were performed with previously used electrodes, no such phenomena were observed in the investigators' practice, and most occurred in the posterior vagina. No other reports of such cases involving surgery performed by an experienced hysteroscopic surgeon have appeared in the literature, before or since.

Various explanations have been offered that suggest a mechanism involving either direct or capacitive coupling. Separate in vitro experiments by Vilos and colleagues[31] and Munro,[32] however, cast doubt that capacitive coupling can produce sufficient current density to cause a vaginal or vulvar burn. It also is doubtful that direct coupling can produce any but the smallest burns.

Nevertheless, it is the responsibility of the operator to inspect the electrode and its insulation at all times during the course of surgery. Electrodes containing frayed insulation should be immediately discarded and replaced.

Clearly, however, vaginal and vulvar burns have occurred. By what mechanism do they occur? A more likely explanation for these reported burns involves something much more mundane—spatial disorientation and operator error. Spatial disorientation may ensue when an inexperienced surgeon inadvertently places the resectoscope *past* the cervix into one of the vaginal fornices. The posterior vaginal mucosa has, in my teaching experience, been confused with the endometrial cavity and might be ablated without the careful supervision of a nescient gynecologist. More commonly, an inexperienced practitioner forgets to inactivate the electrosurgical generator after bringing the resectoscope out through the endocervical canal. The results can be painful for the unfortunate woman and embarrassing for the gynecologist. The prevention of such errors involves the careful placement of the resectoscope into the uterine cavity and ascertaining that the resectoscope is always surrounded by the cervix. The proper placement of a resectoscope should be confirmed before the activation of the electrosurgical unit Additionally, the physician should be trained to recognize the sights and sounds of the resectoscope as it passes through the endocervical canal. As a rule, the beginning hysteroscopist should never pass an activated resectoscope into the endocervical canal—and never into the vagina!

LATE COMPLICATIONS

Pregnancy after Endometrial Ablation

Although rare, unintended pregnancy after hysteroscopic ablation and resection of the endometrium has been described.[33-39] I am aware of two unintended pregnancies in my own series approaching 2000 patients—one after an endometrial ablation procedure (rollerball technique) and another after an endomyometrial resection. Both women elected to have their pregnancies terminated early in the first trimester.

Edwards and colleagues[33] reviewed the outcomes of 10 pregnancies after endometrial ablation. Only five progressed to the third trimester. Three women underwent elective terminations. One woman[35] presented with a ruptured isthmic ectopic pregnancy. Two of the pregnancies were complicated by placenta accreta. Only one of the pregnancies resulted in a spontaneous vaginal delivery, although two others went to term with delivery by cesarean section. None of the cesarean sections was complicated by placenta accreta.

A review by Rogerson and co-workers[37] revealed that only 11 of 17 women who elected to continue a pregnancy after endometrial ablation carried past 28 weeks. Of these 11 pregnancies there were 2 (18%) perinatal deaths, 5 (45%) pregnancies complicated by intrauterine growth retardation, 3 (27%) complicated by premature rupture of membranes and 7 (64%) involving preterm delivery. Of the 7 premature deliveries, 6 were by emergency cesarean section and 6 were complicated by some element of placenta accreta.

Edwards and colleagues[33] and other investigators recommend that women undergoing endometrial ablation and endomyometrial resection be offered permanent sterilization at the time of hysteroscopic surgery. This appears to be a reasonable approach and constitutes generally accepted practice. One must be mindful, however, that laparoscopic sterilization carries its own risks and consequences. In counseling a woman regarding the need for this additional procedure, a variety of issues need to be considered, including her age, her unintended pregnancy risk, the additional anesthetic risks, and any other factors that might preclude safe abdominal entry. As greater experience is gained with hysteroscopic tubal occlusion, it may become standard practice to offer this alternative to women who are at risk for an unintended pregnancy.

Symptomatic Hematometra

The development of postoperative *symptomatic* hematometra has been reported[22,39] in 1% to 2% of women undergoing endometrial ablation or resection procedures. Symptomatic hematometra requires two things: functioning endometrial glands and the entrapment of blood. Hematometra is easily diagnosed with the use of transvaginal ultrasound examination and appears as an area of echolucency, with or without coexistent endometrium, within the uterine cavity (Fig. 16–9). The hysteroscopic resection of endometrial tissue responsible for the development of a hematometra represents one of the most difficult challenges to a hysteroscopic surgeon. Figure 16–10 depicts the appearance of functioning endometrial tissue discovered at reoperative hysteroscopy. Note that the active endometrial tissue was present in the uterine cornua.

Affected women generally present with cyclic lower abdominal pain, often characterized as sharp or stabbing. The pain may be in the midline or in either lower quadrant. If pain is associated with vaginal bleeding, the diagnosis is straightforward and confirmed on transvaginal ultrasound examination. Unfortunately, hematometra also can develop in women with amenorrhea. In any woman who has undergone an endometrial ablation or resection, the possibility of hematometra should be a consideration in the differential diagnosis of pelvic pain. Moreover, all women who undergo these procedures should be advised of the possibility of the late development of symptomatic hematometra and that unexplained sharp lower abdominal pain, with or without vaginal bleeding, might warrant a call to her gynecologist.

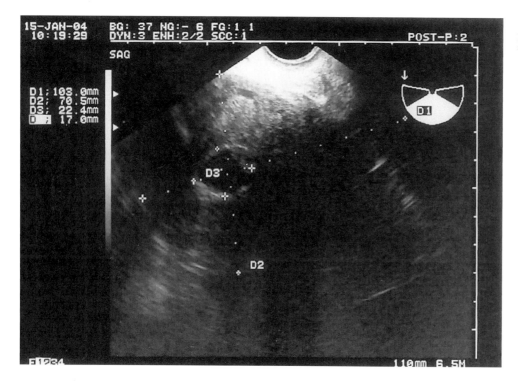

Figure 16–9 ▪ Hematometra depicted on transvaginal ultrasound study.

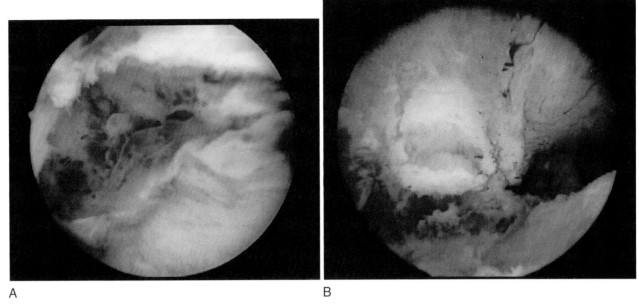

Figure 16–10 ▪ **A,** The hysteroscopic appearance of endometrial regrowth at the uterine cornua. **B,** The hysteroscopic appearance of the endometrial regrowth at the uterine cornua after much of it has been resected.

The incidence of *asymptomatic* hematometra probably is greater than the 2% noted for the symptomatic variety but is unknown because of the lack of published series of women who have undergone endometrial ablations and have been systematically followed with periodic ultrasound examinations. A woman with an asymptomatic hematometra does not require treatment provided that the intrauterine blood collection is not associated with active endometrial glands and that she is willing to undergo periodic ultrasound examination to rule out any neoplastic progression.

Hill and colleagues[22] reported treating 14 of 16 cases of hematometra by cervical dilatation alone. In my experience, relief is short-lived with use of this approach, and many patients have recurrent symptoms. A preferred method of managing hematometra is to perform a reoperative hysteroscopic resection[14] of any endometrial elements that are associated with it. To minimize the risk of uterine perforation or the creation of a false passage, this procedure should be performed under ultrasound guidance.

In my experience, most hematometras occur at the uterine fundus, often near one or both cornual regions of the uterine fundus. Hematometra formation probably involves several different mechanisms, including incomplete resection of areas of endometrium in the cornual region of the uterus, endometrial regrowth, formation of intrauterine synechiae, and cervical stenosis.

Persistent and Recurrent Vaginal Bleeding

Persistent vaginal bleeding follows most endometrial ablation and resection procedures. A majority of patients who are not amenorrheic experience sufficient clinical improvement with reduction in their symptoms that no further surgery is necessary. A significant number of patients, however, experience persistent or recurrent vaginal bleeding, with or without associated pelvic pain. Many of these women will require another

operative procedure. Various authors[10,40-44] report the frequency of further surgery—repeat hysteroscopic surgery or hysterectomy—to be between 9% and 17%.

Counseling patients who are not satisfied with the outcome of endometrial ablation or resection is complex. Among the factors to be considered are the patient's age at the time of her recurrent symptoms, the length of time between initial treatment and recurrence of symptoms, the presence of adenomyosis, the patient's desire to avoid hysterectomy, operator skill, and availability of ultrasound guidance.

I generally reserve reoperative hysteroscopic surgery for women who fulfill the following criteria: age older than 40 years, a period of satisfaction not less than 1 year since her original surgery, and strong patient motivation to avoid hysterectomy. The presence or absence of adenomyosis in the original histologic specimen also should be considered. As a rule I avoid reoperative hysteroscopic surgery whenever the original specimen reveals severe adenomyosis.

In our[45] series of 304 women who underwent hysteroscopic endomyometrial resection, 69 (22.7%) specimens showed evidence of adenomyosis. Of these women, 9 (13%) had subsequent surgery—either a reoperative hysteroscopic resection or hysterectomy. Of the 235 women without adenomyosis (77.3%), 18 (7.7%) required further surgery. Although this finding does not rise to the level of statistical significance ($P = .17$), the presence of severe adenomyosis should certainly be considered sufficient reason not to expose the patient to further hysteroscopic surgery.

For patients who are considered inappropriate candidates for reoperative hysteroscopic surgery, one alternative is the use of an endometrial suppressive agent. I generally prefer the use of danocrine 200 mg per day. Other possible regimens include raloxifene 60 mg per day and depomedroxyprogesterone acetate 150 mg every 3 months. Leuprolide acetate can be used to temporarily suppress endometrial regrowth in some women ▪ but is not recommended for long-term suppression.

For women who are poor operative candidates for repeat surgery and in whom medical therapy is not desired, a subtotal or total hysterectomy is a reasonable alternative.

Postablation Tubal Sterilization Syndrome

Townsend and colleagues[46] first described the development of a focal cornual hematometra with retrograde menstruation into a tube that had been previously occluded by a sterilization procedure or secondary to a disease process. The result is one of a coexistent hematosalpinx (Fig. 16–11), which may cause cyclic or continuous lower abdominal pain.

This syndrome should be suspected whenever a patient with a known or suspected tubal occlusion after endometrial ablation presents with cyclic lower abdominal pain. The diagnosis often is suggested on transvaginal ultrasound studies, which may reveal an area of echolucency adjacent to the uterine cornua or a cystically dilated fallopian tube (Fig. 16–12).

Treatment, at minimum, requires laparoscopic salpingectomy and reoperative hysteroscopy to remove any residual endometrial elements from the uterine cornua. Hysterectomy is a reasonable option in most cases.

The avoidance of postablation tubal sterilization syndrome (PTSS) is similar to the avoidance of subsequent hematometra—careful ablation or resection of the endometrium in the uterine cornua. At first glance, the uterine cavity may appear normal, until the surgeon searches for the tubal ostium. During the course of endomyometrial resection, whose success is dependent on the careful identification and removal of all endometrial elements, the surgeon frequently discovers deeply recessed uterine cornua and tubal ostia (Fig. 16–13) that in haste would have been overlooked only to cause recurrent vaginal bleeding, hematometra or, in women with previous sterilization procedures, PTSS.

Immediate and Delayed Diagnosis of Endometrial Cancer

Valle and Baggish[47] surveyed the peer-reviewed literature and reported eight cases of endometrial cancer diagnosed 5 months to 5 years after endometrial ablation or resection. Five of the eight women had preoperative endometrial biopsies that revealed endometrial adenomatous hyperplasia. One of

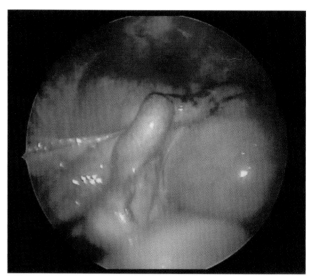

Figure 16–11 ▪ The postablation sterilization syndrome: a hematosalpinx seen at laparoscopy. The patient is the same as in Figure 16–10.

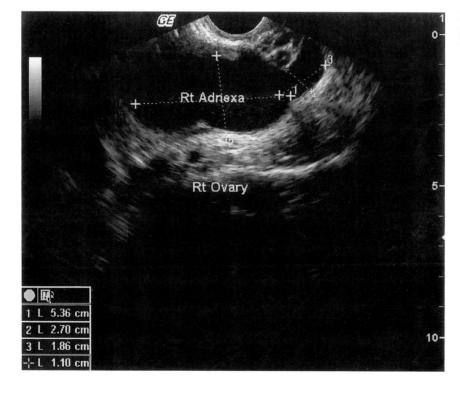

Figure 16–12 ▪ The postablation sterilization syndrome: Sonographic appearance of a hematosalpinx.

Figure 16–13 ▪ Demonstration of deeply recessed cornual regions of the uterus—the kind that are easily overlooked.

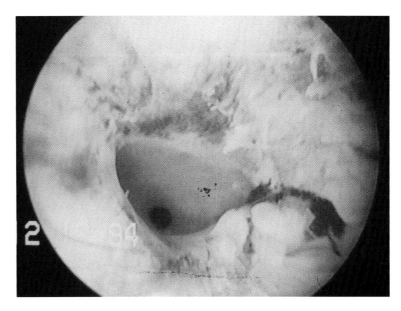

the five had cytologic atypia and a second had architectural atypia. All five patients were obese and diabetic. One had polycystic ovarian disease.

In our own series of 304 women,[45] 3 patients were found to have adenocarcinoma of the endometrium at the time of endomyometrial resection. Preoperative biopsies revealed that 1 of the 3 had focal complex hyperplasia, a second had focal areas of complex adenomatous hyperplasia without atypia, and a third had a benign endocervical polyp. The first 2 patients had well-differentiated adenocarcinoma of the endometrium, which was treated with hysterectomy and bilateral salpingo-oophorectomy. They both remain free of disease at 1 and 2 year follow-up evaluation, respectively. The third patient was diagnosed with a FIGO stage Ib grade II adenocarcinoma of the endometrium infiltrating into the superficial one third of the myometrium after an endomyometrial resection and polypectomy. Her incapacitating medical problems precluded surgery and she was treated with radiation therapy alone. A year later she presented with a large pelvic mass consistent with a poorly differentiated adenocarcinoma of the endometrium and died a year after that. Most of these women had multiple risk factors for developing adenocarcinoma of the endometrium, notably endometrial hyperplasia. Only one was thought to have a benign endometrial polyp. Other important risk factors for endometrial cancer are obesity, hypertension, diabetes, nulliparity, delayed menopause, chronic anovulation, and unopposed estrogen therapy.

Women with multiple risk factors for endometrial cancer should be counseled about the benefits of hysterectomy compared with those of endometrial ablation or endomyometrial resection. Additionally, it is my strong recommendation that any woman who undergoes endometrial ablation or resection in the presence of two or more risk factors for endometrial cancer should have a transvaginal ultrasound examination as part of her annual evaluation. The development of asymptomatic hematometra, with or without endometrial gland proliferation, may indicate early-stage endometrial cancer and requires further investigation. If these areas cannot be ade-

quately biopsied or excised, the patient should be advised to undergo hysterectomy unless it is medically contraindicated.

Physicians who perform endometrial ablation are strongly advised to resect any suspicious areas of the endometrium before an endometrial destructive technique. The histologic diagnosis of a previously unsuspected lesion will dramatically affect the patient's postoperative care and may persuade the physician or the patient that a more aggressive approach to her postoperative care is warranted.

References

1. Serden SP, Brooks PG. Treatment of abnormal uterine bleeding with the gynecologic resectoscope. J Reprod Med 1991;36:697.
2. Townsend DE, Richart RM, Paskowitz RA, Wolfork RE. "Rollerball" coagulation of the endometrium. Obstet Gynecol 1990;76:310.
3. Wortman M. Diagnostic and operative hysteroscopy. In: Penfield AJ, ed. Outpatient gynecologic surgery. Baltimore: Williams & Wilkins, 1997;65.
4. Gomez PI, Gaitan H, Nova C, Paradas A. Paracervical block in incomplete abortion using manual vacuum aspiration: Randomized clinical trial. Obstet Gynecol 2004;103:943.
5. Thomas JA, Leyhland N, Duranel N, Windrim RD. The use of oral misoprostol as a cervical ripening agent in operative hysteroscopy: A double-blind, placebo-controlled trial. Am J Obstet Gynecol 2002;186:876.
6. Preutthipan S. Herabutya Y. Vaginal misoprostol for cervical priming before operative hysteroscopy: A randomized controlled trial. Obstet Gynecol 2000;96:890.
7. Phillips DR, Nathanson HG, Milim SJ, Haselkorn JS. The effect of dilute vasopressin solution on the force needed for cervical dilatation: A randomized controlled trial. Obstet Gynecol 1997;89:507.
8. Wortman M, Daggett A. Hysteroscopic endocervical resection. J Am Assoc Gynecol Laparosc 1996;4:63.
9. Jansen FW, Vredevoogd CB, Ultzen K, et al. Complications of hysteroscopy: A prospective, multicenter study. Obstet Gynecol 2000;96:266.
10. Magos AL, Baumann R, Lockwood GM, Turnbull AC. Experience with the first 250 endometrial resections for menorrhagia. Lancet 1992;337:1074.
11. Scottish Hysteroscopy Audit Group. A Scottish audit of hysteroscopic surgery for menorrhagia: Complications and follow up. Br J Obstet Gynaecol 1995;102:249.
12. Brooks PG. Complications of operative hysteroscopy: How safe is it? Clinical Obstet Gynecol 1992;35:256.
13. Wortman M, Daggett A. Hysteroscopic myomectomy. J Am Assoc Gynecol Laparosc 1995;3:39.

14. Wortman M, Daggett A. Reoperative hysteroscopic surgery in the management of patients who fail endometrial ablation and resection. J Am Assoc Gynecol Laparosc 2001;8:272.
15. Baggish MS, Brill AI, Rosensweig B, et al. Fatal acute glycine and sorbitol toxicity during operative hysteroscopy. J Gynecol Surg 1993;9:137.
16. Propst AM, Liberman RF, Harlow BL, Ginsburg ES. Complications of hysteroscopic surgery: Predicting patients at risk. Obstet Gynecol 2000;96:517.
17. Arieff AI. Hyponatremia, convulsions, respiratory arrest, and permanent brain damage after elective surgery in healthy women. N Engl J Med 1986;314:15.
18. Arieff AI, Ayus JC. Endometrial ablation complicated by fatal hyponatremic encephalopathy. JAMA 1993;270:1230.
19. Indman PD, Brooks PG, Cooper JM, et al. Complications of fluid overload from resectoscopic surgery. J Am Assoc Gynecol Laparosc 1998; 5:63.
20. Hamou J, Fryman R, McLucas B, Garry R. A uterine distention system to prevent fluid intravasation during hysteroscopic surgery. Gynaecol Endosc 1996;5:131.
21. Corson SL, Brooks PG, Serden SP, et al. Effects of vasopressin administration during hysteroscopic surgery. J Reprod Med 1994;39:419.
22. Hill D, Maher P, Wood C, et al. Complications of operative hysteroscopy. Gynaecol Endosc 1992;1:185.
23. Adcock J, Martin D. Air embolus associated with tubal insufflation. J Am Assoc Gynecol Laparosc 1999;6:505.
24. Karandy EJ, Dick HJ, Dwyer RP, et al. Fatal air embolism. A report of two cases including a case of paradoxical air embolism. Am J Obstet Gynecol 1959;78:96.
25. Crozier TA, Luger A, Dravecz M, et al. Gas embolism with cardiac arrest during hysteroscopy. A case report on 3 patients. Anesthesiol Instensvmed Notfallmed Schmerzther 1991;25:412.
26. Perry PM, Baughman VL. A complication of hysteroscopy: Air embolism. Anesthesiology 1990;73:546.
27. Brooks PG. Venous air embolism during operative hysteroscopy. J Am Assoc Gynecol Laparosc 1997;4:399.
28. Munro MG, Weisberg M, Rubinstein E. Gas and air embolization during hysteroscopic electrosurgical vaporization: Comparison of gas generation using bipolar and monopolar electrodes in an experimental model. J Am Assoc Gynecol Laparosc 2001;8:488.
29. Martin JD, Shenk LG. Intraoperative myocardial infarction after paracervical vasopressin infiltration. Anesth Analg 1994;79:1201.
30. Vilos GA, D'Souza I, Huband D. Genital tract burns during rollerball endometrial coagulation. J Am Assoc Gynecol Laparosc 1997;4:273.
31. Vilos GA, Brown S, Graham G, et al. Genital tract burns during hysteroscopic endometrial ablation: Report of 13 cases in the United States and Canada. J Am Assoc Gynecol Laparosc 2000;7:141.
32. Munro MG. Factors affecting capacitive current diversion with a uterine resectoscope: An in vitro study. J Am Assoc Gynecol Laparosc 2003;10:450.
33. Edwards A, Tippett C, Lawrence M, Tsaltas J. Pregnancy outcome following endometrial ablation. Gynaecol Endosc 1996;5:349.
34. Goldberg JM. Intrauterine pregnancy following endometrial ablation. Obstet Gynecol 1994;83:836.
35. Lam AM, Al-Jumaily RY, Holt EM. Ruptured ectopic pregnancy in an amenorrhoeic woman after transcervical resection of the endometrium. Aust N Z J Obstet Gynaecol 1992;32:81.
36. Mongelli JM, Evans AJ. Pregnancy after transcervical endometrial resection. Lancet 1991;338:578.
37. Rogerson L, Gannon B, O'Donnovan P. Outcome of pregnancy following endometrial ablation. J Gynecol Surg 1997;13:155.
38. Whitlaw NL, Garry R, Sutton CJ. Pregnancy following endometrial ablation: Two case reports. Gynaecol Endosc 1992;1:129.
39. Wood C, Rogers P. A pregnancy after planned partial endometrial resection. Aust N Z J Obstet Gynaecol 1993;33:316.
40. Chullapram T, Song JY, Fraser I. Medium-term follow-up on women with menorrhagia treated by rollerball endometrial ablation. Obstet Gynecol 1996;88:71.
41. Paskowitz RA. "Rollerball" ablation of the endometrium. J Reprod Med 1995;40:333.
42. Rankin L, Steinberg LH, Transcervical resection of the endometrium: A review of 400 consecutive patients. Br J Obstet Gynaecol 1991;99:911.
43. Wortman M, Daggett A. Hysteroscopic management of intractable uterine bleeding: A review of 103 cases. J Reprod Med 1993;38:505.
44. Wortman M, Daggett A. Hysteroscopic endomyometrial resection: A new technique for the treatment of menorrhagia. Obstet Gynecol 1994;83:295.
45. Wortman M, Daggett A. Hysteroscopic endomyometrial resection. J Laparoendosc Surg 2000;4:197.
46. Townsend DE, McCausland A, Fields G, et al: Postablation tubal sterilization syndrome. Obstet Gynecol 1993;82:422.
47. Valle RF, Baggish MS. Endometrial carcinoma after endometrial ablation: High-risk factors predicting its occurrence. Am J Obstet Gynecol 1998;179:569.

Complications Related to Hysteroscopic Distention Media

17

Liza M. Swedarsky and Keith Isaacson

Because the uterus is a potential space, the cavity must be distended in order to visualize the entire space and treat any pathologic condition encountered. Distention media can be in the form of gas or liquid. Liquid media can be viscous or nonviscous. Nonviscous media can either contain electrolytes or be electrolyte free.

This chapter reviews all of the uterine distention media that have been used to date. The etiology, prevention, recognition, and management of associated complications are described for each distention medium.

TYPES OF UTERINE DISTENTION MEDIA

Gas

Carbon Dioxide

Carbon dioxide (CO_2) is the only gas distention medium used in gynecologic endoscopy. It has the same refraction as that of air and yields a clear, accurate image of the endometrial cavity. It is easy to infuse, does not clog essential instrumentation, is inexpensive and readily available, and is well tolerated by patients when compared with other liquid distention media used with local anesthesia. CO_2 is regarded as a safe uterine distention medium because it is rapidly absorbed in the blood and is readily released during pulmonary ventilation.[1] It was used as early as 1925 as an intrauterine distention medium, with minimal success.[2]

CO_2 is considered an excellent choice to use with small (3-mm) diagnostic sheaths. It has been considered best suited for office diagnostic hysteroscopy and least advantageous for operative hysteroscopy. CO_2 hysteroscopy should be abandoned in the presence of submucosal uterine bleeding because the foaming interaction between blood and gas will make visibility difficult.[3] It also has a tendency to flatten the endometrium, thereby obscuring pathologic features and occasionally reflux through the cervix in multiparous patients. These drawbacks make CO_2 a poor candidate for operative procedures. As well, use of this medium entails a learning curve: Experience and skill are necessary to clear out mucous bubbles, and this step is essential to ensure adequate visualization of the entire cavity and tubal ostia.

Prevention of CO_2 Gas Complications. If CO_2 is to be used for uterine distention, it is imperative that specialized hysteroscopic insufflators allowing precise control of flow (in cubic centimeters per minute or similar-scale units) and pressure be used, to minimize complications. These insufflators electronically monitor the intrauterine pressure and flow rates. Flow rates may be adjusted for specific intrauterine pressures that allow for optimal visualization. Laparoscopic insufflators should not be used that allow gas to flow at rates of liters per minute. Minimal risks exist from extravasation of CO_2 when the recommended maximum pressure of 100 mm Hg and maximum flow rate of 100 mL per minute are not exceeded.[4] Lindeman and Mohr reported adequate visualization at flow rates of 40 to 60 cc (mL) per minute and pressures of 40 to 80 mm Hg.[5] Complications, described next, typically are secondary to improper regulation of flow and pressure. It also is a common mistake for endoscopists to use flow rates that are too high, resulting in obstructive gas bubbles.

Complications Associated with CO_2 Use. Complications associated with CO_2 use (Table 17–1) have been attributed mostly to improper use and selection of insufflators resulting in higher pressure and flow rates. Most often, equipment was used that was not designed for hysteroscopy. Under these circumstances, large volumes of CO_2 may be intravasated, resulting in metabolic changes, embolization, and death.[6] Excessive intravasation of CO_2 may result in an increase in the partial pressure of CO_2 and a decrease in the partial pressure of O_2, leading to metabolic acidosis and consequent cardiac arrhythmias or cardiac arrest. In 1991 a survey from the American Association of Gynecologic Laparoscopists (AAGL) reported the incidence of CO_2 embolism to be as low as 0.1 case per 1000 procedures. Embolization of small volumes of CO_2 is not dangerous and occurs in 52% of patients undergoing hysteroscopy.[7] Loffer reports intravasation rates of 57.7% at instillation pressures of 60 to 120 mm Hg, compared with 14.7% at pressures less than 60 mm Hg.[8]

Management of Complications. Treatment of excessive CO_2 intravasation consists of immediate termination of the procedure, patient ventilation, and pulmonary and vascular supportive measures. In the setting of significant embolization

Table 17–1 ▪ Laparoscopic Complications Associated with Use of Carbon Dioxide

Category	Examples
Metabolic	Increase in partial pressure of CO_2
	Decrease in partial pressure of O_2
	Hypercarbia
	Metabolic acidosis
CO_2 or air embolus	Respiratory collapse
	Cyanosis
	Cardiac arrest
Mechanical	Tubal rupture
	Rupture of hydrosalpinx
	Diaphragmatic rupture

Table 17–2 ▪ Laparoscopic Complications Associated with Use of Dextran 70 (Hyskon)

Noncardiogenic pulmonary edema
Anaphylactic shock
Disseminated intravascular coagulation
Acute renal failure
Oliguria
Coagulopathies
Allergic reactions
Factitious laboratory results

with accumulation of CO_2 in the right side of the heart, blood flow to that side may be increased by turning the patient on her left side. (See the discussion of management of gas embolization in Chapter 2.)

Liquid Distention Media

Viscous Media

Dextran 70

Dextran 70 (Hyskon, from Pharmacia Laboratories, Piscataway, New Jersey) is discussed for historical purposes only. Before the introduction of continuous-flow hysteroscopes in the mid-1980s, viscous distention media were necessary to permit intrauterine visualization in the presence of bleeding. Dextran 70 is not immiscible with blood and was the medium of choice for operative hysteroscopy. Currently, low-viscosity fluids and CO_2 have largely replaced this agent for use in diagnostic and operative hysteroscopy.

Dextran was first introduced as a uterine distention medium by Edström and Fernström.[9] Dextrans initially were discovered in the 1940s and were used in clinical medicine as plasma expanders. Dextran 70 (Hyskon) is a viscous, colorless, electrolyte-free, nonconductive, and biodegradable polysaccharide liquid. Its immiscibility with blood made this agent a valuable candidate for use in operative hysteroscopy. Hyskon is composed of 32% dextran in 10% dextrose. Dextran 70 is composed of D-glucose polymers, with molecular weights averaging 70,000 daltons (Da). It is a product of bacterial polymerization of glucose on cell surfaces.

Because of its hyperosmolarity, Hyskon is a rapid plasma expander. The molecular weight of dextran causes it to increase plasma oncotic pressure, because it is limited to the intravascular space. Fluids and electrolytes then are drawn intravascularly from interstitial and third spaces. For every 100 mL absorbed, the plasma volume is expanded by an additional 860 mL.[10] Therefore, the absorption of only 100 mL of Hyskon into the circulation can expand the intravascular volume by nearly 10 times the amount of the absorbed fluid.

Prevention of Complications from Hyskon. In most circumstances, Hyskon is administered through a 60-mL syringe

through tubing to the operative hysteroscope. A Hyskon pump was developed by DeCherney but was used in only a small percentage of hysteroscopic procedures in the late 1980s and early 1990s.

In diagnostic procedures, the risk of intravasation is low because myometrial vessels typically are not open or entered, the procedure is brief, and usually no more than 50 to 100 mL of Hyskon is used. Operative procedures may require up to 200 mL of media, thus increasing the risk of intravasation.[11] Manufacturers suggest limiting the volume used to 500 mL per procedure. It also has been suggested that operative hysteroscopic procedures be limited to 45 minutes when this agent is used.[12] Many clinicians well versed in hysteroscopy believe that the amount of absorbed fluid is key in determining complication risks, rather than time or volume limitations. Ruiz and colleagues, however, studied the incidence of complications with use of Hyskon in 1783 patients; their findings supported the volume restrictions suggested by manufacturers. When recommendations were exceeded, a 1.1% frequency of pulmonary edema and a 0.5% frequency of disseminated intravascular coagulation were found.[13]

One major disadvantage related to the highly viscous nature of Hyskon is its tendency to harden and "caramelize" onto hysteroscopic equipment when it dries. Therefore, instruments must be immediately soaked in hot water after completion of the procedure, to prevent clogging of the equipment secondary to solidification of the dextran. Likewise, because of its viscous nature, Hyskon cannot be used with flexible hysteroscopes or instrumentation designed for continuous flow.

Many adverse reactions have been reported with the intravasation of Hyskon (Table 17–2). Case reports have described anaphylactic shock in the setting of Hyskon use even when the patient was exposed to very small volumes. The incidence has been reported to be 4 in 1000.[14] Dextrans have been known to be immunogenic. It has been theorized that some patients have an immediate histamine response to Hyskon as a result of previous sensitization to naturally occurring antigens from either oral exposure to sugar beets, which are metabolized to dextrans, or to commercial sugars contaminated with dextrans, or because of cross-reactivity with bacterial antigens such as streptococci, pneumococci, or salmonellae.[15,16] It does not appear that atopic patients are at increased risk. Ahmed and colleagues reported three cases of anaphylaxis over a 6-month period. In all cases, the volume used was less than 100 mL. Several patients with anaphylactic responses were later skin tested and found to be seronegative for dextran allergy.[17]

Noncardiogenic pulmonary edema has also been a reported complication associated with the use of Hyskon. Although exact volumes are not clearly reported, it appears that larger volumes of Hyskon, ranging from 600 to 1200 mL, were used.[18-22] The pathomechanism for the pulmonary edema appears to be significant expansion of plasma volume and hence intravascular volume overload. Unfortunately, the effects are long lasting, because the plasma half-life of high-molecular-weight dextrans is several days.[16]

Some reports suggest that pulmonary edema after the use of Hyskon may be attributed to direct toxic effects on the pulmonary vasculature.[18,19,21] This type of toxicity has been described with other drugs such as ritodrine, methadone, and salicylates, and with other dextrans such as dextran 40.[18,23] The proposed mechanism involves increased capillary leakage, leading to the development of pulmonary edema. This concept of a direct toxic effect has not been fully accepted, and animal studies have failed to demonstrate direct pulmonary toxicity.[12]

Dextran also has been associated with coagulation disorders. Disseminated intravascular coagulation has been reported after hysteroscopic use of Hyskon.[22] Dextrans have been used in the past as thromboprophylactic agents as an alternative to heparin. Dextran molecules have several antithrombotic properties, such as decreased platelet adhesiveness to endothelium coated with dextran. Dextran also may alter fibrin clot structure, making it more amenable to lysis. It also has been shown to decrease fibrinogen and clotting factors V, VIII, and IX, and the factor VIII–von Willebrand complex. Rapid expansion of plasma volume also has been postulated to contribute to dilution of clotting factors.[16]

Rhabdomyolysis has been reported in one patient after using Hyskon for the treatment of Asherman's syndrome.[24] A 12-fold increase was noted in the patient's serum creatine kinase level over 24 hours. This patient's clinical picture also was complicated by pulmonary edema and coagulopathy.

Intravascular absorption of dextran also has been associated with oliguria and acute renal failure. Dextran 40 has been reported by Moran and Kapsner to cause anuria when given to a patient postoperatively.[25] These investigators also hypothesized that glomerular filtration may decrease as a result of increased intravascular oncotic pressure. Hydrostatic pressure, which normally favors movement of fluid from the capillary into Bowman's capsule, suddenly becomes disrupted within the capillary bed. This disturbance may cause low-molecular-weight dextrans to precipitate in renal tubules, causing mechanical obstruction within renal nephrons and constriction of the renal arteries. This phenomenon lowers glomerular perfusion pressure and, in the setting of an elevated plasma oncotic pressure, induces renal insufficiency. Owing to their large molecular weight, dextrans are poorly cleared from the bloodstream. Typically, polymers greater than 50,000 Da are largely cleared by the reticuloendothelial system.

Dextrans also have been shown to cause falsely elevated laboratory values, such as elevated glucose levels. They also may interfere with the measurement of serum bilirubin concentrations, protein levels, and blood cross-matching. Transfusion mismatching may occur if the specimen for blood type and screen studies is obtained after intravasation occurs.

Recognition of Dextran Toxicity. Patients with dextran toxicity may present with a plethora of symptoms caused by the aforementioned complications. Patients may present in respiratory distress caused by pulmonary edema and with arterial blood gases suggestive of hypoxemia. Presenting symptoms may include hemoptysis, fluid from the endotracheal tube, and bleeding from the vagina or intravenous sites. Chest radiography reveals patchy bilateral infiltrates and prominent pulmonary vasculature suggestive of pulmonary edema. Laboratory values in the setting of coagulopathy or disseminated intravascular coagulopathy may reveal elevated prothrombin and partial thromboplastin times, decreased hematocrit, platelets, and fibrinogen. Patients experiencing anaphylaxis can present with shortness of breath or a diffuse erythematous rash.

Treatment of Dextran Toxicity. Management involves treatment of fluid overload and pulmonary edema by means of diuresis and respiratory support. Appropriate treatment has not been clearly defined, because diuresis alone will not fully address the underlying problem of increased plasma oncotic pressure. Plasmapheresis may be considered in the setting of intractable pulmonary edema and renal failure. Dialysis is not effective in removing dextrans and therefore should not be instituted. Coagulopathies may require a blood transfusion, especially if the patient is actively bleeding. Often coagulopathies can be corrected with diuresis.

The Hyskon infusion should be immediately ceased in the setting of suspected anaphylaxis. Treatment with intravenous or intratracheal epinephrine may be necessary. Steroids may be administered during serious or prolonged reactions, to prevent recurrent anaphylactic symptoms. Antihistamines also may be used.

Low-Viscosity Fluids

Low-viscosity crystalloids have virtually replaced all other distention media because of their excellent safety profile and the advent of continuous-flow hysteroscopes. Low-viscosity fluids are either electrolyte-free media or electrolyte-containing isotonic media. The electrolyte-containing media include normal saline and lactated Ringer's solution. These two media cannot be used with monopolar electrocautery because the power in the electrode will be dispersed, making the electrode ineffective. No injury to the uterus will occur if monopolar energy is mistakenly used in the presence of electrolyte-containing media.

Fluids for operative hysteroscopy using a monopolar resectoscope must be nonconductive and therefore electrolyte free. The most commonly used electrolyte media are 1.5% glycine, 3% sorbitol, and 5% mannitol (Table 17–3). Osmotically active particles have been added to 5% mannitol, which has been suggested to possibly reduce complications from intravasation of hypotonic solutions such as glycine and sorbitol. Table 17–3 compares the osmolality of the most commonly used nonconductive distention media.

These nonviscous, hypotonic solutions are readily available and inexpensive, making them ideal for operative hysteroscopy. They also are well suited for use with the continuous-flow hysteroscope. Intravasation of low-viscosity solutions containing amino acids such as glycine or sugars

Table 17–3 ■ **Osmolality of Serum and Commonly Used Nonconductive Distention Media**

Serum/Medium	Osmolality (mOsm/L)
Normal serum osmolality	290
Glycine 1.5%	200
Sorbitol 3%, mannitol 0.5%	178
Mannitol 5%	280

Data from Indman PD, Brooks PG, Cooper JM, et al. Complications of fluid overload from resectoscopic surgery. J Am Assoc Gynecol Laparosc 1998;5:63.

such as glucose and sorbitol-mannitol can cause complications virtually identical to those initially described by urologists in the 1940s. Hemolytic reactions resulted from using sterile water during transurethral resection of the prostate (TURP). *Post-TURP syndrome* has been used to describe the clinical picture in which the patient presents with nausea, vomiting, headache, visual disturbances, agitation, confusion, and lethargy. Transient hypertension also may occur, followed by hypotension or bradycardia. This constellation of symptoms results from dilutional hyponatremia, hypervolemia, and decreased serum osmolality. Without treatment, patients have experienced seizures, cardiac arrest, coma, and death.[27] Because gynecologists are now faced with the same side effect profile resulting from intravasation of electrolyte-free and hypotonic media, an appreciation of the basic physiology involved is important to the ability to prevent, recognize, and treat complications.

ISOTONIC, ELECTROLYTE-CONTAINING MEDIA

Normal Saline and Lactated Ringer's Solution

Normal saline and lactated Ringer's solution both are isotonic distention fluids used in operative hysteroscopic procedures when monopolar electrosurgery is not required. Both solutions preferentially conduct electrocurrent; therefore, initiation of cutting and tissue coagulation will be difficult during monopolar electrosurgery because of energy dispersion. Accordingly, electrolyte-containing media are used in diagnostic procedures; in procedures using instrumentation such as biopsy forceps, polyp forceps, or scissors; and in procedures using bipolar electrosurgery. Normal saline is 0.9% sodium chloride solution, and lactated Ringer's contains sodium chloride, sodium lactate, calcium chloride, and potassium chloride in distilled water. Because they are isotonic, osmotic gradients are not created across cell membranes; therefore, intravasation is not complicated by hemolysis or hyponatremia. Fluid overload resulting in pulmonary and laryngeal edema may still occur when large volumes are used; however, diuresis of these fluids can be performed easily.

ELECTROLYTE-FREE MEDIA

Glycine

Glycine is a simple amino acid that is mixed in water and is supplied in 3-L bags as a 1.5% solution. It is electrolyte free, nonhemolytic, nonimmunogenic, and hypo-osmolar (200 mOsm/L). It commonly is used in operative hysteroscopy when monopolar current is utilized. Intravasation of glycine media may lead to hyperammonemia with encephalopathic symptoms, hyponatremia, hypervolemia, hypo-osmolarity, and central pontine myelinolysis (CPM). The pathophysiology, diagnosis, and treatment of each of these potential complications are described in detail.

Hyperammonemia. Glycine is metabolized into glyoxylic acid and ammonia through oxidative deamination in the liver and kidneys. Some persons may metabolize glycine more rapidly. Patients with hyperammonemia present with a constellation of symptoms notable for nausea, vomiting, altered mental status, muscle aches, and decreased visual acuity. Decreased visual acuity results from the secondary inhibitory neurotransmitter effects of glycine in the retina on the horizontal and ganglion cells.[16] Ammonia toxicity should be considered in all patients with severe central nervous system deficits otherwise unexplained by the degree of hyponatremia or hypo-osmolarity.

L-Arginine may be given to stimulate the metabolism of ammonia by the urea cycle in the setting of severe ammonia toxicity.

Hypervolemic, Hypo-osmolar Hyponatremia. Glycine medium may be intravasated through large uterine vessels during operative hysteroscopy. With the half-life for glycine approximating 85 minutes, initial serum osmolality remains unchanged owing to the osmotic activity of the absorbed glycine molecules. Eventually, the glycine is absorbed intracellularly, resulting in a surplus of intravascular free water. If this surplus is not rapidly eliminated, hypo-osmolar hyponatremia results. The stress of surgery results in the release of antidiuretic hormone, which further exacerbates the effects of the intravasated medium, now appearing to be free water, by inhibiting diuresis. It appears that women are more prone to suffer from this mechanism—estrogen and progesterone have been proved to inhibit the cellular sodium-potassium adenosine triphosphatase, which allows sodium to be excreted extracellularly.[28,29]

The potential effects of hypervolemic, hypo-osmolar hyponatremia include irreversible brain damage due to hyponatremic encephalopathy. The pathophysiology is caused by acute hypo-osmolality and also is a function of hyponatremia. Water readily navigates through cellular membranes during a rapid equilibration that takes place to correct the hypo-osmolar hyponatremia. It also traverses the blood-brain barrier freely. Hence, a rapid increase in intravascular free water will shift water into the brain, causing cerebral edema. As the brain swells, it may be injured by compression against the bony skull. As intracranial pressure increases, cerebral blood flow decreases, resulting in hypoxemic neurons and pressure necrosis. Arieff and Ayus reported that an increase in intracranial volume of as little as 5% may lead to brain herniation.[30] Brain herniation will result in respiratory arrest, which will lead to further decreases in cerebral blood flow and ischemic injury.

Treatment for water intoxication should consist of removing excess fluid by means of diuresis and correction of hyponatremia. Expectant management and spontaneous diuresis are not an option. Arieff reported on a series of 15 patients in whom hyponatremia developed after elective surgery. Eight of the 15 women experienced the onset of seizures and ultimately respiratory arrest without warning signs. Each became symptomatic after a period of less than 10 minutes of lucidity.[28]

No strict guidelines or clear standards exist for treatment. Both the degree to which the sodium should be corrected and the rate of correction are controversial. Rapid sodium resuscitation may obscure CPM or cause demyelination. Slow correction prevents demyelination. As a rule of thumb, if the hyponatremia is acute and is recognized, the correction with diuretics and hypertonic saline should be done acutely. If the deficit occurs over a more chronic period (longer than 24 hours), correction should be slow in order to prevent CPM.

Guidelines have been suggested by the AAGL and are included at the end of the chapter. These guidelines specify the maximum amount of media that may be absorbed before operative hysteroscopic procedures should be aborted. Generally, serum sodium levels decrease by 10 millimoles per liter (mmol/L) for every liter of hypotonic fluid absorbed.[14] A patient probably will absorb at least 1 L of medium before demonstrating symptoms; however, this may depend on the preoperative sodium level. Most patients with low sodium are not symptomatic because they are young and healthy. Those with symptoms are hyponatremic, however (Table 17–4).

Assessment of the patient's electrolyte status and symptoms should be initiated at fluid deficits of 1 L. At a deficit of 1.5 L, the procedure should be aborted. Elderly patients with a history of cardiovascular disease or liver disease or with preexisting central nervous system (CNS) deficits and patients on chronic diuretics should be thoroughly assessed; at deficits of 750 mL in these patients, the procedure should be discontinued. Symptom profiles may vary depending on the amount of absorbed media (see Table 17–4).

Acute and Chronic Hyponatremia. Mortality rates for untreated acute hyponatremia are greater than those for chronic hyponatremia. Hyponatremia is considered chronic if it has lasted for longer than 48 hours. If the hyponatremia occurs with rapid intravasation into the bloodstream, the correction should be rapid. Rapid resuscitation is first accomplished with loop diuretics such as 10 mg of furosemide given intravenously when a deficit of 1 L is reached. With deficits of greater than 1.5 L and moderate to severe hyponatremia, hypertonic sodium chloride (514 mmol/L), in combination with the use of loop diuretics, can safely be used to increase serum sodium levels by 1 to 2 mEq/L per hour, to a maximum of 6 to 12 mEq/L in the first 24 hours. A total dose of 20 mg of furosemide should be adequate to initiate diuresis unless the patient has a history of renal insufficiency. It is recommended to monitor serum electrolytes every 4 hours during replacement.[16] Small increases in plasma osmolarity diminishes the risk of encephalopathy. Special attention should be given to prevent overcorrection. In fact, the end point should initially be slightly hyponatremic serum levels to avoid overcorrection, which could lead to permanent brain injury. The same repletion after 3 days of hyponatremia could potentially lead to brain dehydration, myelinolysis, and death. In patients with chronic hyponatremia, it has been recommended that serum sodium levels be increased by no greater than 25 mEq/L in a 48-hour period, or 12 mEq/L per 24 hours.[16,31]

Central Pontine Myelinolysis. CPM represents brain injury resulting from brain desiccation due to too-rapid correction of serum hyponatremia. Sterns also described this insult as the "osmotic demyelinating syndrome."[32] The brain responds to changes in serum osmolality by shunting sodium and fluid into the cerebrospinal fluid (CSF). Initially the brain is resistant to osmotic swelling; however, its ability to avoid osmotic swelling is time limited. Within 3 to 4 hours, the brain's secondary mechanism of extruding potassium and water ensues. If hyponatremia and hypo-osmolarity persist, neurons extrude cytoplasmic organic osmolytes such as taurine, myoinositol, glutamine, glutamate, and phosphocreatine.[33] Because it takes several days for neurons to replete these osmolytes, increases in serum osmolarity due to rapid correction with sodium result in further extrusion of water out of neurons, leading to dehydration. Therefore, serum osmolarity must not be corrected too rapidly because the rate of return and regeneration of intracellular osmols is much slower than the rate at which they were extruded.

Sorbitol

Sorbitol is a 6-carbon alcohol that is metabolized by the liver to fructose and glucose and ultimately into CO_2 and water. A nonconductive 3% solution has been used in resectoscopic procedures. Because sorbitol is hypo-osmolar (see Table 17–3), complications from intravasation will be similar to those encountered with glycine. Hence, treatment measures are similar to those used for water intoxication, such as use of furosemide and normal saline solution for replacement of urinary salt loss and maintenance of intravascular volume.[16]

Sorbitol and Mannitol

Solutions containing 2.7% sorbitol and 0.5% mannitol have been used for both TURP procedures and endometrial

Table 17–4 ■ Signs and Symptoms of Hyponatremia	
Serum Sodium (mEq/L)	**Associated Signs and Symptoms**
135-142	Normal serum sodium
130-135	*Mild hyponatremia*: apprehension, disorientation, vomiting, irritability, twitching, shortness of breath, nausea
125-130	*Mild to moderate hyponatremia*: dilute urine, moist mucous membranes, moist skin, pitting edema, polyuria, pulmonary rales
<120	*Severe hyponatremia* and possible hyponatremic encephalopathy: congestive heart failure, lethargy, confusion, muscular twitching, focal weakness, convulsions, death
<115	Possible brainstem herniation; grand mal seizures, coma, respiratory arrest coma; mortality rates up to 85%

Data from Morrison D. Management of hysteroscopic surgery complications. AORN J 1999;69:194.

ablation performed with the rollerball technique.[34] Such media were largely developed to reduce the hemolysis and hyponatremia seen with use of glycine. The sorbitol-mannitol solution is supplied in 3-L bags. The indications for its use and complication profile are similar to those for glycine. Theoretically, risks from water intoxication secondary to fluid overload may be decreased, because sorbitol and mannitol both are diuretics.

Mannitol

Mannitol also is a 6-carbon alcohol. In fact, sorbitol and mannitol are alditol isomers.

Mannitol 5% solution also is nonconductive, but it is isotonic as a result of the presence of osmolytes other than electrolytes (see Table 17–3). Its osmolarity (280 mOsm/L) is very similar to that of serum, thus decreasing the risks of hypo-osmolality if intravasated. Only 6% to 10% of the absorbed mannitol is metabolized. Mannitol is cleared by the kidneys and is excreted largely unchanged in the urine. The half-life of mannitol in blood plasma is approximately 15 minutes in patients with normal renal function.[34] It has been suggested that because mannitol is isotonic, its intravasation is less likely to cause cerebral edema and its subsequent consequences.[26] It has been shown in animals, however, that cerebral edema can occur from hyponatremia even in the presence of normal serum osmolality. Therefore, with use of 5% mannitol for uterine distention, the same fluid management guidelines are recommended as those for use of 1.5% glycine or 3% sorbitol.

PREVENTION OF FLUID-RELATED COMPLICATIONS

Adherence to five key principles to optimize surgical intervention is key to the prevention of fluid-related complications[26]:

1. Select distention media least likely to cause complications. Use only electrolyte-containing media when monopolar energy is not being used.
2. Accurate measurements of the difference between intake and ouput are key to preventing excessive intravasation. This is best accomplished using one of a number of commercial weighted fluid management systems that track the weight of the fluid going in and of the fluid recovered. Equipped with data on the specific gravity of each distention medium, these machines will calculate and display the fluid deficit in real time. These machines are accurate to within 1% to 2%.
3. Recognize fluid deficits promptly.
4. Treat hyponatremia and hypervolemia.
5. Develop a fluid management protocol within each institution that is agreed on by the anesthesia team, the nursing team, and the surgeon.

SUGGESTED HYSTEROSCOPIC FLUID MONITORING GUIDELINES

Suggested hysteroscopic fluid monitoring guidelines are presented next. These guidelines were published in 2000 by the AAGL.[35]

Media

1. High-viscosity 32% dextran 70 has been largely replaced by CO_2 and low-viscosity fluids in diagnostic and operative hysteroscopy.
2. Use of CO_2 in operative hysteroscopy is limited at this time. It is used primarily for diagnostic purposes.
3. Saline and Ringer's lactate solutions are recommended for diagnostic hysteroscopy or in surgical procedures in which mechanical, laser, or bipolar energy is used.
4. When using monopolar energy, consider using 5% mannitol, rather than glycine or sorbitol. Remember that the same fluid management guidelines apply to 5% mannitol as for 1.5% glycine and 3% sorbitol.

Delivery of Distention Media

1. Before beginning distention, air should be flushed from all hysteroscopic tubing.
2. Only CO_2 insufflators designed for hysteroscopy should be used.
3. Pressure cuffs on low-viscosity-fluid bags generally are not appropriate except for short procedures in which diagnostic hysteroscopes with narrow-diameter inflow channels are used.
4. Adequate visualization generally can be obtained with a maximum delivery pressure of 7 to 100 mm Hg when either a hysteroscopic pump or a gravity system is used. Minimum pressures should be used for adequate visualization to minimize fluid intravasation.
5. The height of the highest portion of the continuous-flow column of fluid to the level of the uterus is used to measure pressure from gravity systems when low-viscosity fluids are used—1 foot equals approximately 25 mm Hg.
6. Fluid pumps for low-viscosity media do not guarantee safety, and their use is a matter of convenience.

Risks of Excessive Intravasation

1. Excessive intravasation of CO_2 should not occur if appropriate flow rates (maximum 100 mL per minute) and pressures (less than 100 mm Hg) are used.
2. The primary risk associated with use of electrolyte-containing solutions such as Ringer's lactate and normal saline is fluid overload. The magnitude of risk depends on the patient's cardiovascular status.
3. Nonelectrolyte solutions such as sorbitol and 1.5% glycine carry the risks of fluid overload, hyponatremia, hypo-osmolality, cerebral edema, and death.
4. Mannitol 5% acts as its own diuretic. It may cause hyponatremia but not hypo-osmolality. Currently, the effects of mannitol in procedures in which patients are exposed to large loads are not entirely known. The recommended guidelines for fluid management are the same for 1.5% glycine, 3% sorbitol, and 5% mannitol.

Limits of Intravasation

1. The anesthesiologist should be encouraged to closely monitor and limit hydration of patients preoperatively and intraoperatively when uterine distention media are used.

2. Completion of the procedure should be planned to coincide with intravasation of 750 mL to 1 L of electrolyte-free medium.

3. If fluid intravasation reaches approximately 1500 mL of a nonelectrolyte solution or 2500 mL of normal saline, the procedure should be brought to a conclusion, electrolytes assessed, administration of diuretics considered, and further diagnostic and therapeutic interventions (such as diuretic therapy) begun as indicated.

4. Management of hyponatremia is not standardized at present. We recommend giving 10 mg of intravenous furosemide once the fluid deficit reaches 1 L. Blood specimens for determining serum electrolyte levels are drawn at that time, and the procedure is discontinued when the deficit reaches 1.5 L.

Monitoring

1. Mechanical monitoring using a system that weighs the fluid going in and the fluid collected is highly desirable because it removes the human error factor in measuring fluid deficit. Such monitoring systems provide early warning of excessive intravasation in real time and indicate the rapidity with which the loss is occurring. These systems typically are accurate within 1% to 2% of the actual deficit so long as all of the effluent fluid is collected. This requires an adequate collection drape placed along the small of the patient's back extending below the buttocks.

2. If mechanical monitoring is not available, a designated member of the operating room staff should record frequent measurements of intake, output, and deficit.

3. A designated member of the operating room staff should inform both the anesthesiologist and the surgeon of the fluid deficit frequently—typically, every 5 minutes during the procedure.

References

1. Salat-Baroux J, Hamou JE, Maillard G, et al. Complications from microhysteroscopy. In: Siegler AM, Lindemann HJ, eds. Hysteroscopy: Principles in practice. Philadelphia: JB Lippincott, 1984;112.
2. Rubin JC. Am J Obstet Gynecol 1925;10:313.
3. Baggish MS, Barbot J, Valle RF. Diagnostic and operative hysteroscopy. Chicago: Year Book, 1989;163.
4. Siegler AM, Kemmann E. Hysteroscopy. Obstet Gynecol Surv 1975;30:567.
5. Lindeman HJ, Mohr J. CO$_2$ hysteroscopy: Diagnosis and treatment. Am J Obstet Gynecol 1976;124:129.
6. Salat-Baroux J, Hamou JE, Maillard G, et al. Complications from microhysteroscopy. In: Siegler AM, Lindemann HJ, eds. Hysteroscopy: Principles in practice. Philadelphia: JB Lippincott 1984;112.
7. Rythen-Alder E, Brundin J, Notini-Gudmarsson A, et al. Detection of carbon dioxide embolism during hysteroscopy. Gynaecol Endosc 1992;1:207.
8. Loffer FD. Complications of hysteroscopy—their cause, prevention, and correction. J Am Assoc Gynecol Laparosc 1995;3:11.
9. Edström K, Fernström I. The diagnostic possibilities of a modified hysteroscopic technique. Acta Obstet Gynecol Scand 1970;49:327.
10. Lukacsko P. Noncardiogenic pulmonary edema secondary to intrauterine instillation of 32% dextran 70. Fertil Steril 1985;54:560.
11. Pellicer A, Diamond M. Distending media for hysteroscopy. Obstet Gynecol Clin North Am 1988;15:23.
12. Schingl EF. Hyskon (32% dextran 70), hysteroscopic surgery, and pulmonary edema. Letter to the editor. Anesth Analg 1990;70:223.
13. Ruiz JM, Neuwirth RS. The incidence of complications associated with the use of Hyskon during hysteroscopy: Experience in 1783 consecutive patients. J Gynecol Surg 1992;8:219.
14. Isaacson KB. Complications of hysteroscopy. Obstet Gynecol Clin North Am 1999;26:39.
15. Bailey G, Strub RL, Klein RC, Salvaggio J. Dextran-induced anaphylaxis. JAMA 1967;200:889.
16. Witz CA, Silverberg KM, Burns WN, et al. Complications associated with the absorption of hysteroscopic fluid media. Fertil Steril 1993;60:745.
17. Ahmed N, Falcone T, Tulandi T, Houle G. Anaphylactic reaction because of intrauterine 32% dextran-70 instillation. Fertil Steril 1991;55:1014.
18. Leake JF, Murphy AA, Zacur HA. Noncardiogenic pulmonary edema: A complication of operative hysteroscopy. Fertil Steril 1987;48:497.
19. Zbella EA, Moise J, Carson SA. Noncardiogenic pulmonary edema secondary to intrauterine instillation of 32% dextran 70. Fertil Steril 1985;43:479.
20. Golan A, Seidner M, Bahar M, et al. High-output left ventricular failure after dextran use in an operative hysteroscopy. Fertil Steril 1990;54:939.
21. Mangar D, Gerson JI, Constantine RM, Lenzi V. Pulmonary edema and coagulopathy due to Hyskon (32% dextran 70) administration. Anesth Analg 1989;68:686.
22. Jedeikin R, Olsfanger D. Disseminated intravascular coagulopathy and adult respiratory distress syndrome: Life-threatening complications of hysteroscopy. Am J Obstet Gynecol 1990;12:44.
23. Kaplan AI, Sabin S. Dextran 40: Another cause of drug-induced noncardiogenic pulmonary edema. Chest 1975;68:376.
24. Brandt RR, Dunn WF, Ory SJ. Dextran 70 embolization: Another cause of pulmonary hemorrhage, coagulopathy, and rhabdomyolysis. Chest 1993;104:631.
25. Moran M, Kapsner C. Acute renal failure associated with elevated plasma oncotic pressure. N Engl J Med 1987;317:150.
26. Indman PD, Brooks PG, Cooper JM, et al: Complications of fluid overload from resectoscopic surgery. J Am Assoc Gynecol Laparosc 1998;5:63.
27. Bernstein GT, Loughlin KR, Gittes RF. The physiologic basis for the TURP syndrome. J Surg Res 1989;46:135.
28. Arieff AI. Hyponatremia, convulsions, respiratory arrest, and permanent brain damage after elective surgery in healthy women. N Engl J Med 1986;314:1529.
29. Berl T. Treating hyponatremia: What is all the controversy about? Ann Intern Med 1990;113:417.
30. Arieff AI, Ayus JC. Treatment of symptomatic hyponatremia: Neither haste nor waste. Crit Care Med 1991;19:748.
31. Morrison D. Management of hysteroscopic surgery complications. AORN J 1999;69:194.
32. Sterns RH. The treatment of hyponatremia: First do no harm. Am J Med 1990;88:557.
33. Sterns RH. The management of symptomatic hyponatremia. Semin Nephrol 1990;10:503.
34. Townsend DE, et al: "Rollerball" coagulation of the endometrium. Obstet Gynecol 1990;76:310.
35. Loffer FD, Bradley LD, Brill AI, et al. Hysteroscopic fluid monitoring guidelines: From the Ad Hoc Committee on Hysteroscopic Fluid Guidelines of the American Association of Gynecologic Laparoscopists. J Am Assoc Gynecol Laparosc 2000;7:167.

Complications of Endometrial Ablation

18

Ellis Downes and Madhavi Manoharan

Since endometrial ablation was first introduced by such pioneers as Milton Goldrath and Thierry Vancaillie in the early 1980s,[1] it has become an important component of the surgical armamentarium of the gynecologist in treating menorrhagia. Initially the surgical procedures were hysteroscopic transcervical endometrial resection and rollerball ablation. These became known as the first-generation ablative procedures.

These operations were extensively investigated in well-designed robust studies[2] that confirmed their efficacy and safety. Although these are good operations, however, they were relatively slow to be taken up by gynecologists. This lag in application may be due in part to the technical problems and challenges of performing the surgery safely but also was due to the small but significant numbers of complications, some of which caused postoperative death, as evidenced in the U.K. Mistletoe Audit of hysteroscopic surgery.[3] The main complications were uterine perforation causing bleeding or bowel damage, bleeding, and problems with fluid overload. To overcome these problems, meticulous attention was encouraged, with training and medical devices designed to reduce the incidence of fluid overload problems by more accurately measuring fluid loss or even adding a sheath over the hysteroscope, which meant that saline could be used.[4]

Despite these innovations, the numbers of hysteroscopic procedures remained relatively low compared with hysterectomy rates. Increasingly, however, a number of different investigators looked at delivering energy in different forms into the uterus to destroy the endometrium for treatment of menorrhagia. Some of these ablative techniques were very effective but had an unacceptably high incidence of complications—for example, radiofrequency endometrial ablation (RAFEA), introduced by the late Geoff Phipps in the United Kingdom. This technique was found unfortunately to have a relatively high risk of bladder complication. It is no longer used as a result of this and other reasons.

The last 10 years have seen a dramatic increase in both the number and type of endometrial ablations being performed. Table 18–1 lists the current ablative techniques available, although not all techniques are commercially available or approved worldwide. Complications of these procedures are the subject of this chapter. Of note, all of these ablative procedures are inherently safer than hysterectomy, the operation they replace. No surgical procedure is completely complication free, but ablative techniques are much safer than hysterectomy—a fact that should never be forgotten by patients and their lawyers as well. As the numbers of hysterectomies continue to slowly fall, in concert with the increase in ablation rates, the hope is that the accumulating experience and continued refinements in technique and instrumentation will result in the safest and most effective operation possible for treatment of menorrhagia by endometrial ablation.

WHY DO COMPLICATIONS OCCUR?

Table 18–2 summarizes the factors contributing to the development of complications during endometrial ablative procedures.

Medical Conditions

One of the reasons why endometrial ablation is so useful is that it can be used in women with menorrhagia who are not fit enough for hysterectomy. Indeed, this was the initial indication for use of this technique, according to a pioneering historical case report.[5] Therefore, it is not surprising that complications related to medical conditions are more likely to occur. This consideration highlights the need for careful preoperative assessment and close liaison with an experienced anesthetist.

Poor Surgical Training

One of the regrettable issues in modern surgery is that medical device companies have to sell equipment to physicians, and on occasion a fine line may exist between training surgeons and selling to them. It may be difficult for a relatively young sales representative to proffer advice or even criticism regarding less than optimal technique to a senior surgeon. Reputable medical device companies are now developing training programs separate from the sales process, and in some countries, regulatory authorities make it a condition of device approval

Table 18–1 ■ Endometrial Ablation Techniques

Energy Form	Type of Ablation	Device*
Freezing	Global	HerOption
Diathermy	Global	Novasure
Microwave	Global, iterative	Microsulis
Open heated saline	Hysteroscopic, global	HydroThermAblator
Closed heated saline	Global	Thermachoice Cavaterm
Laser	Global	Endometrial laser intrauterine thermo-therapy

*Commercial name.

Table 18–2 ■ Potential Causes of Endometrial Ablation Complications

Medical condition of patient
Poor training of surgeon
Inappropriate patient selection
Problems related to dilation of cervix
Inherent device-related problems
Postoperative problems

that robust training programs are in place, some of them conducted by specialist medical societies. The onus must always remain with the surgeon, bound by professional standards and personal integrity, to ensure that the practitioner attempts procedures only within the level of training and personal competence. In the event of a complication leading to litigation, the plaintiff's lawyers will be only too keen to examine all details of the surgeon's training.

Inappropriate Patient Selection

Much of this relates to surgical training as discussed above. Key points to consider are uterine size and the presence of myoma. If the uterine cavity is too big, not only is a poor result more likely, but the complication rate may be higher. Likewise, with a small cavity (less than 7 cm), it may be more difficult to satisfactorily deploy some ablative devices such as the Novasure or the Cavaterm and Thermachoice balloons. Similar problems may occur with myomectomy. The balloon devices (Thermachoice and Cavaterm), Novasure, and ELITT cannot be used with myoma because of the difficulty in satisfactorily placing them. Microwave endometrial ablation (MEA) can be used to ablate submucous myomas up to 4 cm in size. Complications also are more likely to occur with repeat ablations because of the presence of scarring and possible intrauterine synechiae. Such ablations should be performed only by experienced surgeons, who may feel that hysteroscopic resection of adhesions and subsequent transcervical resection of endometrium possibly under laparoscopic control is a more feasible option.

Dilation of Cervix

It is self-evident that the cervix has to be dilated to allow passage of the ablative device before an endometrial ablation

can begin. Dilation often can be surprisingly difficult, particularly in a nulliparous patient or one who received a luteinizing hormone–releasing hormone (LH-RH) agonist (Lupron or Zoladex) to prepare the endometrium, and there is a risk of a cervical tear which, given the vascular supply to the cervix, can result in brisk bleeding. Pressure studies have shown the cervix is far less compliant after LH-RH administration than after danazol. Because cervical dilation can be extremely painful, we perform local anesthetic ablations with endometrial preparation after progestogen stimulation (Provera 10 mg TDS for 2 to 3 weeks before surgery) or using menstrual scheduling. The risk of a cervical tear also is reduced if the force to dilate the cervix is applied using two cervical grasping instruments such as Littlewood or Vulsellum graspers, rather than one, at two different points on the cervix.

Device-Related Problems

Device-related problems obviously are specific to the actual ablation procedure performed. A key concern in delivering energy to destroy the endometrium is ensuring that the device is actually in the uterine cavity before the energy is delivered. If it is not, the possibility of damaging bowel or other abdominal organs is very high. Many of the devices have safety features to confirm this. For example, Thermachoice has a pressure transducer to confirm that the intrauterine pressure is high enough for the procedure to begin; low pressure may indicate the device is outside the uterine cavity. Likewise, the microwave endometrial ablation applicator has thermocouples at its tip and half-way along that measure the temperature rise at the commencement of the procedure. A temperature curve analyzing thousands of MEAs allows the development of software which terminates the microwave heating procedure in the rare event of a possible uterine perforation not detected hysteroscopically.

Postoperative Problems

All the ablation devices, by destroying the endometrium, cause superficial tissue necrosis. A postoperative serosanguineous discharge is very common; indeed in our experience a prolonged discharge is usually associated with a good postoperative result. It is essential in preoperative counseling to warn the patient about this and also to warn her that occasionally the discharge can become infected, needing antibiotics. Cramping postoperatively is very common and can be effectively treated with non-steroids; rectal diclofenac is particularly effective (100 mg PR 1 hour preprocedure, especially for local anesthetic procedures). No patient should be discharged home with anything other than minimal discomfort. Increasing lower abdominal pain after a period of relatively minimal abdominal discomfort should be taken very seri-ously and the patient admitted for urgent investigation to exclude the rare possibility of uterine perforation and intra-abdominal mishap.

DEVICE-SPECIFIC ENDOMETRIAL ABLATION COMPLICATIONS

A more detailed examination of specific ablation devices follows. It is extremely difficult to analyze complication data.

Do surgeons report all complications? If they do so, to whom—a statutory agency such as the American Federal Device Authority, the device manufacturers, or the surgeon's own hospital authorities? Publishing such data may be in conflict with commercial considerations, and complications undoubtedly are underreported. Relatively few studies in the literature are concerned with endometrial ablation complications, and it is impossible with the current status of complication reporting to say that device A is safer or more dangerous than device B.

The American Federal Device Authority insists, as a condition of device approval, that manufacturers notify this body of all serious adverse events. These are published in the public domain on the Authority's Web site through the Manufacturers and User Facility Device Experience (MAUDE) database (i.e., Manufacturers Adverse Untoward Events) of the U.S. FDA (Food and Drug Administration). The MAUDE database represents reports of adverse events involving medical devices. The data consist of all voluntary reports since 1993, user facility reports since 1991, distributor reports since 1993 and manufacturers' reports since 1996. The data are upgraded on a quarterly basis.

Some attempts have been made to create league tables of complication rates, to examine trends,[6] although these have been criticized[7] because of the problem of accurately determining incidence levels. If uterine perforation occurs in 30 procedures using device A and in only 5 procedures using device B, without knowing the total number of cases being undertaken one cannot comment on the relative safety or danger of the two devices. Nevertheless, notwithstanding these problems, the MAUDE database has a useful role in determining incidence trends and may allow surgeons and others, including device manufacturers, to change device design or procedure in an attempt to further reduce complications—a philosophy of practice similar to air accident reporting in the aviation industry.

We recently conducted a search of the MAUDE database for all of the adverse events reported with the use of endometrial ablation techniques.

The five FDA-approved endometrial ablation devices and techniques are

- HydroThermAblator
- Microwave endometrial ablation
- HerOption Uterine Cryoablation Therapy System
- Thermachoice
- Novasure Impedance-Controlled Endometrial Ablation

A search of the MAUDE database for adverse events reported from 2000 to 2004 revealed a total of 65 adverse events associated with use of these devices and techniques, including 1 death.

The distribution of adverse events by *device* was as follows:

- HydroThermAblator: 21
- Microwave endometrial ablation: 4
- HerOption Uterine Cryoablation Therapy System: 5
- Thermachoice: 14
- Novasure Impedance-Controlled Endometrial Ablation: 21

The distribution of adverse events by *type of injury* was as follows: 2 cases of hemorrhage; 20 cases of bowel injury; 3 cases of endometritis; 1 case of post–tubal sterilization syndrome; 3 cases of pelvic inflammatory disease; 1 case of ureteral injury; 3 cases of hematometra; 4 cases of hematoma of the uterus; 21 cases of second- and third-degree burns to cervix, vagina, perineum, or buttocks; 2 cases of uterine perforation; 1 case of cervical laceration; and 1 case of constipation and abdominal discomfort.

HydroThermAblator

With the HydroThermAblator, 20 cases of second- and third-degree burns to cervix, vagina, perineum, and buttocks were reported that required treatment.

Bowel injury became evident in one patient. In this case, uterine perforation was suspected before use of the ablation device. Nevertheless, the surgeon went ahead with the procedure, and the patient required laparotomy with bowel resection.

Microwave Endometrial Ablation

The technique of MEA has been recently approved by the FDA. A total of four adverse events were reported in the MAUDE database. Three of them involved perforation of the uterus with bowel injury, which required resection of the bowel. The fourth adverse event reported was peritonitis secondary to pyosalpinx after MEA. The patient required laparotomy and hysterectomy.

HerOption Uterine Cryoablation Therapy System

A total of five adverse events were reported with the HerOption Uterine Cryoablation Therapy System. In two patients, excessive bleeding occurred after cryoablation, and both patients required hysterectomy. The third adverse event was bowel injury necessitating resection.

In one patient, severe abdominal pain developed nearly a month after the procedure. On laparotomy, she was found to have perforation of the uterus with perforation of the colon and formation of pelvic abcess. She required a hysterectomy with colostomy.

One case of endometritis was reported. Foul-smelling vaginal discharge developed, and the patient had to be treated with antibiotics.

Thermachoice

A total of 14 adverse events were reported with use of the Thermachoice device. Bowel injury occurred in three procedures; in one, the patient required resection of bowel, and another patient required a sigmoid colostomy for sigmoid abcess. The third patient required laparotomy with resection of bowel and colostomy.

One case of post–tubal sterilization syndrome was reported; tubo-ovarian abscess necessitating removal of the adnexa developed in another patient; and damage to the pelvic sidewall and ureteral injury occurred in still another patient, who required ureteral stenting for management. Hematometra developed in three patients after endometrial ablation with Thermachoice; management required dilation and curettage (D&C), release of the hematometra, and antibiotics.

Three additional patients presented with severe abdominal pain and on laparotomy were found to have hematoma of the uterus, which required hysterectomy. Broad ligament hematoma developed in one patient, who needed hysterectomy. Severe vaginal and urethral burn due to leakage of hot fluid also was reported in one patient. This patient required urethral catheterization and referral for urologic consultation.

Novasure Impedance Controlled Endometrial Ablation

Twenty-one adverse events, including one death, were reported with use of the Novasure Impedance Controlled Endometrial Ablation technique. Two cases of uterine perforation were reported; in one patient, the site of perforation was cauterized at laparoscopy. Thirteen cases of uterine perforation with injury to bowel were reported; the one death was due to this complication.

The patient who died had an undiagnosed 6-cm submucous fibroid and underwent late-evening D&C, hysteroscopy, and endometrial ablation procedure. Sounding length at the time of operative visit was documented as 10 cm (actual sounding length of the autopsy specimen was 6 cm). Multiple cavity integrity assessment (CIA) tests performed with two devices indicated the possibility of uterine perforation. Eventually the patient "passed" the CIA test, most likely as a result of occlusion of the perforation with the fibroid, allowing the ablation to proceed. Postoperative hysteroscopy revealed uterine cavity blanching, and the fibroid was still undiagnosed. The patient remained hospitalized overnight. Three hours after discharge, the patient sought treatment at a different hospital for severe abdominal pain and was given painkillers and antiemetic medications. The patient continued to experience pain the next day, and the doctor prescribed alternate pain and antiemetic medications by telephone. Three days after the procedure, the patient was admitted to the hospital and diagnosed with peritonitis and septic shock. Subsequent laparotomy revealed uterine and small bowel perforations. Small bowel resection and appendectomy were performed. The patient was unstable during and after surgery and expired shortly thereafter in the intensive care unit.

The county medical examiner reported that the patient had a previously undiagnosed, large submucous 6-cm fibroid occupying the entire uterine cavity. The size of the uterine and bowel perforations was consistent with uterine sound diameter, indicating that the perforations had been caused by the sound instrument. The reported intraoperative 10-cm sounding length compared with the 6-cm autopsy sounding length also indicates that the perforations were caused by the uterine sound instrument. No indication that the larger-diameter Novasure device had exited the uterine cavity was present. The CIA alarm correctly identified the presence of uterine perforation on multiple occasions. It is believed that after multiple manipulations, the fibroid was temporarily pressed against the perforation site, allowing for occlusion and ablation initiation.

Tubo-ovarian abscess was reported in one patient, with development of septicemia. The patient required hysterectomy with removal of the affected adnexa.

Endometritis developed in two patients. One of these patients had severe endometritis with *Escherichia coli* infection and required hysterectomy.

Cervical laceration, reported in one patient, was due to injury by the Novasure device and was treated by cauterization with silver nitrate and Monsel's paste.

One of the patients presented with constipation and abdominal discomfort. She underwent laparoscopy, but no bowel or uterine perforation was found.

CONCLUSIONS

The MAUDE database does not, for numerical data reasons, allow any medical device company to claim that its product is any safer than any other, nor allow any such company to claim that another's device is more dangerous. Worldwide, considerable underreporting of endometrial ablation complications is likely. The prudent gynecologist looking to offer endometrial ablation procedures to patients will do so only after having acquired complete familiarity with the technique and related principles, including patient selection and careful theoretical and practical clinical training, which responsible manufacturers of relevant instrumentation are very happy to provide. In this way, the complication rate can be kept to a minimum, and women can benefit from the advantages of the endometrial ablation approach to management, avoiding hysterectomy.

References

1. Goldrath MH, Fuller TA, Segal S. Laser photovaporization of endometrium for the treatment of menorrhagia. Am J Obstet Gynecol 1981;140:14.
2. Cooper KG, Jack SA, Parkin DE, Grant AM. Five-year follow up of women randomised to medical management or transcervical resection of the endometrium for heavy menstrual loss: Clinical and quality of life outcomes. Br J Obstet Gynaecol 2001;108:1222.
3. Overton C, Hargreaves J, Maresh M. A national survey of the complications of endometrial destruction for menstrual disorders: The MISTLETOE study. Minimally invasive surgical techniques—laser, endothermal or endoresection. Br J Obstet Gynaecol 1997;104:1351.
4. Isaacson KB, Olive DL. Operative hysteroscopy in physiologic distention media. J Am Assoc Gynecol Laparosc 1999;6:113.
5. Cherney AH, Diamond MP, Lavy G, Polan ML. Endometrial ablation for intractable uterine bleeding: Hysteroscopic resection. Obstet Gynecol 1987;70:668.
6. Gurtcheff SE, Sharp HT. Complications associated with global endometrial ablation: The utility of the MAUDE database. Obstet Gynecol 2003;102:1278.
7. Gardner S, Schultz DG. Complications associated with global endometrial ablation: The utility of the MAUDE database. Obstet Gynecol 2004;103(5 Pt 1):995.

Laparoscopic Training and Education

19

Charles R. Rardin and Gary Frishman

Classic surgical training is derived essentially from apprenticeship: Junior residents observe and assist faculty surgeons, and increasing responsibility is given and complexity of assigned surgery increases as the trainees progress. The surgical experience available in traditional surgery has been shown to vary widely among accredited residency programs; one questionnaire study showed that the number of hysterectomies performed by an individual trainee ranged from 50 to 133, and caselogs for incontinence procedures showed totals ranging from 1 to 20.[1]

Experience in laparoscopy varies even more widely; surgical innovations and new developments in instrumentation have rendered training more complex, and other demands on resident time and reduction in resident work hours curtail available training opportunities. The breadth of surgical repertoires also varies widely: Training in salpingostomy and tubal ligation are nearly universally available, whereas advanced laparoscopic pelvic reconstruction and gynecologic oncology are available only at selected centers. Formal laparoscopic training curricula are provided at a minority of residency programs.[1] Financial and temporal pressures are serving to drive gynecologists from the role of instructor back into the role of surgeon, relegating the trainee to the role of camera holder. Some programs may be resistant to support laparoscopic education, because the introduction of minimally invasive techniques has been shown, in some programs, to take "basic" cases out of the hands of junior trainees by converting such cases to more advanced, laparoscopic procedures.[2]

Assessment of an individual trainee's surgical skills also has been widely variable. Despite the importance of such evaluation, it traditionally occurs in an unstructured and variable manner. This type of assessment has been shown to be vulnerable to bias and poor reliability.[3,4] Often, only the most severely deficient trainees receive feedback that improvement is required; specific areas of improvement and methods of remedy may not be made clear.

THE LEARNING CURVE

The process of learning technical and surgical procedures often is described in terms of a *learning curve*, a tool introduced in the 1930s. The first learning curves (also known as progress functions) depicted estimates of the cost of building airplanes as a function of the number of airplanes built; cost per unit decreased over number of units produced, up to a point. With regard to surgical procedures, a learning curve generally reflects some measure of efficacy (e.g., operative time, complication rate, success rate, survival curve) measured as a function of the number of times the learner has repeated the procedure. When the incremental benefit of performing additional cases approaches zero, the curve reaches its plateau, and the learning curve can be described. A common misconception is that a comparison of data obtained at two different points in time—for instance, a surgeon's first 10 cases compared with his or her last 10 cases—is adequate to describe the learning curve. Until plateau is reached, however, the learning process must be assumed to be ongoing, with corresponding changes in the learning curve, and any statements regarding a minimum number of procedures required to achieve proficiency are likely to be premature. Similarly, the term *steep learning curve* often is used to characterize a procedure that is difficult and requires many repetitions to achieve competency—but a procedure with a steep learning curve is, in fact, mastered in very few repetitions. The presumption is made that, before plateau is attained, performance has not been optimized, and patients are at increased risk for adverse outcomes (regarding the measured parameter). The learning curve for a particular procedure is an estimate of the resources required to achieve proficiency, and of the number of patients at increased risk while proficiency is being attained. Such considerations are important in the planning and allocation of surgical training resources.

Another consideration is that two learning curves can be applied to any particular procedure—the first is the efficacy of the procedure itself, measured among the researchers who developed the procedure; the second describes the "teachability" of the procedure as it is measured among new trainees. Published reports claiming to describe the learning curve may reflect only one or the other of these concerns. Another caveat of published estimates of learning curves, particularly retrospective analyses, is selection bias. A surgeon may be more likely to be more selective in choosing candidates for a procedure new to his or her repertoire; as experience grows, selection may become broader, and more difficult cases undertaken. This effect is not included in the data on which the learning curve is based, so that the minimum number of cases to achieve proficiency is underestimated.

Clinical experience has suggested that the learning curve for endoscopic procedures is shallower than for analogous open procedures, indicating that greater experience is required to maximize surgeon performance. As previously discussed, teaching and experience in laparoscopic surgery vary widely between training programs but generally are more limited than with the traditional approaches. The combination of an extended learning curve and less experience often provides the "double whammy" that may lead a surgeon to choose traditional over endoscopic procedures.

Estimates of the Learning Curve

In one study, laparoscopic splenectomy among pediatric patients was characterized by a learning curve for a single attending surgeon; the conclusion was that operative time, and cost, continued to decrease steadily until the 20th case.[5] A curriculum based on use of a video trainer determined that trainees reached the 90th percentile of peak performance (an approximation of plateau) after 30 to 35 repetitions, irrespective of training level.[6] An evaluation of laparoscopic sigmoid resection yielded a plateau of 70 to 80 cases.[7] Kreiker and co-workers described their findings in a prospective assessment of a single surgical team learning laparoscopically assisted vaginal hysterectomy (LAVH), specifically with regard to operative time, and found that plateau was reached after 80 cases; all major complications in their study occurred before plateau was attained.[8]

Of interest, a population-based assessment of the learning curve for LAVH reached very different conclusions: The rate of conversion to laparotomy stabilized after 5 cases, and complication rates did not improve at all with increasing experience.[9] These findings might have been influenced by the fact that the median surgical experience for all trainees was only 2 cases, with a wide range (1 to 107 cases), and that 80% of all cases included represented the individual surgeon's first 20 procedures. Thus, it is probable that plateau was reached by only a handful of surgeons, and that a majority of cases included in the study represented early experience. These factors would be likely to attenuate the shape of the described learning curve.

Indeed, it is very likely (as well as intuitive) that the factors influencing the learning curve will prevent the development of universal estimates: A review of the literature for general surgery laparoscopic procedures concluded that outcomes measures were too subjective, and findings too disparate, to permit clear calculation of a learning curve.[10]

One model that may serve to estimate the learning curve in a more precise fashion involves the technique of laparoscopic retroperitoneal lymph node dissection for gynecologic malignancies. In addition to traditional surgical outcomes such as operative time, estimated blood loss, duration of hospitalization, and disease-free interval, lymph node sampling provides an immediate measure of technical adequacy: lymph node yield. Spirtos and associates reported on an initial group of 10 patients undergoing laparoscopic lymph node sampling at the time of type III radical hysterectomy and described a mean lymph node yield of 24.8 nodes.[11] Several years later, the same investigators reported on a larger series of 78 patients undergoing type III radical hysterectomy; the mean lymph node count had improved to 34.1 among this group, and in the final 20 patients of the series, the mean was 44 nodes, a number that compares favorably with that observed with laparotomy.[12] Again, as noted previously, the fact that the final group of patients demonstrated continued improvement in the outcomes of interest suggests that the learning curve data set is not yet complete. It is not infrequent for publications to assert calculation of a learning curve; if plateau has not been reached, however, such reports serve instead to demonstrate simply the number of procedures when improvement is first seen, not when it is maximized.[13-16]

Factors Influencing the Learning Curve

It generally is accepted that surgical experience is, to some degree, cumulative and transferable—that lessons and skills learned in one procedure can be of benefit to a surgeon learning a new procedure. The effect of previous surgical experience on the development of new skills has been assessed with regard to laparoscopic surgery. An evaluation of surgeon performance before and after the Yale Laparoscopic Boot Camp course confirmed the intuitive supposition that post-training experience and visuospatial aptitude enhanced the rate at which new, laparoscopic technical skills were acquired.[17] More specifically, with regard to newly developed laparoscopic gastric bypass procedures, the completion of a fellowship conferred improved performance and shortening of the learning curve for the laparoscopic modification.[18]

Grantcharov and associates, reporting on the effect of laparoscopic experience on the performance of structured laparoscopic simulation exercises, found that surgical experience had a significant effect on performance.[19] In this model, surgeons of various levels of experience with laparoscopic cholecystectomy were assessed in their performance of structured exercises, performed repeatedly over time. Experienced surgeons (who had performed greater than 100 procedures) reached plateau in time, error, and economy of movement assessments after 1 procedure; surgeons of intermediate experience (15 to 80 procedures) reached plateau after 5 repetitions of the exercise; and beginners (fewer than 10 procedures) required 7 repetitions to complete the learning curve.

A study using a model of laparoscopic nephrectomy in rabbits demonstrated more rapid progress and fewer severe complications among experienced gynecologists than among medical students.[20] By contrast, however, a study evaluating performance on laparoscopic knot-tying exercises found that surgeons experienced in open techniques (but without laparoscopic experience) fared no better than interns; only residents with current and ongoing laparoscopic instruction showed improved performance.[21] Although these findings do not support the assertion that traditional surgical experience can translate directly to shorter learning curves in laparoscopy, the study measured only a single, technical aspect of the surgery (knot tying); clearly, technical expertise is only one component of surgical competency, and experience is likely to play an important role in the safe and efficacious performance of surgical procedures.

Neurophysiologic research has focused on the possibility that surgeons may possess different levels of innate aptitude. A study investigating predictors of surgical skill determined that neurophysiologic testing of complex visuospatial organization, stress tolerance (or the ability to prioritize essential and nonessential details), and psychomotor abilites were positively correlated with surgical skills, as determined by faculty preceptors.[22] By contrast, variables including standardized test scores (National Board, Medical College Admission Test) and also pure motor characteristics (such as speed and precision) did not predict skill rating.

A systematic assessment of basic human performance has been described as a more objective alternative to the subjective evaluations that make up the traditional residency experience. Gettman and colleagues described their findings in the investigation of the relationship between surgeons' scores in a series of Basic Performance Resource Measures and their aptitude and performance in learning laparoscopic skills.[23]

Scoring in Basic Element of Performance measures such as central processing and upper extremity motor control, isometric strength, and steadiness versus tremor correlated with surgical performance of laparoscopic nephrectomy in the porcine model. These assessments accurately predicted performance in 13 of the 20 surgeons evaluated with this model; of importance, the model demonstrated particularly high accuracy regarding the poorest surgical performers. Scientific modeling such as this may, say proponents, represent a way to help predict surgical aptitude for the selection of surgical training candidates, and to match trainees with training resources most effectively.

MODELS OF LAPAROSCOPIC TEACHING

Despite the limitations in resources for endoscopic training, the nature of video endoscopy makes it amenable to education in ways not easily applicable to laparotomy. In traditional surgery, the view is optimized for the primary surgeon, and perhaps for the assistant; all other participants are given a suboptimal view. In video endoscopy, all participants share the same view; moreover, videotaping and other forms of archiving make sharing endoscopic experience much more productive. In addition, the suitability of simulations is much higher for endoscopic procedures; indeed, simulation is the backbone of most published laparoscopic curricula. In the era of early development of operative laparoscopy, traditional apprenticeship-type training programs were common; more recently, formal curricula in endoscopic training have been developed and published.

Mechanical simulators are the most common type of trainer. Several authors have published their experience demonstrating that mechanical simulators provide training that improves performance of the trainees, as well as reliable assessment tools regarding skill levels of trainees.[24-27] Although commercially available simulators are available, one study demonstrated that simulations can be created in a much more

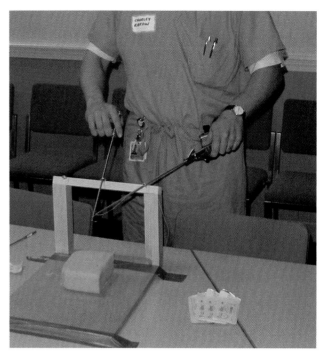

Figure 19–1 ▪ Simple pelvic trainer.

cost-effective manner using simple materials, reducing the per-resident cost from a range of $4000 to $6000 to only $40 (Fig. 19–1).[28]

The impact of such formal, simulation-based laparoscopic curricula is the subject of several reports. Some published studies focus on skill development: One study reported that a formal seminar in laparoscopic suturing and knot tying resulted in improvements in dominant, nondominant, and two-handed skills.[29] A randomized study of residents in training demonstrated that participation in a video-based simulator program enhanced skill acquisition, both in simulator tasks and in operative performance (as assessed by blinded faculty members).[30] Another report described experience with a curriculum involving simulator and animal (rat) models; performance of 5 specific tasks in the simulators was significantly improved among participants of the curriculum compared with controls.[31] A 7-week program involving didactics, simulators, and animal laboratories resulted in enhancement in operative time, increased skills assessments (both self-assessment and faculty evaluation), and a dramatic increase in the satisfaction with training.[32] A session of laparoscopic dissection of fresh cadavers demonstrated a trend toward improvement in faculty skill evaluation and test performance, although the sample size limited the statistical strength of these findings.[33]

Other studies focus on the impact of training programs on clinical outcomes. One program that included six 4-hour sessions per year, including didactics, bench exercises, and animal laboratory experience demonstrated that participants showed improvements in operative time, blood loss, hospital stay, and conversion rate.[34] An evaluation of a curriculum involving laboratory-based drill and video observation resulted in enhanced acquisition of laparoscopic skill and proficiency.[35]

SURGICAL SKILLS ASSESSMENT TOOLS

If the surgical mentoring and experience that a trainee in a residency program receives are variable and unpredictable in quantity and quality, likewise the evaluation and assessment of that trainee's skills and aptitude typically have been erratic, biased, and poorly reliable.[36] Incorporation of specific guidelines and checklists into the assessments of resident trainees has been shown to increase interobserver reliability and discrimination between senior and junior residents.[37] Development of tools such as the Objective Structured Assessment of Technical Skills (OSATS) has provided a much more reliable and reproducible method of evaluating trainee performance, using bench-station simulator or animal models.[38-40] In this model, use of global assessment tools provided more reliable measures of skill than did use of task-specific checklists, particularly when bench models were used. This model has been shown to perform with a high degree of reliability in a cost-effective manner whether the examiners were blinded or were familiar with the examinee.[41,42] Tools such as these use as their measure of construct validity the ability to discriminate between post-graduate year levels; clearly, other measures of the validity of the assessment tool will be useful (such as correlation with clinical outcomes, complication rates, or operative time). The development and implementation of objective tools such as OSATS are vital, however, not only for assessing the surgical competency of trainees but, even more important, to provide a means to measure and thereby improve the quality of training programs. Moreover, early identification of surgeons with skill deficiencies may serve to address some of the disparity in skill levels on completion of training, and to better allocate educational resources.

LAPAROSCOPIC SURGERY ASSESSMENT TOOLS

In addition to the skills assessment tools such as OSATS, which include laparoscopic modules, some additional tools have been developed specifically for the evaluation of laparoscopic skills. The Interactive Voice Response (IVR) system was developed at the University of Ottawa; this tool involves use of a telephone-based rating system, by both the precepting attending surgeon and the trainee, immediately after completion of each procedure, to rate trainee performance. As with OSATS, performance was enhanced with advancing level of training, and reliability was demonstrated after 12 evaluated cases.[43]

Several published laparoscopic curricula have included a description of the assessment systems incorporated into the curricula, along with an evaluation of the performance of that assessment system. Many of these programs primarily base the assessment of surgical skill on time required to complete assigned tasks.[24,44-46] One study, which used a computer-based method of accuracy and economy-of-movement evaluation, demonstrated that although the time-to-completion reached plateau quickly, more sophisticated measures of accuracy continued to improve over additional repetitions.[47] A mechanical simulator–based curriculum included skills assessments of the trainees, videotaped as they executed laparoscopic tasks.[28] Two different sets of skills were assessed: Participants were assessed by blinded faculty surgeons on the basis of performance in the global skills categories of clinical judgment, spatial orientation, serial complexity (appropriate "flow" of components of the procedures), and dexterity. They also were assessed by nonclinicians according to a specific scorecard that catalogued events such as number of times instruments were out of control, number of attempts for main procedural elements, and so on. This method of evaluation demonstrated high reliability and construct validity.

As was found in using the OSATS model, the McGill Inanimate System for Training and Evaluation of Laparoscopic Skills (MISTELS) demonstrated that global or general skills assessments were superior to task-specific assessments in discriminating among experience levels of participants.[48] MISTELS also is superior to subjective, in-training evaluation reports in the identification of residents with below-average skills.[49] Simulation systems also have been shown to demonstrate and quantify the effect of sleep deprivation on surgeon performance indices.[50] Assessment methods such as these are important to the enhancement of unbiased and accurate assessment of surgical trainees, the importance of which increases with the increasing technical advancements of surgical techniques.

INTEGRATION OF NEW TECHNOLOGIES

The suitability of video endoscopy training systems for application in computer-based models and curricula has lead to increased popularity of these designs. Participants of programs on CD-ROM or available over the Internet can observe videos and then complete training and assessment modules at their own pace. Such programs have been shown to boost intern performance to the level of a second-year resident, and post-test improvement is seen in all participants.[51] Multimedia-based interactive programs also have demonstrated enhanced self-reported comfort levels among residents and were preferred over printed materials, lectures, videos, and animal laboratories by the trainees.[52]

Virtual reality (VR) represents a computer-based simulation system coupled with a mechanical interface and offers the benefits of infinite variation in simulation, as well as computer-based objective performance assessment and identification of areas of deficiency (Fig. 19–2). VR training has been successfully integrated into a number of sectors and industries, including the military and law enforcement, as well as aviation and aeronautics. A growing number of endoscopy-based VR systems have been developed (Fig. 19–3). Although superiority of VR over mechanical simulators in the acquisition of skills has not been verified, VR offers the advantage of automated, real-time, objective assessment of performance. One model, known as the Computer-Enhanced Laparoscopic Training System (CELTS), employs cognitive and psychomotor learning theory in its customizable set of tasks.[53] This system allows for a sophisticated set of performance analyses, such as for depth perception, motion smoothness, and instrument orientation; these parameters were successful in discriminating between experts and trainees. Learning curves associated with task-specific skills using VR have shown that plateau generally is reached in 21 to 30 repetitions.[54] Some data suggest that VR training may result in greater improvement in operative performance than that achieved with video trainers.[55]

The development of robot-based surgery clearly has implications for the training of laparoscopic surgeons. The robot systems have several main advantages, these including motion scaling (converting large movements of the surgeon to very fine movements of the instruments), capability of an additional degree of motion (by means of a type of instrument known as an endo-wrist), and the enhancement of psychomotor performance (through tremor-stabilizing algorithms). Some systems also employ three-dimensional video, enhancing depth perception. In addition, the robotic systems seem uniquely suited to telesurgery, which could enhance the availability of expert surgeons. The performance of these systems in the training of residents is in the early stages. One study demonstrated a steeper learning curve (i.e., more rapid acquisition of skills), among both experienced and inexperienced surgeons, in the performance of drills using a robotic system.[56] Another study demonstrated that laparoscopic drills were completed more quickly with the robotic system than with traditional laparoscopy, and that novice surgeons using the robot performed as quickly as, and in some cases more quickly than, expert surgeons did using traditional laparoscopy.[57] The continued development and refinement of these systems may, in some measure, serve to redress some of the current deficiencies in laparoscopic training by improving skill acquisition.

LAPAROSCOPIC CREDENTIALING

Background and Definitions

Before the 1980s, the act of obtaining staff privileges at a hospital typically permitted a surgeon to perform any and all procedures with any equipment and without any specific procedural or subspecialty requirements or restrictions. Although there is no one uniform policy throughout the United States, the credentialing process has evolved substantially. Multiple objectives are behind these changes, including quality assurance and patient protection as well as the goal of reducing medicolegal risk. The concept of corporate negligence states that the corporation (hospital) owes clients (patients) due care in selection of surgeons allowed to practice under its jurisdiction. If due care in the credentialing process is not performed, then the hospital may be liable for bad outcomes. Each hospital typically develops its own guidelines for certification and granting privileges using available resources and existing guidelines.

The Council on Resident Education in Obstetrics and Gynecology (CREOG) defines credentialing and licensure as the following:

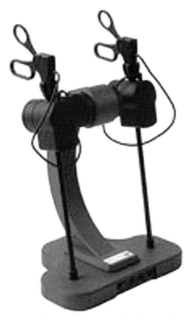

Figure 19–2 ▪ Virtual laparoscopic interface. (Reproduced by permission of Immersion Corporation, copyright ©2006 Immersion Corporation. All rights reserved.)

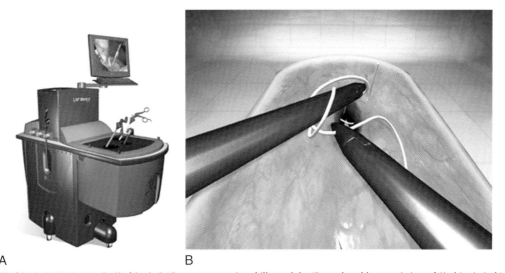

A   B

Figure 19–3 ▪ **A,** Simbionix LAP Mentor. **B,** Simbionix LAP mentor suturing skills module. (Reproduced by permission of Simbionix Ltd.)

Credentialing is the process of obtaining information, verifying the information, and evaluating applicants who want to obtain or renew medical staff privileges within a health institution or organization. During the credentialing process, the types of medical credentials that are evaluated include state medical licenses, documentation of completion of training, and evidence of medical professional liability insurance. The credentialing process also may entail the gathering of additional information, such as continuing medical education and work history records.

Licensure is a requirement for the practice of medicine in the United States. A medical license is one of the components of the information gathered during the credentialing process. In each of the 50 states, the District of Columbia, and the U.S. territories, boards of medical licensure regulate the ability of physicians to practice medicine. Because licenses are specific to individual states, a physician must obtain a license in each state in which he or she practices.[58]

The On-Line Medical Dictionary provided by Cancerweb offers the following definitions:

Certification: Compliance with a set of standards defined by nongovernmental organizations. Certification is applied for by individuals on a voluntary basis and represents a professional status when achieved, for example, certification for a medical specialty.

Standards and guidelines: Bounds or constraints within which all practices in a given area are carried out in achieving the goals and objectives for that area. Standards and guidelines provide environmental safeguards and also describe constraints prescribed by law.[59]

Credentialing Overview

There are different categories of hospital privileges that may vary in description and terminology from institution to institution. New practitioners to an institution typically obtain *probationary privileges*. Probationary privileges may require various degrees of oversight by other staff and/or mandatory assistance with hospital-run or resident-run patient clinics or similar activities. Typically, a temporary or probationary privilege is granted for a period of time (e.g., 1 year), during or at the end of which the surgeon's performance is reviewed before unrestricted or full privileges are granted. *Courtesy privileges* are given to physicians who have minimal activity at a hospital but who wish to be able to practice there as needed. *Emergency privileges* may be granted to physicians who cannot wait for the routine credentialing process, for example, a surgeon who needs to operate at a particular hospital on a semiemergency basis because of a need for his or her particular skills or because he or she needs instruments or technology available at that hospital. An outreach surgeon is a surgeon who typically commutes to perform needed surgery, often to a rural area. *Active* or *attending privileges* are the typical privileges granted to physicians who have met the hospital's requirements. These privileges may require admitting a certain number of patients per year as well as annual renewal of privileges. If physicians are semiretired or no longer admit patients, they may be given *emeritus privileges*.

The credentialing process has several facets. To withstand legal scrutiny and to be fair and consistent, uniform standards should be developed that are applicable to all practitioners

who seek privileges. Privileges should be specific rather than global. Most obstetric and gynecology departments have a general, category I credential (e.g., routine vaginal delivery, hysterectomy, cesarean section) and additional, more specific credentials for more advanced procedures (e.g., use of laser, operative resectoscopic surgery). It is the responsibility of each health care facility to oversee the credentialing process; each chief of service typically supervises the process for the department.

A credentialing committee, set up under the department chair, initially reviews an applicant's request, verifying its accuracy regarding education, residency, and work records. An applicant's references should be checked and questions should be asked concerning competence, background, experience, health, and ethics. These interviews do not have to be limited to an applicant's list of references. Physicians typically qualify for the most basic set of privileges by virtue of having completed a residency or providing documentation of previous training. A probationary period is still common, however. Furthermore, a graduating resident may not have achieved expertise (warranting credentialing) in more difficult or complicated procedures during training. Although it is easy to document that a physician applying for staff privileges has completed a residency, it is often challenging to ascertain which specific advanced procedures he or she is qualified to perform. Having a residency program director "sign off" a resident on a specific procedure no longer automatically guarantees the resident privileges to perform that procedure at a new institution. To obtain credentials to perform more advanced procedures, documentation of didactic exposure, such as a course, along with hands-on exposure provided by the completion of a number of procedures (supported by copies of operative notes or similar documentation) may be necessary. Alternatively, completion of a fellowship may suffice in a similar fashion as a residency would for basic privileges. Depending on the complexity of the procedure and the available documentation of prior experience, preceptorships may also be utilized, with the supervising physician signing off on completion of the procedure.

The number of procedures required for both documentation and prior experience as well as the requirements for supervised surgery may vary based on the institution and the complexity of the procedure. Some procedures may parallel others so that a physician may get credit by doing one or the other. For example, a physician may be able to get privileges for a salpingectomy if he or she documents the ability to perform an oophorectomy.

A physician's ability to perform procedures that are performed infrequently is more difficult to assess. It is not always realistic to request documentation or preceptorship for uncommon procedures such as the repair of a bladder laceration because of its unpredictable and infrequent occurrence. Credentialing of these procedures is often tied into general privileges granted at a lower level of documentation. As noted earlier, there are no uniform policies concerning how to document adequate training. Even the process of choosing the specific number of procedures to be performed as documentation of competency is challenging.

A prospective randomized study evaluated training and credentialing in gastrointestinal endoscopy.[60] Utilizing objective measures of skill in ERCP and colonoscopy, the authors reported that the previously accepted and published threshold numbers that had been required for credentialing were not adequate for most physicians to achieve confidence. For example, the ability to cannulate the duct of interest successfully in 80% of cases was used as a minimum measure of competency in ERCP. Although 180 supervised procedures were required to achieve this level of competence, the published requirement was only 75 procedures.[60]

When determining competence, a further challenge is documenting adequate clinical judgment in addition to technical ability. Currently, there are no standards for this, although most applications require letters from colleagues bearing witness as to the applicant's character.

It is also important to have continued ongoing credentialing processes. The mechanism for this is typically combined with that for renewal of privileges. Ideally, an ongoing review board evaluates each physician's actual performance before renewing credentials, including the number of procedures performed and any complications that may have occurred, along with whatever other outcomes are available. At a bare minimum, continuing medical education is required. In addition, the credentialing guidelines should be periodically reviewed by each institution to make sure that they are up to date and reflect the current standard of care and technology. Future credentialing guidelines will most likely include a web-based testing and/or documentation of proficiency via a virtual trainer or surgical simulation model.

Credentialing Process

When physicians decide to practice at new institutions, they must decide which procedures and practices as well as what instrumentation and equipment they wish to apply for. The specific protocol for obtaining privileges typically involves choosing from various options, which are often in a menu-type format. For example, at Women & Infants' Hospital of Rhode Island, an incoming surgeon may request general obstetric and gynecologic privileges along with the use of the intraperitoneal laser. This latter privilege requires documentation of successful completion of an approved residency that is signed off by the surgeon's program director (which usually is sufficient for general privileges) along with additional verification of the program director for competence in this specific technique. Alternatively, documentation of completion of a fellowship in reproductive medicine or attendance in an advanced course on laser along with practical experience via a preceptor's supervision is sufficient. The surgeon must also have an operational knowledge of the specific laser used at a hospital. If the surgeon was trained and previously credentialed in the use of the Yag laser, the surgeon would not automatically be eligible for laser privileges with the CO_2 laser. The preceptorship period for laser privileges involves observing or assisting, or both, in at least five laser cases. Following this, the surgeon may proceed as the primary surgeon under the supervision of a preceptor until the precepting surgeon deems the probationary surgeon to be qualified. In recognition of the different levels of complexity of surgical cases, it is also suggested that the mastery of treatment of mild disease such as endometriosis that is not on the bowel or bladder be undertaken before proceeding to the mastery of more extensive disease.

One uniform gray zone in credentialing regulations is how a preceptor determines when to sign off on a surgeon. A specific algorithm is followed for credentialing graduating residents for endoscopic procedures at Women & Infants' Hospital of Rhode Island. In addition to successful completion of the residency, residents must attend the hospital's endoscopy course to be certified. The class is designed to train them in specific endoscopic procedures as well as energy sources, operating room set up, possible complications of the procedure, and the like. Residents must also pass a written and practical (hands-on) endoscopy test before graduation. Lastly, they must be signed off on specific endoscopic procedures by attending physicians. The following criteria are used by the supervising attending physician before signing off on a resident:

1. Knowledge of indication and appropriate patient population for the procedure
2. Knowledge of the procedure (technique)
3. Anticipating steps in surgery
4. Knowledge of anatomy
5. Ability to handle variation of normal surgery (e.g., unusual anatomy, unexpected findings, complications)
6. Familiarity with instrumentation
7. Appropriate speed (not too slow or too fast)

By making these guidelines as specific as possible, the goal of Women & Infants' Hospital of Rhode Island is to provide for a precise and reproducible credentialing mechanism.

Occasionally, a decision is made to begin requiring credentialing for a new technique, instrumentation, or procedure that some physicians are already utilizing or performing. In that case, there is often a provision for the practicing surgeon to be "grandfathered" by documenting the skills in question via some mechanism such as operative notes indicating mastery of a skill or a specific instrument.

Occasionally there are unintended consequences of the credentialing and board certification process. Insurance companies often look at this benchmark and restrict reimbursement for procedures performed to those who have achieved board certification. Since this restriction may dramatically affect amount a newly graduated physician can be reimbursed, the American Board of Obstetricians and Gynecologists has taken a more proactive stance. Recently, the Board's guidelines have been changed to speed the board certification process to allow newly graduated residents an accelerated course to full participation in insurance companies' health care networks.

Available Resources for Credentialing

A number of different organizations and resources are involved in the credentialing process. In addition to information obtained from a residency program and a physician's application, a number of independent data banks are available for hospitals to query. The best known is the National Practitioner Data Bank (NPDB), which is a repository of information on physicians and other health care practitioners. The NPDB was established in 1996 by the Health Care Quality Improvement Act. The NPDB may be contacted by phone (1-800-767-6732) or by accessing their web site (www.npdb.com).

Another resource is the Federal Physician Data Center (http://www.docinfo.org/), a central repository for formal actions taken against physicians by state licensing and disciplinary boards and other agencies. This resource provides information that is publicly available and legally releasable to state medical boards. The Health Care Integrity and Protection Databank (http://www.npdb-hipdb.com/) reports final adverse action taken against health care providers. Its focus is on national health care fraud and abuse data. The Federal Credentials Verification Service (888-275-3287) obtains verification of physicians' professional portfolios, including their medical education, postgraduate training, licensure, board actions, and the like. Physicians may ask this service to forward information to their hospitals, state medical boards, or other agencies or parties. This board speeds the credentialing process because its information has already been verified.

The Joint Commission on Accreditation of Healthcare Organizations (JCAHO) is a nongovernmental, independent, nonprofit organization that participates in the accreditation of tens of thousands of health care organizations in the United States. In addition to hospitals, health care networks and ambulatory and long-term facilities and clinical laboratories are accredited. Although accreditation via JCAHO is not required by law, nearly all hospitals seek it because courts and legislatures typically look at the JCAHO standards as an important guide to minimum hospital standards. For JCAHO accreditation, an organization must ensure that every practitioner providing care possesses the necessary credentials attributable to those specific services.

In the field of obstetrics and gynecology, the American College of Obstetricians and Gynecologists (ACOG) has never attempted to control the credentialing process. The most recent Committee Opinion on Gynecologic Surgery, entitled "Credentialing Guidelines for New Operative Procedures" (number 142), was printed in August 1994 and subsequently was withdrawn. At that time, the committee suggested the following core elements to the credentialing process: (1) applicants must be members in good standing at their institutions; (2) applicants must have documented education and personal experience in the specific requested operative procedure; (3) applicants should be supervised in that procedure by a qualified surgeon who should then make a written recommendation to the department head; and (4) applicants should restrict their activities to equipment for which they are qualified and. procedures for which they are credentialed. In the years since that last committee opinion, ACOG has moved away from formal suggestions and toward letting each local institution determine its own standards. In the section "Evaluating Credentials and Granting Privileges" of ACOG's 2002 publication *Guidelines for Women's Health Care*, it says that "once an applicant is accepted on staff, it becomes the institution's responsibility to determine which privileges should be granted." It goes on to say that "credentialing and granting of privileges are local activities that should be based on training, experience, and demonstrated competence."[61]

Regarding nongynecologic procedures, ACOG has come out with a formal statement via a Committee Opinion (No. 253, March 2001) entitled "Nongynecologic Procedures" that cosmetic procedures (e.g., laser hair removal and liposuction) are not considered gynecologic procedures. Therefore, these are typically not taught in an approved obstetrics and gynecology residency, and it is "inappropriate for the College to establish guidelines for training."

The American Association of Gynecological Laparoscopists established the Accreditation Council for Gynecologic Endoscopy (ACGE) in 1993 to provide standards for operative endoscopic procedures. Although the ACGE does not formally credential surgeons, it does provide documentation of membership. Membership is limited to gynecologic endoscopic surgeons, although physicians outside the United States are eligible to become accredited members. Re-accreditation is necessary via application every 5 years. To become accredited by the ACGE, two letters of recommendation are required. One of these must be from the physician's department head or chief of staff and the other from another physician, preferably not someone in practice with the applicant.

For laparoscopy, three practice levels are defined. Practice level 1 includes minor procedures such as sterilization or treatment of stage 1 endometriosis. Procedures included in practice level 2 are American Fertility Society (AFS) stage 2 with endometriosis, oophorectomy, or moderate adhesiolysis (LAVH is considered within practice level 2). Practice level 3 involves treatment of severe endometriosis, myomectomy for deep tumors, tubal reversal, and similarly challenging procedures. Twenty-five consecutive cases within 2 consecutive calendar years in the practice level or higher are required for each application.

Hysteroscopy is also broken down into three practice levels. Practice level 1 involves diagnostic procedures or polypectomies. Practice level 2 includes tubal canalization, adhesiolysis, and myomectomies for pedunculated fibroids. Practice level 3 encompasses extensive adhesiolysis, resectoscopic endometrial ablation, and metroplasty. Fifteen consecutive cases within 2 practice years are required. Following submission of the cases, seven laparoscopy and five hysteroscopy cases are randomly chosen with additional information required. This additional check is done to document the physician's competence. Surgeons are not alerted as to which cases are selected until after they have submitted their case list. As noted earlier, the ACGE is not a credentialing board. It is merely a way for expert endoscopic gynecologic surgeons to be recognized by their peers. Full credentialing in clinical privileges is necessary before going through this process. For full certification, board certification by the American Board of Obstetrics and Gynecology or the equivalent in the surgeon's home country (e.g., Royal College of Obstetrics and Gynecology in the United Kingdom) is required. The ACGE can be contacted by phone (562-946-4435) or via their web site (http://accreditationcouncil.org).

However, credentialing and certification programs outside the mainstream are not uniformly accepted. *OB/GYN News* quoted ACOG Executive Vice President Dr. Ralph W. Hale's statement that "If 'certification' programs by special interests continue to be accepted by more and more outside groups, we run the risk of devaluing the role of appropriate accrediting and certifying bodies." This controversy extends to the field of ultrasound, in which some insurance companies require credentialing by the American Institute of Ultrasound Medicine or the American College of Radiology before reimbursement for procedures performed by obstetricians and gynecologists.[62]

Credentialing in Other Countries and Specialties

The credentialing process can vary by country, although the basic outline noted earlier is typically followed. The Royal Australian and New Zealand College of Obstetricians and Gynecologists (RANZCOG) has a well thought out process with thorough documentation and extensive guidelines. For example, the requirement for credentialing for hysteroscopic endometrial ablation starts out with a requirement of good diagnostic hysteroscopy skills, which preferably includes more than 100 procedures. Initial training in ablation under supervision with a normal-sized uterus is followed by further cases under supervision and then cases without supervision.

The RANZCOG guidelines differ from many of their American counterparts in their attempt to delineate skill levels for the supervisors, stating that "experienced operators acting as supervisors for endometrial ablations training should have completed at least 50 cases which include technically difficult cases and uterine abnormalities." In addition, it is spelled out that ancillary procedures, such as the treatment of a submucosal fibroid, should not be done concomitantly during an endometrial ablation unless the surgeon is also comfortable with that surgical technique. RANZCOG guidelines also discuss equipment requirements, specifying the use of a hysteroscope with loops and rollerballs and an appropriate energy source that provides an "accurate mix of coagulating and cutting current. High intensity light source. Video camera and monitor. Fluid inflow and outflow systems."

When developing national guidelines, it is important that the goals set forth be achievable by smaller institutions and hospitals. RANZCOG guidelines concerning fluid management for hysteroscopy specify the need for fluid inflow and outflow systems but indicate that they may be via gravity or electronically controlled.[63] This is similar to what happens in the United States when a smaller hospital may not be able to afford an electronically controlled fluid management system and thus must design its guidelines accordingly.

As is true for the existing rules for general medical licensure, being credentialed by another country does not guarantee that credentials will be granted in the United States. An individual hospital's policy may allow for a foreign didactic course, operating room notes, or other source of documentation to be used in their credentialing guidelines. At Women & Infants' Hospital of Rhode Island, a resident taking an elective at a different hospital (inside or outside the United States) may use a report from a precepting surgeon in that hospital as documentation toward endoscopic credentialing only if that specific surgeon's reputation and surgical skills are known to the director of endoscopic credentialing.

Other specialties follow a similar structure for credentialing. Since many areas in a credentialing guideline may be not be clearly spelled out or may be in a gray zone, the Society of American Gastrointestinal Endoscopic Surgeons (SAGES) has been very precise with definitions. SAGES documentation states that " 'must or shall' indicates a mandatory or indispensable recommendation." " 'Should' indicates a highly desirable recommendation." " 'May' or 'could' indicates an optional recommendation; alternatives may be appropriate." The Society also defines the components of a postresidency surgical education and course and specifies that course structures and duration may vary according to objectives. However, each course must have a "stated set of objective(s)." Furthermore, these "objectives must be defined as tasks, the successful completion of which can be quantitatively and qualitatively assessed." The SAGES guidelines specify that the course director and faculty members must have appropriate skills. The course "must have a written policy on disclosure of faculty/industry relationships." In addition, there should be an "appropriate ratio of faculty to participants," and the course site should be physically adequate to meet the objectives and accommodate the enrollees. The guidelines also attempt to define a preceptor and a proctor. A preceptor is "an expert surgeon who undertakes to impart his/her clinical knowledge and skills in a defined setting to a preceptee." A preceptor must be fully qualified in the field. A preceptorship typically involves the acquisition of "additional skill and/or judgment to improve his/her performance of a specific medical or surgical technique and/or procedures." A proctor is a "person who supervises or monitors students. A proctor differs from a consultant or a preceptor in that (s)he functions as an observer and evaluator, does not directly participate in patient care, and receives no fees from the patient."[64]

Occasionally a procedure may be used by more than one specialty (e.g., both general surgeons and gynecologists may perform an appendectomy). Typically, the chair of each department determines the guidelines through the department's own committee, which might or might not follow the existing guidelines and/or accept any previous credentialing by the other department. As expected, this process may involve politics as much as medicine.

Another issue is the use and credentialing of a specific instrument (as opposed to the procedure itself). Sometimes the system's oversight fails with dramatic and catastrophic results. A well-publicized case involved a young woman undergoing a resectoscopic myomectomy in New York City. The pump and fluid monitoring device used by the surgeon had not been approved by the hospital and was utilized in the operating room without biomedical or budget department sanction. Furthermore, the surgeons did not have any formal training with this device and used it for the first time on the patient. Although the nurses in the operating room stated that they were not familiar with the device and had not been trained to use it, the physicians chose to proceed with the procedure. In addition, they permitted the device's salesperson to physically operate the controls. The patient suffered excessive fluid overload and ultimately went into cardiac arrest and died.[65] Presumably, this tragic outcome could have been prevented if the relevant personnel had had a basic understanding of the procedure and instrumentation and standard credentialing guidelines had been followed.

The U.S. Food and Drug Administration often requires training requirements in labeling as part of a premarket approval for a class III device (more complex pieces of equipment such as implantable pacemakers). However, these devices represent a small percentage of all Food and Drug Administration approvals. Furthermore, from the perspective of a hospital's requirements for approval, it may be not always be clear when credentialing or preapproval is needed. Clearly, a new energy source that is a complex piece of machinery should require some extra caution, whereas a different Kocher clamp would not require the same level of diligence.

The resectoscopic myomectomy case previously mentioned also illustrated failures in the supervision of the salesperson. The surgeons stated that they assumed that the sales representative had been approved to enter the operating room.[65] This case clearly points out that the credentialing guidelines committee should work closely with any group overseeing hospital operating room policies concerning instrumentation and equipment use as well as the participation of the manufacturing company's sales force. Many hospitals have systems in place to prevent this type of tragedy because it is often difficult for a nurse in the operating room to refuse a senior surgeon the use of a device or make the surgeon stop a procedure because of a perceived lack of surgical experience. At Women & Infants' Hospital of Rhode Island, no new instrumentation is allowed in the operating room without preapproval (including an in-service demonstration with the nurses). Also, physicians' specific credentials and approved procedures are built into the operating room booking system so they may not schedule surgeries for which they lack credentials.

References

1. Mandel LP, Lentz GM, Goff BA. Teaching and evaluating surgical skills. Obstet Gynecol 2000;95:783.
2. McCormick PH, Tanner WA, Keane FB, et al. Minimally invasive techniques in common surgical procedures: Implications for training. Ir J Med Sci 2003;172:27.
3. Elliott DL, Hickman DH. Evaluation of physical examination skills. Reliability of faculty observers and patient instructors. JAMA 1987; 258:3405.
4. Warf BC, Donnelly MB, Schwartz RW, et al. Interpreting the judgment of surgical faculty regarding resident competence. J Surg Res 1999;86:29.
5. Cusick RA, Waldhausen JH. The learning curve associated with pediatric laparoscopic splenectomy. Am J Surg 2001;181:393.
6. Scott DJ, Young WN, Tesfay ST, et al. Laparoscopic skills training. Am J Surg 2001;182:137.
7. Dinçler S, Koller MT, Steurer J, et al. Multidimensional analysis of learning curves in laparoscopic sigmoid resection: Eight-year results. Dis Colon Rectum 2003;46:1371.
8. Kreiker GL, Bertoldi A, Larcher JS. Prospective evaluation of the learning curve of laparoscopic-assisted vaginal hysterectomy in a university hospital. J Am Assoc Gynecol Laparosc 2004;11:229.
9. Visco AG, Barber MD, Myers ER. Early physician experience with laparoscopically assisted vaginal hysterectomy and rates of surgical complications and conversion to laparotomy. Am J Obstet Gynecol 2002;187:1008.
10. Dagash H, Chowdhury M, Pierro A. When can I be proficient in laparoscopic surgery? A systematic review of the evidence. J Pediatr Surg 2003;38:720.
11. Spirtos NM, Schlaerth JB, Kimball RE, et al. Laparoscopic radical hysterectomy (type III) with aortic and pelvic lymphadenectomy. Am J Obstet Gynecol 1996;174:1763.
12. Spirtos NM, Eisenkop SM, Schlaerth JB, et al. Laparoscopic radical hysterectomy (type III) with aortic and pelvic lymphadenectomy in patients with stage I cervical cancer: Surgical morbidity and intermediate follow-up. Am J Obstet Gynecol 2002;187:340.
13. Bencini L, Sánchez LJ. Learning curve for laparoscopic ventral hernia repair. Am J Surg 2004;187:378.
14. Holub Z, Jabor A, Bartos P, et al. Laparoscopic surgery in women with endometrial cancer: The learning curve. Eur J Obstet Gynecol Reprod Biol 2003;107:195.
15. Wattiez A, Soriano D, Cohen SB, et al. The learning curve of total laparoscopic hysterectomy: Comparative analysis of 1647 cases. J Am Assoc Gynecol Laparosc 2002;9:339.
16. Gaston KE, Moore DT, Pruthi RS. Hand-assisted laparoscopic nephrectomy: Prospective evaluation of the learning curve. J Urol 2004;171:63.
17. Risucci D, Geiss A, Gellman L, et al. Surgeon-specific factors in the acquisition of laparoscopic surgical skills. Am J Surg 2001;181:289.
18. Oliak D, Owens M, Schmidt HJ. Impact of fellowship training on the learning curve for laparoscopic gastric bypass. Obes Surg 2004;14:197.
19. Grantcharov TP, Bardram L, Funch-Jensen P. Learning curves and impact of previous operative experience on performance on a virtual reality simulator to test laparoscopic surgical skills. Am J Surg 2003;185:146.
20. Molinas CR, Binda MM, Mailova K, et al. The rabbit nephrectomy model for training in laparoscopic surgery. Hum Reprod 2004;19:185.
21. Figert PL, Park AE, Witzke DB, et al. Transfer of training in acquiring laparoscopic skills. J Am Coll Surg 2001;193:533.
22. Schueneman AL, Pickleman J, Hesslein R, et al. Neuropsychologic predictors of operative skill among general surgery residents. Surgery 1984;96:288.
23. Gettman MT, Kondraske GV, Traxer O, et al. Assessment of basic human performance resources predicts operative performance of laparoscopic surgery. J Am Coll Surg 2003;197:489.
24. Derossis AM, Fried GM, Abrahamowicz M, et al. Development of a model for training and evaluation of laparoscopic skills. Am J Surg 1998;175:482.
25. Fried GM, Derossis AM, Bothwell J, et al. Comparison of laparoscopic performance in vivo with performance measured in a laparoscopic simulator. Surg Endosc 1999;13:1077.
26. Hamilton EC, Scott DJ, Kapoor A, et al. Improving operative performance using a laparoscopic hernia simulator. Am J Surg 2001;182:725.
27. Sammarco MJ, Youngblood JP. A resident teaching program in operative endoscopy. Obstet Gynecol 1993;81:463.
28. Adrales GL, Chu UB, Hoskins JD, et al. Development of a valid, cost-effective laparoscopic training program. Am J Surg 2004;187:1573.
29. Melvin WS, Johnson JA, Ellison EC. Laparoscopic skills enhancement. Am J Surg 1996;172:377.
30. Scott DJ, Young WN, Tesfay ST, et al. Laparoscopic skills training. Am J Surg 2001;182:137.
31. Gutt CN, Kim ZG, Krähenbühl L. Training for advanced laparoscopic surgery. Eur J Surg 2002;168:172.
32. Cundiff GW. Analysis of the effectiveness of an endoscopy education program in improving residents' laparoscopic skills. Obstet Gynecol 1997;90:854.
33. Cundiff GW, Weidner AC, Visco AG. Effectiveness of laparoscopic cadaveric dissection in enhancing resident comprehension of pelvic anatomy. J Am Coll Surg 2001;192:492.
34. Whitted RW, Pietro PA, Martin G, et al. A retrospective study evaluating the impact of formal laparoscopic training on patient outcomes in a residency program. J Am Assoc Gynecol Laparosc 2003;10:484.
35. Coleman RL, Muller CY. Effects of a laboratory-based skills curriculum on laparoscopic proficiency: A randomized trial. Am J Obstet Gynecol 2002;186:836.
36. Reznick RK. Teaching and testing technical skills. Am J Surg 1993; 165:358.
37. Winckel CP, Reznick RK, Cohen R, et al. Reliability and construct validity of a structured technical skills assessment form. Am J Surg 1994;167:423.
38. Martin JA, Regehr G, Reznick R, et al. Objective structured assessment of technical skill (OSATS) for surgical residents. Br J Surg 1997;84: 273.
39. Goff BA, Lentz GM, Lee D, et al. Development of an objective structured assessment of technical skills for obstetric and gynecology residents. Obstet Gynecol 2000;96:146.
40. Goff BA, Lentz GM, Lee D, et al. Development of a bench station objective structured assessment of technical skills. Obstet Gynecol 2001;98:412.
41. Lentz GM, Mandel LS, Lee D, et al. Testing surgical skills of obstetric and gynecologic residents in a bench laboratory setting: Validity and reliability. Am J Obstet Gynecol 2001;184:1462.
42. Goff BA, Nielsen PE, Lentz GM, et al. Surgical skills assessment: A blinded examination of obstetrics and gynecology residents. Am J Obstet Gynecol 2002;186:613.
43. Fung Kee Fung K, Fung Kee Fung M, Bordage G, et al. Interactive voice response to assess residents' laparoscopic skills: An instrument validation study. Am J Obstet Gynecol 2003;189:674.
44. Hanna GB, Drew T, Clinch P, et al. Computer-controlled endoscopic performance assessment system. Surg Endosc 1998;12:997.
45. Rosser JC, Rosser LE, Salvagi RS. Skill acquisition and assessment for laparoscopic surgery. Arch Surg 1997;132:200.
46. Shapiro S, Paz-Partlow M, Daykhovsky L, et al. The use of a modular skills center for the maintenance of laparoscopic skills. Surg Endosc 1996;10:819.

47. Smith CD, Farrell TM, McNatt SS, et al. Assessing laparoscopic manipulative skills. Am J Surg 2001;181:547.

48. Powers TW, Murayama KM, Toyama M, et al. Housestaff performance is improved by participation in a laparoscopic skills curriculum. Am J Surg 2002;184:626.

49. Feldman LS, Hagarty SE, Ghitulescu G, et al. Relationship between objective assessment of technical skills and subjective in-training evaluations in surgical residents. J Am Coll Surg 2004;198:105.

50. Eastridge BJ, Hamilton EC, O'Keefe GE, et al. Effect of sleep deprivation on the performance of simulated laparoscopic surgical skill. Am J Surg 2003;186:169.

51. Schell SR, Flynn TC. Web-based minimally invasive surgery training: Competency assessment in PGY 1-2 surgical residents. Curr Surg 2004;61:120.

52. Ramshaw BJ, Young D, Garcha I, et al. The role of multimedia interactive programs in training for laparoscopic procedures. Surg Endosc 2001;15:21.

53. Stylopoulos N, Cotin S, Maithel SK, et al. Computer-enhanced laparoscopic training system (CELTS): Bridging the gap. Surg Endosc 2004;18:782.

54. Brunner WC, Sierra R, Massarweh N, et al. Novice learning curves for laparoscopic virtual reality training: Implications for competency. J Surg Res 2003;114:259.

55. Hamilton EC, Scott DJ, Fleming JB, et al. Comparison of video trainer and virtual reality training systems on acquisition of laparoscopic skills. Surg Endosc 2002;16:406.

56. Prasad SM, Maniar HS, Soper NJ, et al. The effect of robotic assistance on learning curves for basic laparoscopic skills. Am J Surg 2002;183:7027.

57. Sarle R, Tewari A, Shrivastava A, et al. Surgical robotics and laparoscopic training drills. J Endourol 2004;18:63.

58. CREOG Transitions: Prerequisites to Practice: Credentialing and Licensing (July 2001).

59. http://cancerweb.ncl.ac.uk/omd/.

60. Jowell PS, Baillie J, Branch MS, et al. Quantitative assessment of procedural competence. A prospective study of training in endoscopic retrograde cholangiopancreatography. Ann Intern Med 1996;125:983.

61. American College of Obstetricians and Gynecologists. Guidelines for women's health care, 2nd ed. Washington, DC: ACOG, 2002;31.

62. Residency Review Committee, The Accreditation Council for Medical Graduate Medical Education, and The American Board of Obstetrics and Gynecology. ACOG Today 2001;1:45.

63. RANZCOG Guidelines for endometrial ablations C-Trg 3 July 2002. http://www.ranzcog.edu.au/Open/statements/Html/C-trg3.htm.

64. Society of American Gastrointestinal Endoscopic Surgeons. Framework for post-residency surgical education and training. http://www.sages.org/.

65. Prager LO. Unprepped for surgery. AMNews staff. May 24/31, 1999. http://www.ama-assn.org/amednews/1999/pick_99/feat0524.htm.

Index

Note: Page numbers followed by the letter b refer to boxed material, those followed by f refer to figures, and those followed by t refer to tables.

225